THE NEURONAL CODES
OF THE CEREBELLUM

THE NEURONAL CODES OF THE CEREBELLUM

Edited by

DETLEF H. HECK

University of Tennessee Health Science Center
Department of Anatomy & Neurobiology
Memphis, TN, USA

AMSTERDAM • BOSTON • HEIDELBERG • LONDON
NEW YORK • OXFORD • PARIS • SAN DIEGO
SAN FRANCISCO • SINGAPORE • SYDNEY • TOKYO

Academic Press is an imprint of Elsevier

Academic Press is an imprint of Elsevier
125 London Wall, London EC2Y 5AS, UK
525 B Street, Suite 1800, San Diego, CA 92101-4495, USA
225 Wyman Street, Waltham, MA 02451, USA
The Boulevard, Langford Lane, Kidlington, Oxford OX5 1GB, UK

Cover Image: Rat brain cerebellum. Multiphoton photography, 300x. Thomas Deerinck and
Mark Ellisman, National Center for Microscopy and Imaging Research, University of California
San Diego, CA, USA. Second Prize, 2014 Olympus BioScapes Digital Imaging Competition®.
www.OlympusBioScapes.com.

Notices
Knowledge and best practice in this field are constantly changing. As new research and
experience broaden our understanding, changes in research methods, professional practices,
or medical treatment may become necessary.

Practitioners and researchers must always rely on their own experience and knowledge in
evaluating and using any information, methods, compounds, or experiments described herein.
In using such information or methods they should be mindful of their own safety and the safety
of others, including parties for whom they have a professional responsibility.

To the fullest extent of the law, neither the Publisher nor the authors, contributors, or editors,
assume any liability for any injury and/or damage to persons or property as a matter of
products liability, negligence or otherwise, or from any use or operation of any methods,
products, instructions, or ideas contained in the material herein.

ISBN: 978-0-12-801386-1

British Library Cataloguing-in-Publication Data
A catalogue record for this book is available from the British Library

Library of Congress Cataloging-in-Publication Data
A catalog record for this book is available from the Library of Congress

For information on all Academic Press publications
visit our website at http://store.elsevier.com/

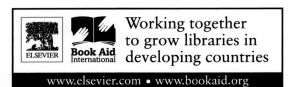

Working together
to grow libraries in
developing countries

www.elsevier.com • www.bookaid.org

Publisher: Mica Haley
Acquisition Editor: Mica Haley
Editorial Project Manager: Kathy Padilla
Production Project Manager: Julia Haynes
Designer: Matt Limbert

Typeset by TNQ Books and Journals
www.tnq.co.in

Printed and bound in the United States of America

Contents

7. Cerebellar Neuronal Codes—Perspectives from Intracellular Analysis In Vivo
HENRIK JÖRNTELL

8. The Role of the Cerebellum in Optimizing Saccades
ZONG-PENG SUN, SHABTAI BARASH AND PETER THIER

9. Coordination of Reaching Movements: Cerebellar Interactions with Motor Cortex
ERIC J. LANG

Contributors

Dora E. Angelaki Department of Neuroscience, Baylor College of Medicine, Houston, TX, USA

Shabtai Barash Department of Neurobiology, Weizmann Institute, Rehovot, Israel

H.J. Boele Department of Neuroscience, Erasmus MC, Rotterdam, The Netherlands

M.M. ten Brinke Department of Neuroscience, Erasmus MC, Rotterdam, The Netherlands

Stefano Casali Department of Brain and Behavioral Sciences, University of Pavia, Pavia, Italy

Richard Courtemanche FRQS Groupe de Recherche en Neurobiologie Comportementale (CSBN), Concordia University, Montréal, QC, Canada; Department of Exercise Science, Concordia University, Montréal, QC, Canada; PERFORM Centre, Concordia University, Montréal, QC, Canada

Egidio D'Angelo Department of Brain and Behavioral Sciences, University of Pavia, Pavia, Italy; Brain Connectivity Center, C. Mondino National Neurological Institute, Pavia, Italy

C.I. De Zeeuw Department of Neuroscience, Erasmus MC, Rotterdam, The Netherlands; Netherlands Institute for Neuroscience, Royal Academy of Arts and Sciences (KNAW), Amsterdam, The Netherlands

Timothy J. Ebner Department of Neuroscience, University of Minnesota, Minneapolis, MN, USA

Ariana Frederick FRQS Groupe de Recherche en Neurobiologie Comportementale (CSBN), Concordia University, Montréal, QC, Canada; Department of Biology, Concordia University, Montréal, QC, Canada

Henrik Jörntell Neural Basis of Sensorimotor Control, Department of Experimental Medical Science, Lund University, Lund, Sweden

Kamran Khodakhah Dominick P. Purpura Department of Neuroscience, Albert Einstein College of Medicine, Bronx, NY, USA

Eric J. Lang Department of Neuroscience & Physiology, New York University School of Medicine, New York, NY, USA

Jean Laurens Department of Neuroscience, Baylor College of Medicine, Houston, TX, USA

Clément Léna Institut de Biologie de l'ENS (IBENS), Inserm U1024, CNRS 8197, École Normale Supérieure, Paris, France

Stefano Masoli Department of Brain and Behavioral Sciences, University of Pavia, Pavia, Italy

Daniela Popa   Institut de Biologie de l'ENS (IBENS), Inserm U1024, CNRS 8197, École Normale Supérieure, Paris, France

Laurentiu S. Popa   Department of Neuroscience, University of Minnesota, Minneapolis, MN, USA

Davide Reato   Dominick P. Purpura Department of Neuroscience, Albert Einstein College of Medicine, Bronx, NY, USA

Martina Rizza   Department of Brain and Behavioral Sciences, University of Pavia, Pavia, Italy

Volker Steuber   Science and Technology Research Institute, University of Hertfordshire, Hatfield, UK

Martha L. Streng   Department of Neuroscience, University of Minnesota, Minneapolis, MN, USA

Zong-Peng Sun   Department of Cognitive Neurology, Hertie Institute for Clinical Brain Research, University of Tübingen, Tübingen, Germany;   Graduate School of Neural and Behavioural Sciences and International Max Planck Research School, University of Tübingen, Tübingen, Germany

Esra Tara   Dominick P. Purpura Department of Neuroscience, Albert Einstein College of Medicine, Bronx, NY, USA

Peter Thier   Department of Cognitive Neurology, Hertie Institute for Clinical Brain Research, University of Tübingen, Tübingen, Germany

Foreword

The cerebellar field has usually led the way in systems neuroscience. From the foundational work of Eccles, Ito, and Szentáothai (1967), the cerebellum was the first brain system for which the basic circuitry was established. Two years later (not coincidently), with the publications of David Marr's seminal "A theory of cerebellar cortex" (1969), the cerebellum appears to have been the first brain system to be considered in terms of the computation it accomplishes—and in terms of how its cells and synapses produce this computation. With behaviors like adaptation of the vestibular–ocular reflex and eyelid conditioning, the cerebellum for several decades was the only brain system for which it was possible for experimenters to control inputs while monitoring outputs, or at least good proxies for outputs. These factors also yielded the great advantage of being able to relate output relatively directly to measurable behaviors. With this volume the reader is given a snapshot of where the field stands in terms of understanding the neural codes employed by the cerebellum. With so much known about its synaptic organization and synaptic physiology, and with so much known about rules for converting inputs to output, the cerebellum seems like a great system to make groundbreaking progress on neural codes and their purposes.

One of the hallmark features of cerebellar research, one that arises in part from the seminal accomplishments described above, is how remarkably specific and concrete questions can be framed. The chapters of this volume are rife with examples. From efforts to understand single neurons or properties of single neurons (Popa et al., Chapter 1; Reato et al., Chapter 2; Steuber, Chapter 5; Jörntell, Chapter 7), to projects using computer simulations of the cerebellum (Boele, Chapter 3; D'Angelo, Chapter 11), to attempts to understand interactions between the cerebellum and other brain structures (Léna and Popa, Chapter 6; Lang, Chapter 9), the reader will encounter ideas concrete and specific enough that they can be put to the test experimentally. This is the hallmark of great theories and ideas, that they are expressed concretely enough that they could be disproven if they are wrong. This volume also presents the reader with a healthy sample of work that connects cerebellar processing quite directly to well-characterized behaviors (Popa et al., Chapter 1; Reato et al., Chapter 2; Boele et al., Chapter 3; Laurens and Angelaki, Chapter 4; Sun et al., Chapter 8; Lang, Chapter 9).

Ultimately what we hope to accomplish in the category of neural codes is this: we will have a list of well-characterized coding schemes with specific ideas about the circumstances under which each is useful or applicable. To view it another way, if we were imagining the construction of a new brain system with particular computational properties, we would know which collection of codes to employ, and why. Here is a list of codes considered (in both positive and negative lights) in this volume.

- The chapter by Popa et al. (1) considers that Purkinje cell simple spikes represent a sort of multiplexed code, with one signal leading and another lagging movement and one signal representing prediction and the other feedback input.
- The Reato et al.'s Chapter 2 offers consideration of the rebound excitation code often attributed to deep cerebellar nucleus neurons. Although these neurons clearly have the conductances that make them apt to fire following release from inhibition, these authors find no evidence of this code in use in vivo.
- The Boele et al.'s Chapter 3 describes the (now commonplace) use of computer simulations of the cerebellum to investigate certain structure–function properties of cerebellar computation.
- The Laurens and Angelaki's Chapter 4 describes a detailed model of how various neural codes allow the cerebellum to encode self-motion.
- Chapter 5 (Steuber) again picks up the question of rebound excitation in deep nucleus neurons in the broader context of considering the various ways in which Purkinje cell inhibition of these neurons influences cerebellar output.
- Recurrent or loop-like connectivity is encountered often in the brain. Chapter 6 (Léna and Popa) considers the important cerebellar output that returns to the cerebral cortex in the form of cerebrocerebellar loops.
- The Jörntell's Chapter 7 offers interesting (and I believe quite important) insights from another angle by considering the key holes in our current understanding. He offers, among other things, that a better understanding of mossy fiber input codes is urgently needed.
- The Sun et al.'s Chapter 8 uses cerebellar control of saccades to consider both codes within the cerebellum (and how plasticity alters them) and how cerebellar output interacts with downstream brainstem codes to produce saccadic eye movements.
- The Lang's Chapter 9 considers the interesting question of codes used by cerebellar outputs that influence descending motor pathways versus those used by outputs that project back to motor cortex.
- Oscillations are everywhere, even in the cerebellum. The Courtemanche and Frederick's Chapter 10 offers new ideas on the computational properties of the 4- to 25-Hz oscillations seen in the granule layer of the cerebellar cortex.

- Finally, the D'Angelo's Chapter 11 describes work spanning single-neuron physiology to biophysical modeling of neurons to expanding network models of the cerebellum to applications in robotics.

Although most cerebellar researchers are accustomed to such concreteness in the expression of ideas and theories, most systems neuroscientists working on other systems covet it. I believe it remains the case that one of the main things our field has to offer is road maps to a better and more specific understanding of all brain systems. If you are a cerebellar researcher this volume will update you on the very latest ideas on cerebellar codes. If you study another region of the brain and are considering whether this book will be worth your time, I offer to you that your time investment will return rich dividends.

Michael Mauk, Ph.D.
University of Texas at Austin
Austin, Texas
May 18, 2015

Preface

The cerebellum takes a special place among brain structures, if only because of its gross anatomical appearance as a "small brain" (Kleinhirn) attached to the "large brain" (Großhirn), which earned it its name. But the uniqueness of the cerebellum also extends to the structure of its neural network, whose basic wiring diagram—first described by R. y Cajal in 1911—seems so charmingly simple that it seduced generations of experimentalists and theoreticians to anticipate the complete translation of its structure into function in the not-too-distant future.

One hundred years after Cajal, we can confidently say that, although we have not yet reached that critical level of understanding, we have made great strides toward this goal. Along the way, many deeply rooted assumptions about cerebellar structure and function were overturned and critical new insights gained. The chapters in this book summarize many of the crucial advancements toward understanding the neuronal coding of information in the cerebellum and are written by scientists who were key drivers of the dramatic progress of cerebellar research over the past two or three decades.

The idea for this book evolved from a symposium on neural coding in the cerebellum, which I organized at the 2013 Annual Meeting of the Society for Neuroscience in San Diego, California. The fact that the symposium met with great interest, together with the realization that the topic had never been comprehensively addressed in book form, led to the decision to generate this book. The lines of research relevant to the topic of neuronal coding in the cerebellum are too numerous and diverse to be comprehensively represented in a single volume. The focus of this book is on experimental, theoretical, and modeling research relevant to cerebellar control of behavior in vivo.

I thank all the authors who took valuable time away from pressing work in their labs to contribute their excellent chapters to this book. With funding levels on a continual decline, science has become an increasingly competitive enterprise, which makes it that much more laudable for researchers to make time for activities that benefit the community, as I am confident this book will.

Unfailing support throughout the many months it took to complete this book came from two superb editors at Elsevier, Kathy Padilla and Mica Haley, to whom I am very grateful.

Detlef H. Heck
University of Tennessee Health Science Center
Memphis, Tennessee
May 18, 2015

1

Signaling of Predictive and Feedback Information in Purkinje Cell Simple Spike Activity

Laurentiu S. Popa[a], Martha L. Streng[a], Timothy J. Ebner

Department of Neuroscience, University of Minnesota, Minneapolis, MN, USA

INTRODUCTION

It is widely acknowledged that the cerebellum is essential for the production of smooth, continuous movements. To understand the precise role of the cerebellum in the control of movements, it is necessary to understand how information is encoded and processed in the cerebellar circuitry. This includes understanding the signals present in cerebellar neurons and the transformation of those signals from the afferent input stage through the cerebellar cortex and then to the cerebellar nuclei. Unfortunately, this level of insight still evades the field and a description of how the circuit operates is far from complete. At present, the bulk of available information is about how Purkinje cells signal and process behavioral information. As the only output neurons of the cerebellar cortex, Purkinje cells are a key node in the network and, therefore, are integral to understanding cerebellar function. This chapter focuses on the signals found in the discharge of Purkinje cells during movements and what those signals tell us about cerebellar function.

[a] Both authors contributed equally.

PURKINJE CELL DISCHARGE SIGNALS MANY FEATURES OF MOVEMENTS

The discharge of Purkinje cells modulates with a host of movement-related parameters. Kinematic signaling in the simple spike discharge has been reported across a wide range of motor behaviors involving various effectors. During arm movements, the simple spike firing of Purkinje cells in the intermediate zone of lobules IV–VI of awake monkeys is correlated with limb position, direction, speed, and movement distance (Coltz, Johnson, & Ebner, 1999; Fortier, Kalaska, & Smith, 1989; Fu, Flament, Coltz, & Ebner, 1997; Harvey, Porter, & Rawson, 1977; Hewitt, Popa, Pasalar, Hendrix, & Ebner, 2011; Mano & Yamamoto, 1980; Marple-Horvat & Stein, 1987; Pasalar, Roitman, Durfee, & Ebner, 2006; Roitman, Pasalar, Johnson, & Ebner, 2005; Thach, 1970). The importance of kinematic signaling in the cerebellar cortex is evident in that limb position and velocity are found in the simple spike discharge during passive limb movements in anesthetized or decerebrate cats and rats (Giaquinta et al., 2000; Kolb, Rubia, & Bauswein, 1987; Rubia & Kolb, 1978; Valle, Bosco, & Poppele, 2000). During the vestibulo-ocular reflex (VOR), smooth pursuit, ocular following, or saccades, eye movement kinematics have been documented in the simple spike activity of Purkinje cells in the floccular complex and oculomotor vermis (Dash, Catz, Dicke, & Thier, 2012; Gomi et al., 1998; Laurens, Meng, & Angelaki, 2013; Lisberger, Pavelko, Bronte-Stewart, & Stone, 1994; Medina & Lisberger, 2009; Miles, Braitman, & Dow, 1980; Miles, Fuller, Braitman, & Dow, 1980; Shidara, Kawano, Gomi, & Kawato, 1993; Stone & Lisberger, 1990).

Others have suggested that Purkinje cells specify the motor command, that is, the forces or muscle activity needed to generate movements (Holdefer & Miller, 2009; Kawato & Wolpert, 1998; Kobayashi et al., 1998; Shidara et al., 1993; Yamamoto, Kawato, Kotosaka, & Kitazawa, 2007). Observations favoring this hypothesis include reciprocal simple spike discharge during joint flexion/extension movements (Frysinger, Bourbonnais, Kalaska, & Smith, 1984; Smith, 1981; Thach, 1968), simple spike correlation to electromyographic activity (Holdefer & Miller, 2009), and the reconstruction of simple spike and complex spike firing from eye-movement dynamics during the ocular following response (Gomi et al., 1998; Kobayashi et al., 1998; Shidara et al., 1993). However, whether simple spikes encode movement dynamics independent of kinematics remains controversial (Ebner, Hewitt, & Popa, 2011; Pasalar et al., 2006; Roitman et al., 2005; Yamamoto et al., 2007).

The cerebellum in general and Purkinje cell output specifically have been postulated to play a role in movement timing (Braitenberg & Atwood, 1958; Keele & Ivry, 1990; O'Reilly, Mesulam, & Nobre, 2008; Welsh, Lang, Suglhara, & Llinas, 1995). In the flocculus, the duration of pauses in simple spike output prior to movement onset is linearly correlated with saccade duration (Noda & Suzuki, 1979), whereas vermal Purkinje cell simple spike discharge is timed to saccade initiation (Waterhouse & Mcelligott, 1980), and saccade onset/offset is encoded at the population level (Thier, Dicke, Haas, & Barash, 2000). Additionally, the observations of complex spike rhythmicity and the ability of climbing fibers to evoke synchronous activity in Purkinje cells have led to the hypothesis that complex spikes serve as an internal clock necessary for the regulation of movement timing (Llinas, 2013; Llinas & Sasaki, 1989; Sasaki, Bower, & Llinas, 1989; Welsh et al., 1995).

Purkinje cell simple spike discharge has also been associated with parameters related to task performance. For example, induced dissociation between cursor and hand movement by coordinate transformation shows that in some Purkinje cells, simple spikes encode the cursor position independent of hand kinematics (Liu, Robertson, & Miall, 2003). Simple spike discharge modulates with target motion during both reaching and tracking tasks (Cerminara, Apps, & Marple-Horvat, 2009; Ebner & Fu, 1997; Miles, Cerminara, & Marple-Horvat, 2006). These observations suggest that, in addition to a robust encoding of movement parameters, simple spike discharge also contains representations of task-specific parameters relevant to the behavioral goal.

PURKINJE CELL DISCHARGE AND MOTOR ERRORS

For several decades, the dominant view has been that motor errors are signaled by complex spike discharge (Gilbert & Thach, 1977; Ito, 2000, 2013; Kawato & Gomi, 1992; Kitazawa, Kimura, & Yin, 1998; Stone & Lisberger, 1986;). This view is a central tenet of the Marr–Albus–Ito hypothesis in which long-term depression (LTD) of parallel fiber–Purkinje cell synapse results from coactivation of parallel fiber and climbing fiber inputs (Albus, 1971; Ito & Kano, 1982; Marr, 1969). This framework for understanding the role of the climbing fiber input and complex spikes is supported by numerous studies. Complex spike discharge is coupled with errors during saccades, smooth pursuit, and ocular following (Barmack & Simpson, 1980; Graf, Simpson, & Leonard, 1988; Kobayashi et al., 1998; Medina & Lisberger, 2008; Soetedjo & Fuchs, 2006). Undoubtedly, complex spike discharge in response to retinal slip provides one of the strongest demonstrations of error encoding (Barmack & Shojaku, 1995; Graf et al., 1988; Kobayashi et al., 1998). During arm movements, complex spikes modulate with perturbations (Gilbert & Thach, 1977; Wang, Kim, & Ebner, 1987), adaptation to visuomotor transformations (Ojakangas & Ebner, 1994), and end-point errors (Kitazawa et al., 1998).

However, other studies found limited support for the classical view, suggesting that error processing in the cerebellum is more multifaceted than originally proposed. Perturbations and performance errors during reaching in cats do not evoke responses in inferior olive neurons, the origin of the climbing fiber projection (Horn, van Kan, & Gibson, 1996). Complex spike modulation could not be related to direction or speed errors during reaching (Ebner, Johnson, Roitman, & Fu, 2002; Fu, Mason, Flament, Coltz, & Ebner, 1997). Even when climbing fiber input is associated with errors during reaching movements, the complex spikes occur only in a small percentage of trials (Kitazawa et al., 1998; Ojakangas & Ebner, 1994). In both saccadic and smooth pursuit adaptation, complex spike discharge in the oculomotor vermis increases late in adaptation when errors have greatly decreased (Catz, Dicke, & Thier, 2005; Dash, Catz, Dicke, & Thier, 2010; Prsa & Thier, 2011). A similar dissociation between complex spike modulation and error amplitude occurs during reach adaptation (Ojakangas & Ebner, 1992). In a 2015 study in which monkeys adapted to a transient mechanical perturbation during reach, the rather weak complex spike modulation evoked could not account for either the learning or the changes in simple spike firing (Hewitt, Popa, & Ebner, 2015). In the oculomotor vermis, complex spike error modulation with saccades appears limited to direction errors, and whether they encode error magnitude is unclear (Soetedjo & Fuchs, 2006; Soetedjo, Kojima, & Fuchs, 2008). Therefore, the precision, specificity, and extent to which complex spikes encode error information remain unknown.

It has also been suggested that the low frequency of the complex spike discharge limits their bandwidth, which is inconsistent with the error monitoring required for fast or continuous movements. The limitations of the low-frequency discharge could be mitigated by findings that complex spikes evoke graded changes in Purkinje cells and the wide range of response latencies (Najafi, Giovannucci, Wang, & Medina, 2014a, 2014b; Rasmussen et al., 2013; Yang & Lisberger, 2014). Complex spike synchrony at the population level has also been argued to provide a finer temporal resolution for encoding information compared to the activity of individual Purkinje cells (Jacobson, Lev, Yarom, & Cohen, 2009). An additional factor to consider is that both complex spike probability and synchrony are modulated by the local simple spike activity (Chaumont et al., 2013; Marshall & Lang, 2009; Witter, Canto, Hoogland, de Gruijl, & De Zeeuw, 2013), suggesting that the climbing fiber activity is highly dependent on the behavioral and experimental context. Together, these observations suggest a need for reevaluating the classical hypothesis that complex spike discharge is the only or primary channel carrying motor error information in the cerebellum.

Although few studies have explicitly tested whether simple spikes provide error information, there is evidence for this concept. For example, the changes in simple spike output following smooth pursuit adaptation appear sufficient to drive learning (Kahlon & Lisberger, 2000). In the posterior vermis, simple spike firing provides a neural correlate of retinal slip

(Kase, Noda, Suzuki, & Miller, 1979). Cerebellar-dependent VOR adaptation can be driven by instructive signals in the simple spike firing in the absence of climbing fiber input (Ke, Guo, & Raymond, 2009). Increasing VOR gain appears to be dependent on complex spike-driven LTD, while gain decrease depends on noncomplex spike-driven long-term potentiation mechanisms (Boyden, Katoh, & Raymond, 2004; Boyden & Raymond, 2003). Moreover, while optogenetic activation of climbing fibers can induce VOR adaptation (Kimpo, Rinaldi, Kim, Payne, & Raymond, 2014), similar findings result from optogenetically driven increases in simple spike discharge (Nguyen-Vu et al., 2013). Simple spike discharge modulates with trial success or failure in a reaching task (Greger & Norris, 2005) and with direction and speed errors during manual circular tracking (Roitman, Pasalar, & Ebner, 2009). However, in the latter study performance errors were strongly coupled with kinematics. Here we review our studies demonstrating that performance errors are encoded in the simple spike discharge independent of kinematics and challenge the long-held assumption that error signaling in Purkinje cells is completely climbing-fiber-dependent (Popa, Hewitt, & Ebner, 2012, 2014).

COMPUTATIONAL FRAMEWORK FOR CEREBELLAR INFORMATION PROCESSING

The broad range of signals observed in the discharge of Purkinje cells makes constructing a unified theory of the cerebellar cortical function elusive. One theoretical framework that can account for the various signals is that Purkinje cells serve as the output of a forward internal model (Kawato & Wolpert, 1998; Miall & Wolpert, 1996; Pasalar et al., 2006; Shadmehr, Smith, & Krakauer, 2010). A forward internal model predicts the sensory consequences of a motor command. If Purkinje cells are the output of a forward model, multiple types of behavioral signals are integrated to predict the consequences of movement commands. In this view, information about movement kinematics, kinetics, timing, and errors is all relevant to generating predictions about the upcoming motor behavior.

It was initially postulated that error correction was achieved primarily by sensory feedback. However, there are numerous problems with relying on sensory feedback alone to correct for motor errors. Closed-loop control is subject to significant delays and can be unstable (Kawato, 1999; Miall & Wolpert, 1996; Shadmehr et al., 2010; Wolpert & Ghahramani, 2000). Movement correction occurs on a faster time scale (Flanagan & Wing, 1997) and even in the absence of sensory feedback (Golla et al., 2008; Shadmehr et al., 2010; Wagner & Smith, 2008; Xu-Wilson, Chen-Harris, Zee, & Shadmehr, 2009). These findings lead to the realization that the motor system must be making motor predictions to allow for the rapid detection and correction of errors. Typically, these predictions have been thought to be in the kinematic domain, for example, the position or velocity of the limb (Miall & Wolpert, 1996; Wolpert & Ghahramani, 2000). However, the central nervous system is likely to acquire internal models for task-specific performance (Todorov & Jordan, 2002; Wolpert, Miall, & Kawato, 1998) or the physical properties of the environment, such as the gravitational field (Laurens et al., 2013). In this view, multiple internal models are implemented to fully monitor movement kinematics and performance as well as to eliminate sensory ambiguity based on the overall behavioral goal(s).

The cerebellum has been hypothesized to serve as a forward internal model (Kawato & Wolpert, 1998; Pasalar et al., 2006; Shadmehr & Krakauer, 2008; Shadmehr et al., 2010; Wolpert et al., 1998). Predictive control of movement is reduced in patients with cerebellar damage (Horak & Diener, 1994; Martin, Keating, Goodkin, Bastian, & Thach, 1996; Nowak, Hermsdorfer, Rost, Timmann, & Topka, 2004; Smith & Shadmehr, 2005). In healthy subjects, disruption of cerebellar activity by transcranial magnetic stimulation results in inaccurate reaches toward a target (Miall, Christensen, Cain, & Stanley, 2007). Intriguingly, the subjects' reaches would have been accurate if made at earlier time points (e.g., arm position prior to the stimulation onset). These results suggest that disrupting cerebellar activity impaired the generation of internal predictions, requiring that the motor commands be planned and initiated using delayed sensory feedback information about the arm position. Consistent with the view that forward internal models are integral for adaptation, the cerebellum plays a central role in motor learning. Patients with cerebellar damage have deficits in eye-movement adaptation (Golla et al., 2008; Xu-Wilson et al., 2009). Learning to adapt to regularly occurring perturbations during eye movements is also degraded (Muller & Dichgans, 1994). In split-belt walking, healthy subjects learn to adjust stride length and step timing to adapt to treadmill belts moving at different speeds, whereas cerebellar patients do not. Importantly, online, reactive control remains intact, suggesting selective deficits to forward internal model-mediated adaptation (Morton & Bastian, 2006). In healthy subjects, increased cerebellar activation is associated with motor learning, such as adaptation to visuomotor transformations (Imamizu et al., 2000; Kawato et al., 2003; Krakauer et al., 2004; Shadmehr & Holcomb, 1997) or predictable changes in target location during reaching (Diedrichsen, Hashambhoy, Rane, & Shadmehr, 2005).

Effective control of movement requires not only making predictions about the upcoming behavior but also the continuous monitoring of performance and corrections for errors (Berniker & Kording, 2008; Shadmehr et al., 2010; Todorov & Jordan, 2002; Wolpert & Ghahramani, 2000). Error signals are integral to a forward internal model in which the predicted sensory consequences of a movement are compared to the actual sensory feedback (Held & Freedman, 1963; Jordan & Rumelhart, 1992; Miall & Wolpert, 1996; Shadmehr et al., 2010; Wolpert, Ghahramani, & Jordan, 1995). This integration of prediction and feedback, known as a sensory prediction error, serves as a measure of accuracy used both to improve subsequent predictions and to guide future actions. Extensive evidence suggests that humans use sensory prediction errors, particularly during learning and adaptation (Mazzoni & Krakauer, 2006; Morton & Bastian, 2006; Noto & Robinson, 2001; Wallman & Fuchs, 1998; Xu-Wilson et al., 2009). Although other error-related signals such as the actual corrective movements (Kawato, 1996; Miles & Lisberger, 1981) or sensory feedback at the end of a movement contribute (Cameron, Franks, Inglis, & Chua, 2010; Magescas & Prablanc, 2006), sensory prediction errors appear to have a dominant role in controlling movement and motor learning (Gaveau, Prablanc, Laurent, Rossetti, & Priot, 2014; Held & Freedman, 1963; Izawa & Shadmehr, 2011; Mazzoni & Krakauer, 2006; Taylor & Ivry, 2012; Wolpert & Ghahramani, 2000).

If the cerebellum acts as a forward internal model, then it must also process sensory prediction errors. Patients with cerebellar damage show a variety of deficits in learning and adaptation. For example, saccades are too brief in duration to allow for sensory input in flight (Guthrie, Porter, & Sparks, 1983; Keller & Robinson, 1971) and thus must be controlled by internal, sensory prediction error-mediated mechanisms (Chen-Harris, Joiner, Ethier, Zee, & Shadmehr, 2008; Robinson, 1975; Shadmehr et al., 2010). Patients with cerebellar damage, including those with spinocerebellar ataxia type 6, primarily results in Purkinje cell degeneration, are unable to adapt to variability in saccade motor commands (Golla et al., 2008; Xu-Wilson et al., 2009). Sensory prediction error-dependent adaptation of arm movements during visuomotor transformations is also impaired (Tseng, Diedrichsen, Krakauer, Shadmehr, & Bastian, 2007). In healthy subjects, increases in cerebellar activation are observed during errors (Diedrichsen et al., 2005; Ide & Li, 2011; Imamizu et al., 2000), such as the divergence between movement goal and the actual consequences induced by an unexpected force field (Schlerf, Ivry, & Diedrichsen, 2012). Evidence for cerebellar processing of sensory prediction errors also extends to the sensory domain. Increased cerebellar activation occurs with omission of an expected somatosensory stimulus (Tesche & Karhu, 2000). On a single-cell level, neurons in the cerebellar nuclei, the targets of Purkinje cells, encode temporal aspects of stimulus omission (Ohmae, Uematsu, & Tanaka, 2013).

Despite the wealth of behavioral, imaging, and patient studies supporting the hypothesis that the cerebellum acquires and implements forward internal models, little is known about how the components are represented at the cellular level. Of particular interest is whether Purkinje cells encoding the sensory prediction error signals are necessary for learning and adaptation.

PREDICTIVE AND FEEDBACK SIGNALING IN PURKINJE CELL SIMPLE SPIKE FIRING

As reviewed above, Purkinje cells encode rich representations of effector kinematics. Consistent with a forward internal model, simple spike discharge tends to lead effector kinematics during movements (Dash, Dicke, & Thier, 2013; Fu, Flament, et al., 1997; Gomi et al., 1998; Hewitt et al., 2011; Marple-Horvat & Stein, 1987; Roitman et al., 2005; Shidara et al., 1993; Stone & Lisberger, 1990). However, the timing of simple spike modulation in relation to kinematics is very broad, including providing feedback of effector states. This wide timing of distribution, together with kinematic signals during passive limb movements (Giaquinta et al., 2000; Kolb et al., 1987; Rubia & Kolb, 1978; Valle et al., 2000), suggests that simple spikes encode both feed-forward and feedback kinematic signals.

Controlling movements also requires task-specific performance information (Todorov, 2004). These two classes of information can be quite different in the typical paradigms used to study neuronal discharge during reaching movements, in which the subject is monitoring task instructions and performance on a computer screen. More detailed characterizations of both kinematic and performance representations in the discharge of cerebellar neurons are needed as only a few studies of cerebellar neurons have attempted to dissociate these variables (Cerminara et al., 2009; Ebner & Fu, 1997; Liu et al., 2003; Miles et al., 2006).

Most previous studies relied on highly predictable tasks, confounding predictions of motor commands with trial planning and generating stereotypical and time-locked movements that result in highly correlated kinematic parameters (Ebner et al., 2011; Paninski, Fellows, Hatsopoulos, & Donoghue, 2004). Also, task performance and errors are typically highly correlated with kinematics. These constraints limit a thorough understanding of the kinematic and error signals in cerebellar neurons. To address these concerns, Purkinje cells were recorded in nonhuman primates during a manual, pseudo-random tracking task. The advantages of pseudo-random tracking include minimizing coupling among behavioral parameters, allowing for dissociation of feed-forward and feedback signals and providing a more thorough exploration of the behavioral work space (Hewitt et al., 2011; Paninski et al., 2004). Also, tracking a pseudo-randomly moving target is challenging and requires continuous evaluation of motor performance and implementation of corrective movements.

During pseudo-random tracking, both kinematic and performance error signaling were evaluated in the simple spike firing of Purkinje cells (Hewitt et al., 2011; Popa et al., 2012). The kinematic parameters included position (X and Y), velocity (V_x and V_y), and speed (S) of the arm/hand. Performance errors were defined as the divergence between the current movement goal, approximated by the target center, and the consequences of the motor commands, indicated by cursor movement. Performance errors evaluated included the cursor position relative to the target center (XE and YE), distance between the cursor and target center (RE), and angular direction necessary to move from the current position to the target center (PDE). The error parameters provide a continuous measure of the difference between cursor movement relative to the target center rather than discrete errors, such as when the cursor strays outside the target boundaries. Not only are these "natural" measures of motor performance for this tracking task, but the behavior shows that the monkeys strive to minimize these errors and maintain the cursor in the target center (Hewitt et al., 2011; Popa et al., 2012).

Temporal linear regressions were used to fit the simple spike firing to the behavioral parameters to determine the lead/lag (τ value) between Purkinje cell activity and each parameter (Hewitt et al., 2011; Popa et al., 2012). Although this type of regression analysis has been used previously (Ashe & Georgopoulos, 1994; Gomi et al., 1998; Medina & Lisberger, 2009; Roitman et al., 2009), a novel refinement was incorporated such that for each parameter the simple spike variability associated with the other kinematic and error parameters was removed. This was done for each parameter by first determining the firing residuals from a multilinear model of simple spike firing that included the kinematic and error parameters not being evaluated. The firing residuals were then regressed against the parameter of interest, determining the coefficient of determination (R^2) and regression coefficient (β) as functions of time independent of other parameters.

The first of two major findings is that the simple spike discharge of individual Purkinje cells can both lead and lag kinematics and errors. These leads and lags can be appreciated from maps of the simple spike firing in relation to the parameters at different temporal shifts. To construct the maps at different leads and lags, the firing is shifted relative to a behavioral parameter for a series of time intervals (τ values), either before (negative τ) or after a parameter (positive τ). For example, the map of simple spike firing in relation to hand velocity at −120 ms in Fig. 1(A) was computed by averaging the discharge that occurred 120 ms prior to the observed velocity, binned into equal partitions of V_x and V_y. Over the span of τ values, the maps for this example Purkinje cell reveal a modulation pattern in which the simple spike discharge leads velocity with higher firing in the left half of the work space that emerges at approximately −300 ms, reaches a maximum near to −120 ms, and then decreases close to 0 ms (Fig. 1(A)). A nearly opposite pattern of modulation with velocity occuring at feedback timing, characterized by high firing in the upper right quadrant that begins at about 100 ms lag, peaks around 200 ms, and then fades as the lag approaches 500 ms. In the same population of Purkinje cells, bimodal representations of the error signals occur in the simple spike firing. As shown

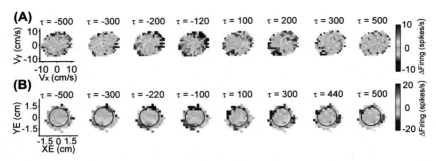

FIGURE 1   Time course of the simple spike modulation with kinematics and performance errors. (A) Simple spike activity of a Purkinje cell in relation to hand velocity (V_x and V_y) at different leads and lags (τ). The 24×24 cm/s velocity work space (−12 to 12 cm/s in both V_x and V_y directions) is partitioned into equal bins at a resolution of 4.8×4.8 cm/s. Average firing rate across each bin is displayed relative to mean firing and color coded as shown in the pseudo-color scale bar. Above each map is the lead ($\tau < 0$) or lag ($\tau > 0$) time of the firing relative to hand velocity. (B) Similar maps of a single Purkinje cell simple spike firing at different leads and lags in relation to position errors (XE and YE). The 6×6 cm position error work space (−3 to 3 cm relative to target center in both XE and YE directions) is partitioned into equal bins at a resolution of 0.75×0.75 cm. The target boundary is denoted by the black circle.

in the discharge maps of another Purkinje cell (Fig. 1(B)), the simple spike discharge leads position error (XE and YE) from −300 to −100 ms with the highest firing in the lower left quadrant and then lags position error from 300 to 500 ms with the highest firing in the upper right quadrant. Therefore, the simple spike firing of individual Purkinje cells carries both predictive and feedback signals about movement kinematics and task performance.

The R^2 and β temporal profiles capture the predictive and feedback modulation in the simple spike firing. For the velocity-encoding example, the R^2 and β plots for V_x (Fig. 2(A) and (B)) have local maxima at both leads and lags that correspond to the timing of the largest modulation observed in the firing maps (Fig. 1(A)). Similarly, for the position error-encoding example (Fig. 1(B)), the R^2 and β plots for XE exhibit leading and lagging modulation with peaks at −220 and 440 ms (Fig. 2(E) and (F), respectively). Performing the regressions after randomizing the trial order for the firing shows that the correlations are well above chance and confirm the robust signaling of kinematics and errors at both lead and lag times.

Dual temporal encoding was common for both kinematics and performance errors. For kinematics, 70% of Purkinje cells (85 of 122) had at least one bimodal profile. Similarly, bimodal timing was observed for all four performance errors, with 72% of Purkinje cells exhibiting bimodal timing for at least one error parameter. The average timing for lead and lag peaks was symmetrical for both kinematics and errors and nearly uniformly distributed throughout the lead and lag τ-values. Therefore, the simple spike firing not only provides feedback but also predicts kinematics and performance errors.

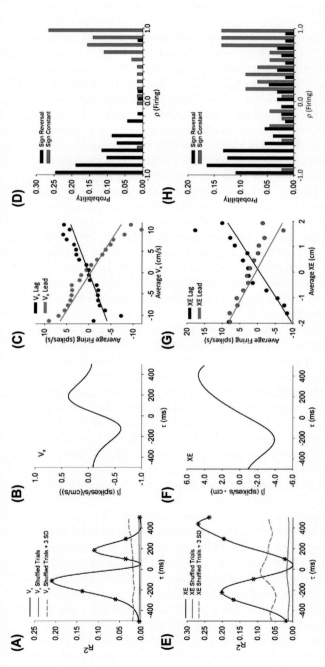

FIGURE 2 Opposing modulation and dual-temporal encoding. (A) R^2 as a function of lead/lag (τ) for V_x for the Purkinje cell shown in Fig. 1(A). Plot shows times of peak modulation with V_x, one at the predictive lead and one at the feedback lag. The red line shows the mean of the control regressions based on shuffling the trial order (100 repetitions) and the dashed line the mean +3 SD. Asterisks (*) on the R^2 line correspond to time points displayed in Fig. 1(A). (B) Plot of the regression coefficients for V_x (β_{V_x}) as a function of τ. Note the change in the sign of the regression coefficient demonstrating the reversal in the firing sensitivity at predictive versus feedback timing. (C) Linear encoding of V_x at the peak lead (−120 ms, in red) and lag (200 ms, in black) timings of simple spike modulation. Individual points denote average simple spike discharge for a given V_x, with the slope constructed from regression coefficients (β_{V_x}) and intercepts (β_0). Note the opposing effects of errors on simple spike modulation at the lead versus lag timing. (D) Distribution of the correlation coefficients (ρ(Firing)) between simple spike firing modulation at the times of lead/lag peaks for each bimodal kinematic profile. (E) R^2 as a function of lead/lag (τ) for XE for the Purkinje cell shown in Fig. 1(B). Plot shows the times of peak modulation with XE, one at the predictive lead and one at the feedback lag. Control regressions based on shuffling the trial order are also shown. (F) Plot of the regression coefficients for XE (β_{XE}) as a function of τ. (G) Linear encoding of XE at the peak lead (−220 ms, in red) and the lag (440 ms, in black) shows the opposing effects of errors on simple spike modulation. (H) Distribution of the correlation coefficients (ρ(Firing)) between simple spike firing modulation at the times of lead/lag peaks for each bimodal error profile. *From Popa et al. (2012) with permission.*

Because of the novel approach to the regression analyses based on firing residuals and concern that the dual representations may be due to "cross-contamination" from other parameters, we undertook several control analyses (Popa et al., 2012). Control regressions show that there is no complementary kinematic or error information remaining in the firing residuals, strongly suggesting that kinematic and error signals obtained from the firing residuals cannot be explained by interactions among parameters. Several analyses also addressed whether the bimodality is generated by an intrinsic temporal structure in either the simple spike firing or the behavioral parameters. For both kinematics and performance errors, the correlations at the times of the peak R^2 values were small or nonexistent. This demonstrates that there is little covariation within a parameter at the times of maximal simple spike modulation. Also, the autocorrelation functions for the simple spike firing and the behavioral parameters lack a temporal structure that can account for the predictive and feedback signals within a single Purkinje cell. Furthermore, shuffling the trial order effectively abolishes the predictive and feedback signals (see Fig. 2(A) and (E)), demonstrating that the regression results are not due to autocorrelated artifacts (Granger & Newbold, 1974). Therefore, the bimodal encoding in the simple spike firing is not an artifact of intrinsic structure within the firing or behavioral parameters.

Decoding analysis tested whether the kinematic and performance error signals predicted by the simple spike firing match the actual values. For each kinematic and error parameter, the correlation coefficient between predicted and observed is 0.99 and the slopes are close to unity. The standard deviations of the decoded estimates are quite small for kinematics and for the errors when the cursor is within the target boundaries, showing that the estimates are relatively invariant to the selection of the training and test trials. Furthermore, the decoding can be performed accurately at a high resolution, supporting the assumption that Purkinje cells can provide continuous kinematic and error representations. Therefore, the Purkinje cell population provides a remarkably accurate prediction of both upcoming kinematics and performance errors.

The second major finding is that the predictive and feedback signals can have opposing effects on the simple spike modulation. The change in the sign of the modulation with V_x is evident in the firing maps (Fig. 1(A)) and in the β temporal profile (Fig. 2(B)). The opposing simple spike modulation can also be appreciated by plotting the firing with respect to V_x (Fig. 2(C)) at the peak lead and lag times. At the peak lead time, V_x has a negative slope (red dots and trend line), and it has a positive slope at the peak lag times (black dots and trend line). Reversal in the simple spike modulation for XE is evident in the firing maps (Fig. 1(B)), temporal profile of the regression coefficient (Fig. 2(E)), and plots of the firing at the peak lead and lag times (Fig. 2(G)).

Reversal of the sign of the simple spike modulation for kinematics and errors was common. The distributions of the correlation coefficients (ρ(Firing)) between simple spike firing modulation at the times of lead/ lag peaks show that Purkinje cells in which the regression coefficients change signs have anticorrelated firing patterns (black bars, Fig. 2(D)) and performance errors (black bars, Fig. 2(H)). The opposing simple spike modulation at the predictive and feedback times with performance errors leads us to suggest that a simple comparison might be used by the motor system to estimate the degree of match between the prediction and the feedback in determining sensory prediction errors (Popa et al., 2012, 2014). However, for the dually encoded kinematic parameters, a large number of Purkinje cells do not reverse sign and instead the simple spike firing patterns at the peak leads and lags are highly positively correlated (red bars, Fig. 2(D)). Although less common, a number of Purkinje cells that dually encode performance errors also exhibit positively correlated firing patterns (red bars, Fig. 2(H)). These two classes of bimodality suggest that a simple subtraction of the opposing modulation at predictive and feedback times is probably not the only mechanism by which the motor system compares predictive and feedback signals in determining sensory prediction errors.

How the motor system weights the information and uncertainty in the predictions and sensory feedback is thought to be essential to computing sensory prediction errors (Shadmehr et al., 2010). A theoretical approach to combining these two sources of information uses a Kalman filter that minimizes the variance of the estimate (Kalman, 1960). This is similar to a Bayesian framework in which the integration of the prediction and the feedback is weighted by their respective uncertainty (i.e., inversely related to the variance) (Kording & Wolpert, 2004). Both the feedback responses to perturbations of reaching movements (Izawa & Shadmehr, 2008; Kording, Ku, & Wolpert, 2004) and the perceptual estimates of position and velocity have been explained using this framework (Ernst & Banks, 2002; Stocker & Simoncelli, 2006). Therefore, while bimodality is hypothesized to serve a well-defined computational purpose linked to the evaluation of sensory prediction errors, we still need to better understand how the predictive and feedback signals are integrated.

One consequence of this hypothesis is that a well-adapted internal model will reduce the simple spike sensitivity to self-generated sensory information in which the signals encoding the consequences of motor commands and those encoding sensory feedback cancel each other out. Consistent with this interpretation, projection targets of Purkinje cells in the rostral fastigial nucleus show greater sensitivity to passive self-motion driven by sensory feedback than to active, self-generated motion driven by both sensory and internal feedback (Brooks & Cullen, 2013). Cancellation of self-generated sensory signals also occurs in cerebellum-like structures owing to anti-Hebbian plasticity at the parallel fiber-principle neuron synapse that sculpts the response to the efferent copy into a negative image of the sensory response (Bell, Han, & Sawtell, 2008; Bell, Han, Sugawara, & Grant, 1997; Han, Grant, & Bell, 2000; Requarth & Sawtell, 2011; Sawtell & Bell, 2008).

Functional imaging studies show similar cerebellar activation patterns in motor and nonmotor tasks. Motor adaptation to constant force fields results in decreased positron emission tomographic activation to motor errors (Nezafat, Shadmehr, & Holcomb, 2001), similar to the reduction in the blood oxygen level-dependent response associated with learning of first-order rules in a cognitive task (Balsters & Ramnani, 2011). Cerebellar activation also decreases during fear conditioning, while both unexpected application and omission of the noxious stimuli triggered increased responses (Ploghaus et al., 2000). These patterns of activation during learning suggest that the cerebellum acquires task-specific internal models that provide predictive signals that oppose the feedback modulation. Adaptation involves minimizing the cerebellar response through cancellation of the predictive and feedback signals.

INTEGRATION OF SIMPLE SPIKE KINEMATIC AND ERROR SIGNALS

An important issue in cerebellar information processing is the signaling capacity of Purkinje cells. Previous studies provided evidence for three to five simultaneous kinematic signals in simple spike firing (Fu, Flament, et al., 1997; Gomi et al., 1998; Hore, Ritchie, & Watts, 1999; Marple-Horvat & Stein, 1987; Medina & Lisberger, 2009; Pasalar et al., 2006; Roitman et al., 2005). However, this level of signaling complexity appears to be simplistic given the physiological and anatomical properties of Purkinje cells. With approximately 200,000 parallel fiber–Purkinje cell synapses (Napper & Harvey, 1988) and fewer than 200 active synapses required to generate a simple spike (Isope & Barbour, 2002), Purkinje cells appear to have a high bandwidth and the capacity to carry a large number of signals. As others have proposed (Albus, 1971; Marr, 1969), Purkinje cells could use plasticity mechanisms to select only the relevant signals from the high number of possible parallel fiber inputs, and these relevant signals maintain consistent relationships to form a representation of the motor behavior. Our studies show that 18 independent signals, five kinematic and four error parameters that can be dually encoded, are represented in the simple spike discharge (Popa, 2013; Popa et al., 2012). Of the 18 possible signals considered, on an average, individual Purkinje cells encode simultaneously 10 of these signals. This level of signal integration is more consistent with the theoretical capabilities.

At the levels of both single Purkinje cells and the population, the strengths of the kinematic and error representations are comparable. Furthermore, accurate decoding of the upcoming behavior can be achieved for both kinematics and errors, which demonstrates that the encoding is equally robust. In addition, the error and kinematic signals are not segregated into subpopulations of Purkinje cells. The presence of both classes of representations in the simple spike discharge of individual neurons raises questions concerning the independence and linearity of the different signals. To address these questions two multilinear models of simple spike firing were evaluated, one with kinematic and the other with error terms. The regression results from the multilinear models were compared to the sum of the individual terms. Both the kinematic and the error signals are highly linear, as the sum of the individual R^2 profiles closely matches the R^2 profiles of the multilinear models (Hewitt et al., 2011; Popa et al., 2012). Therefore, the simple spike kinematic and error signals are largely independent and linear, and these findings support the hypothesis that Purkinje cells linearly integrate parallel fiber input (Walter & Khodakhah, 2006, 2009).

The finding that Purkinje cells simultaneously encode signals from functionally independent classes has two implications. The first implication relates to optimal feedback control theory, in which the integration of multiple classes of signals in Purkinje cells is consistent with utilizing all relevant information to maximize performance (Todorov & Jordan, 2002). The second implication is that associating different signal modalities is an important aspect of the cerebellar function. Functional imaging studies support the view that the cerebellum integrates multiple types of information for both motor and nonmotor domains (for review see Stoodley, 2012; Timmann et al., 2010). The association of information streams across modalities is central to several theories of the cerebellum's role in cognition (Drepper, Timmann, Kolb, & Diener, 1999; Molinari et al., 2008; Timmann et al., 2010).

CONCLUSIONS

This review focuses on the common processing of predictive and feedback signals in the simple spike discharge of Purkinje cells. The ubiquity of the dual encoding of performance errors and kinematics suggests a general principle of how the cerebellar cortex represents and processes motor information. The common signal processing supports the widely held view that the cerebellum provides a uniform computation across functional domains (Ito, 2008; Ramnani, 2006; Schmahmann, 2010; Thach, 2007).

With kinematics and task-specific performance information robustly represented in the simple spike firing, both at predictive and at feedback timings, we postulated that the cerebellar cortex provides two forward internal models. The first model provides accurate information about the arm kinematics that presumably is widely used in various types of movement (Fig. 3), as it has been shown that Purkinje cell kinematic signals generalize across arm movement tasks (Hewitt et al., 2011; Roitman et al., 2005). The second model is task-specific and provides accurate information about the movement consequences relative to the explicit goals of the task (Fig. 3). Although not specifically tested, we speculate that the cursor–target movement signals are learned and reflect the acquisition of a task-specific skill.

There are many questions that remain to understand how the predictive and feedback signals are used downstream either by the cerebellum or beyond. One of the first to consider is the consequences of the convergence of the predicative and feedback signals from tens of Purkinje cells onto neurons in the cerebellar nuclei. It will be essential to understand at the level of nuclear neurons the nature of the transformation of the simple spike signals, whether there is averaging of simple spike activity that minimizes uncorrelated noise (Eccles, 1973; Walter & Khodakhah, 2009) and/or extracts timing of correlated discharge (Person & Raman, 2012).

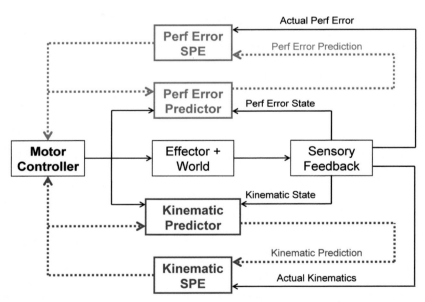

FIGURE 3 Schematic representation of multiple forward internal models for performance error (red) and kinematics (green). The performance and kinematic forward internal models (dashed lines) integrate information about the current performance error and kinematic state, respectively, with a motor command in order to predict the sensory consequences for the given parameter. The respective feed-forward predictions and subsequent sensory prediction errors (SPE) are generated and evaluated in parallel to achieve optimal task performance.

The second question concerns the timing of the kinematic and error signals. Specifically, are the t values the result of a computational process or do they represent sensory system constraints? Successful population decoding of the kinematic and error predictions combines individual Purkinje cell signals at all possible lead times. Therefore, the cerebellar cortex unfurls the predictions throughout a time window of at least 500 ms and could provide a mechanism for the cerebellum's role in coordination among effectors (Bastian, Martin, Keating, & Thach, 1996; van Donkelaar & Lee, 1994; Miall, Reckess, & Imamizu, 2001; Serrien & Wiesendanger, 2000; Thach, Goodkin, & Keating, 1992) and in movement sequences (Braitenberg, Heck, & Sultan, 1997; Molinari et al., 2008; Molinari et al., 1997; Nixon & Passingham, 2000). Another implication for the timing of the signals is in the cerebellum's involvement in working memory (Chen & Desmond, 2005; Hautzel, Mottaghy, Specht, Muller, & Krause, 2009; Marvel & Desmond, 2010). Having predictive and feedback signals over comparable time horizons, the cerebellar cortex may facilitate novel associations between past and current working memory content and among classes of information. Therefore, a major challenge is to understand the functional implications of signal timing for cerebellar function.

Acknowledgments

We thank Lijuan Zhou for technical support and Kris Bettin for manuscript preparation. This work was supported in part by NIH Grants R01 NS18338 and T32 GM008471 and NSF Grant IGERT DGE-1069104.

References

Albus, J. S. (1971). A theory of cerebellar function. *Mathematical Biosciences, 10*, 25–61.

Ashe, J., & Georgopoulos, A. P. (1994). Movement parameters and neural activity in motor cortex and area 5. *Cerebral Cortex, 4*, 590–600.

Balsters, J. H., & Ramnani, N. (2011). Cerebellar plasticity and the automation of first-order rules. *Journal of Neuroscience, 31*, 2305–2312.

Barmack, N. H., & Shojaku, H. (1995). Vestibular and visual climbing fiber signals evoked in the uvula-nodulus of the rabbit cerebellum by natural stimulation. *Journal of Neurophysiology, 74*, 2573–2589.

Barmack, N. H., & Simpson, J. I. (1980). Effects of microlesions of dorsal cap of inferior olive of rabbits on optokinetic and vestibuloocular reflexes. *Journal of Neurophysiology, 43*, 182–206.

Bastian, A. J., Martin, T. A., Keating, J. G., & Thach, W. T. (1996). Cerebellar ataxia: abnormal control of interaction torques across multiple joints. *Journal of Neurophysiology, 76*, 492–509.

Bell, C. C., Han, V., & Sawtell, N. B. (2008). Cerebellum-like structures and their implications for cerebellar function. *Annual Review of Neuroscience, 31*, 1–24.

Bell, C. C., Han, V. Z., Sugawara, Y., & Grant, K. (1997). Synaptic plasticity in a cerebellum-like structure depends on temporal order. *Nature, 387*, 278–281.

Berniker, M., & Kording, K. (2008). Estimating the sources of motor errors for adaptation and generalization. *Nature Neuroscience, 11*, 1454–1461.

Boyden, E. S., Katoh, A., & Raymond, J. L. (2004). Cerebellum-dependent learning: the role of multiple plasticity mechanisms. *Annual Review of Neuroscience, 27*, 581–609.

Boyden, E. S., & Raymond, J. L. (2003). Active reversal of motor memories reveals rules governing memory encoding. *Neuron, 39,* 1031–1042.

Braitenberg, V., & Atwood, R. P. (1958). Morphological observations on the cerebellar cortex. *Journal of Comparative Neurology, 109,* 1–33.

Braitenberg, V., Heck, D., & Sultan, F. (1997). The detection and generation of sequences as a key to cerebellar function: experiments and theory. *Behavioral and Brain Sciences, 20,* 229–245.

Brooks, J. X., & Cullen, K. E. (2013). The primate cerebellum selectively encodes unexpected self-motion. *Current Biology, 23,* 947–955.

Cameron, B. D., Franks, I. M., Inglis, J. T., & Chua, R. (2010). Reach adaptation to explicit vs. implicit target error. *Experimental Brain Research, 203,* 367–380.

Catz, N., Dicke, P. W., & Thier, P. (2005). Cerebellar complex spike firing is suitable to induce as well as to stabilize motor learning. *Current Biology, 15,* 2179–2189.

Cerminara, N. L., Apps, R., & Marple-Horvat, D. E. (2009). An internal model of a moving visual target in the lateral cerebellum. *Journal of Physiology, 587,* 429–442.

Chaumont, J., Guyon, N., Valera, A. M., Dugue, G. P., Popa, D., Marcaggi, P., et al. (2013). Clusters of cerebellar Purkinje cells control their afferent climbing fiber discharge. *Proceedings of the National Academy of Sciences of the United States of America, 110,* 16223–16228.

Chen, S. H., & Desmond, J. E. (2005). Cerebrocerebellar networks during articulatory rehearsal and verbal working memory tasks. *Neuroimage, 24,* 332–338.

Chen-Harris, H., Joiner, W. M., Ethier, V., Zee, D. S., & Shadmehr, R. (2008). Adaptive control of saccades via internal feedback. *Journal of Neuroscience, 28,* 2804–2813.

Coltz, J. D., Johnson, M. T., & Ebner, T. J. (1999). Cerebellar Purkinje cell simple spike discharge encodes movement velocity in primates during visuomotor arm tracking. *Journal of Neuroscience, 19,* 1782–1803.

Dash, S., Catz, N., Dicke, P. W., & Thier, P. (2010). Specific vermal complex spike responses build up during the course of smooth-pursuit adaptation, paralleling the decrease of performance error. *Experimental Brain Research, 205,* 41–55.

Dash, S., Catz, N., Dicke, P. W., & Thier, P. (2012). Encoding of smooth-pursuit eye movement initiation by a population of vermal Purkinje cells. *Cerebral Cortex, 22,* 877–891.

Dash, S., Dicke, P. W., & Thier, P. (2013). A vermal Purkinje cell simple spike population response encodes the changes in eye movement kinematics due to smooth pursuit adaptation. *Frontiers in Systems Neuroscience, 7,* 3.

Diedrichsen, J., Hashambhoy, Y., Rane, T., & Shadmehr, R. (2005). Neural correlates of reach errors. *Journal of Neuroscience, 25,* 9919–9931.

van Donkelaar, P., & Lee, R. G. (1994). Interactions between the eye and hand motor systems: disruptions due to cerebellar dysfunction. *Journal of Neurophysiology, 72,* 1674–1685.

Drepper, J., Timmann, D., Kolb, F. P., & Diener, H. C. (1999). Non-motor associative learning in patients with isolated degenerative cerebellar disease. *Brain, 122*(Pt 1), 87–97.

Ebner, T. J., & Fu, Q. (1997). What features of visually guided arm movements are encoded in the simple spike discharge of cerebellar Purkinje cells? *Progress in Brain Research, 114,* 431–447.

Ebner, T. J., Hewitt, A., & Popa, L. S. (2011). What features of movements are encoded in the discharge of cerebellar neurons during limb movements? *Cerebellum, 10,* 683–693.

Ebner, T. J., Johnson, M. T., Roitman, A., & Fu, Q. (2002). What do complex spikes signal about limb movements? *Annals of the New York Academy of Sciences, 978,* 205–218.

Eccles, J. C. (1973). The cerebellum as a computer: patterns in space and time. *Journal of Physiology, 229,* 1–32.

Ernst, M. O., & Banks, M. S. (2002). Humans integrate visual and haptic information in a statistically optimal fashion. *Nature, 415,* 429–433.

Flanagan, J. R., & Wing, A. M. (1997). The role of internal models in motion planning and control: evidence from grip force adjustments during movements of hand-held loads. *Journal of Neuroscience, 17,* 1519–1528.

Fortier, P. A., Kalaska, J. F., & Smith, A. M. (1989). Cerebellar neuronal activity related to whole-arm reaching movements in the monkey. *Journal of Neurophysiology, 62,* 198–211.

Frysinger, R. C., Bourbonnais, D., Kalaska, J. F., & Smith, A. M. (1984). Cerebellar cortical activity during antagonist cocontraction and reciprocal inhibition of forearm muscles. *Journal of Neurophysiology*, *51*, 32–49.

Fu, Q. G., Flament, D., Coltz, J. D., & Ebner, T. J. (1997). Relationship of cerebellar Purkinje cell simple spike discharge to movement kinematics in the monkey. *Journal of Neurophysiology*, *78*, 478–491.

Fu, Q. G., Mason, C. R., Flament, D., Coltz, J. D., & Ebner, T. J. (1997). Movement kinematics encoded in complex spike discharge of primate cerebellar Purkinje cells. *Neuroreport*, *8*, 523–529.

Gaveau, V., Prablanc, C., Laurent, D., Rossetti, Y., & Priot, A. E. (2014). Visuomotor adaptation needs a validation of prediction error by feedback error. *Frontiers in Human Neuroscience*, *8*, 880.

Giaquinta, G., Valle, M. S., Caserta, C., Casabona, A., Bosco, G., & Perciavalle, V. (2000). Sensory representation of passive movement kinematics by rat's spinocerebellar Purkinje cells. *Neuroscience Letters*, *285*, 41–44.

Gilbert, P. F., & Thach, W. T. (1977). Purkinje cell activity during motor learning. *Brain Research*, *128*, 309–328.

Golla, H., Tziridis, K., Haarmeier, T., Catz, N., Barash, S., & Thier, P. (2008). Reduced saccadic resilience and impaired saccadic adaptation due to cerebellar disease. *European Journal of Neuroscience*, *27*, 132–144.

Gomi, H., Shidara, M., Takemura, A., Inoue, Y., Kawano, K., & Kawato, M. (1998). Temporal firing patterns of Purkinje cells in the cerebellar ventral paraflocculus during ocular following responses in monkeys I. Simple spikes. *Journal of Neurophysiology*, *80*, 818–831.

Graf, W., Simpson, J. I., & Leonard, C. S. (1988). Spatial organization of visual messages of the rabbit's cerebellar flocculus. II. Complex and simple spike responses of Purkinje cells. *Journal of Neurophysiology*, *60*, 2091–2121.

Granger, C. W., & Newbold, P. (1974). Spurious regressions in econometrics. *Journal of Econometrics*, *2*, 111–120.

Greger, B., & Norris, S. (2005). Simple spike firing in the posterior lateral cerebellar cortex of *Macaque mulatta* was correlated with success-failure during a visually guided reaching task. *Experimental Brain Research*, *167*, 660–665.

Guthrie, B. L., Porter, J. D., & Sparks, D. L. (1983). Corollary discharge provides accurate eye position information to the oculomotor system. *Science*, *221*, 1193–1195.

Han, V. Z., Grant, K., & Bell, C. C. (2000). Reversible associative depression and nonassociative potentiation at a parallel fiber synapse. *Neuron*, *27*, 611–622.

Harvey, R. J., Porter, R., & Rawson, J. A. (1977). The natural discharges of Purkinje cells in paravermal regions of lobules V and VI of the monkey's cerebellum. *Journal of Physiology*, *271*, 515–536.

Hautzel, H., Mottaghy, F. M., Specht, K., Muller, H. W., & Krause, B. J. (2009). Evidence of a modality-dependent role of the cerebellum in working memory? An fMRI study comparing verbal and abstract n-back tasks. *Neuroimage*, *47*, 2073–2082.

Held, R., & Freedman, S. J. (1963). Plasticity in human sensorimotor control. *Science*, *142*, 455–462.

Hewitt, A. L., Popa, L. S., & Ebner, T. J. (2015). Changes in Purkinje cell simple spike encoding of reach kinematics during adaptation to a mechanical perturbation. *Journal of Neuroscience*, *35*, 1106–1124.

Hewitt, A., Popa, L. S., Pasalar, S., Hendrix, C. M., & Ebner, T. J. (2011). Representation of limb kinematics in Purkinje cell simple spike discharge is conserved across multiple tasks. *Journal of Neurophysiology*, *106*, 2232–2247.

Holdefer, R. N., & Miller, L. E. (2009). Dynamic correspondence between Purkinje cell discharge and forelimb muscle activity during reaching. *Brain Research*, *1295*, 67–75.

Horak, F. B., & Diener, H. C. (1994). Cerebellar control of postural scaling and central set in stance. *Journal of Neurophysiology*, *72*, 479–493.

Hore, J., Ritchie, R., & Watts, S. (1999). Finger opening in an overarm throw is not triggered by proprioceptive feedback from elbow extension or wrist flexion. *Experimental Brain Research, 125,* 302–312.

Horn, K. M., van Kan, P. L., & Gibson, A. R. (1996). Reduction of rostral dorsal accessory olive responses during reaching. *Journal of Neurophysiology, 76,* 4140–4151.

Ide, J. S., & Li, C. S. (2011). A cerebellar thalamic cortical circuit for error-related cognitive control. *Neuroimage, 54,* 455–464.

Imamizu, H., Miyauchi, S., Tamada, T., Sasaki, Y., Takino, R., Putz, B., et al. (2000). Human cerebellar activity reflecting an acquired internal model of a new tool. *Nature, 403,* 192–195.

Isope, P., & Barbour, B. (2002). Properties of unitary granule cell-->Purkinje cell synapses in adult rat cerebellar slices. *Journal of Neuroscience, 22,* 9668–9678.

Ito, M. (2000). Mechanisms of motor learning in the cerebellum. *Brain Research, 886,* 237–245.

Ito, M. (2008). Control of mental activities by internal models in the cerebellum. *Nature Reviews Neuroscience, 9,* 304–313.

Ito, M. (2013). Error detection and representation in the olivo-cerebellar system. *Frontiers in Neural Circuits, 7,* 1–8.

Ito, M., & Kano, M. (1982). Long-lasting depression of parallel fiber-Purkinje cell transmission induced by conjunctive stimulation of parallel fibers and climbing fibers in the cerebellar cortex. *Neuroscience Letters, 33,* 253–258.

Izawa, J., & Shadmehr, R. (2008). On-line processing of uncertain information in visuomotor control. *Journal of Neuroscience, 28,* 11360–11368.

Izawa, J., & Shadmehr, R. (2011). Learning from sensory and reward prediction errors during motor adaptation. *PLoS Computational Biology, 7,* e1002012.

Jacobson, G. A., Lev, I., Yarom, Y., & Cohen, D. (2009). Invariant phase structure of olivo-cerebellar oscillations and its putative role in temporal pattern generation. *Proceedings of the National Academy of Sciences of the United States of America, 106,* 3579–3584.

Jordan, M. I., & Rumelhart, D. E. (1992). Forward models: supervised learning with a distal teacher. *Cognitive Science, 16,* 307–354.

Kahlon, M., & Lisberger, S. G. (2000). Changes in the responses of Purkinje cells in the floccular complex of monkeys after motor learning in smooth pursuit eye movements. *Journal of Neurophysiology, 84,* 2945–2960.

Kalman, R. E. (1960). A new approach to linear filtering and prediction problems. *Transactions of the ASME – Journal of Basic Engineering, 82,* 35–45.

Kase, M., Noda, H., Suzuki, D. A., & Miller, D. C. (1979). Target velocity signals of visual tracking in vermal Purkinje cells of the monkey. *Science, 205,* 717–720.

Kawato, M. (1996). Learning internal models of the motor apparatus. In J. R. Bloedel, T. J. Ebner, & S. P. Wise (Eds.), *The acquisition of motor behavior in vertebrates* (pp. 409–430). Cambridge: MIT Press.

Kawato, M. (1999). Internal models for motor control and trajectory planning. *Current Opinion in Neurobiology, 9,* 718–727.

Kawato, M., & Gomi, H. (1992). A computational model of four regions of the cerebellum based on feedback-error learning. *Biological Cybernetics, 68,* 95–103.

Kawato, M., Kuroda, T., Imamizu, H., Nakano, E., Miyauchi, S., & Yoshioka, T. (2003). Internal forward models in the cerebellum: fMRI study on grip force and load force coupling. *Progress in Brain Research, 142,* 171–188.

Kawato, M., & Wolpert, D. (1998). Internal models for motor control. *Novartis Foundation Symposium, 218,* 291–304.

Ke, M. C., Guo, C. C., & Raymond, J. L. (2009). Elimination of climbing fiber instructive signals during motor learning. *Nature Neuroscience, 12,* 1171–1179.

Keele, S. W., & Ivry, R. (1990). Does the cerebellum provide a common computation for diverse tasks? A timing hypothesis. *Annals of the New York Academy of Sciences, 608,* 179–207.

Keller, E. L., & Robinson, D. A. (1971). Absence of a stretch reflex in extraocular muscles of the monkey. *Journal of Neurophysiology, 34,* 908–919.

Kimpo, R. R., Rinaldi, J. M., Kim, C. K., Payne, H. L., & Raymond, J. L. (2014). Gating of neural error signals during motor learning. *Elife*, *3*, e02076.

Kitazawa, S., Kimura, T., & Yin, P. B. (1998). Cerebellar complex spikes encode both destinations and errors in arm movements. *Nature*, *392*, 494–497.

Kobayashi, Y., Kawano, K., Takemura, A., Inoue, Y., Kitama, T., Gomi, H., et al. (1998). Temporal firing patterns of Purkinje cells in the cerebellar ventral paraflocculus during ocular following responses in monkeys II. Complex spikes. *Journal of Neurophysiology*, *80*, 832–848.

Kolb, F. P., Rubia, F. J., & Bauswein, E. (1987). Cerebellar unit responses of the mossy fibre system to passive movements in the decerebrate cat. I. Responses to static parameters. *Experimental Brain Research*, *68*, 234–248.

Kording, K. P., Ku, S. P., & Wolpert, D. M. (2004). Bayesian integration in force estimation. *Journal of Neurophysiology*, *92*, 3161–3165.

Kording, K. P., & Wolpert, D. M. (2004). Bayesian integration in sensorimotor learning. *Nature*, *427*, 244–247.

Krakauer, J. W., Ghilardi, M. F., Mentis, M., Barnes, A., Veytsman, M., Eidelberg, D., et al. (2004). Differential cortical and subcortical activations in learning rotations and gains for reaching: a PET study. *Journal of Neurophysiology*, *91*, 924–933.

Laurens, J., Meng, H., & Angelaki, D. E. (2013). Computation of linear acceleration through an internal model in the macaque cerebellum. *Nature Neuroscience*, *16*, 1701–1708.

Lisberger, S. G., Pavelko, T. A., Bronte-Stewart, H. M., & Stone, L. S. (1994). Neural basis for motor learning in the vestibuloocular reflex of primates. II. Changes in the responses of horizontal gaze velocity Purkinje cells in the cerebellar flocculus and ventral paraflocculus. *Journal of Neurophysiology*, *72*, 954–973.

Liu, X., Robertson, E., & Miall, R. C. (2003). Neuronal activity related to the visual representation of arm movements in the lateral cerebellar cortex. *Journal of Neurophysiology*, *89*, 1223–1237.

Llinas, R. R. (2013). The olivo-cerebellar system: a key to understanding the functional significance of intrinsic oscillatory brain properties. *Frontiers in Neural Circuits*, *7*, 96.

Llinas, R., & Sasaki, K. (1989). The functional organization of the olivo-cerebellar system as examined by multiple Purkinje cell recordings. *European Journal of Neuroscience*, *1*, 587–602.

Magescas, F., & Prablanc, C. (2006). Automatic drive of limb motor plasticity. *Journal of Cognitive Neuroscience*, *18*, 75–83.

Mano, N., & Yamamoto, K. (1980). Simple-spike activity of cerebellar Purkinje cells related to visually guided wrist tracking movement in the monkey. *Journal of Neurophysiology*, *43*, 713–728.

Marple-Horvat, D. E., & Stein, J. F. (1987). Cerebellar neuronal activity related to arm movements in trained rhesus monkeys. *Journal of Physiology*, *394*, 351–366.

Marr, D. (1969). A theory of cerebellar cortex. *Journal of Physiology*, *202*, 437–470.

Marshall, S. P., & Lang, E. J. (2009). Local changes in the excitability of the cerebellar cortex produce spatially restricted changes in complex spike synchrony. *Journal of Neuroscience*, *29*, 14352–14362.

Martin, T. A., Keating, J. G., Goodkin, H. P., Bastian, A. J., & Thach, W. T. (1996). Throwing while looking through prisms. I. Focal olivocerebellar lesions impair adaptation. *Brain*, *119*, 1183–1198.

Marvel, C. L., & Desmond, J. E. (2010). Functional topography of the cerebellum in verbal working memory. *Neuropsychology Review*, *20*, 271–279.

Mazzoni, P., & Krakauer, J. W. (2006). An implicit plan overrides an explicit strategy during visuomotor adaptation. *Journal of Neuroscience*, *26*, 3642–3645.

Medina, J. F., & Lisberger, S. G. (2008). Links from complex spikes to local plasticity and motor learning in the cerebellum of awake-behaving monkeys. *Nature Neuroscience*, *11*, 1185–1192.

Medina, J. F., & Lisberger, S. G. (2009). Encoding and decoding of learned smooth pursuit eye movements in the floccular complex of the monkey cerebellum. *Journal of Neurophysiology, 102,* 2039–2054.

Miall, R. C., Christensen, L. O., Cain, O., & Stanley, J. (2007). Disruption of state estimation in the human lateral cerebellum. *PLoS Biology, 5,* e316.

Miall, R. C., Reckess, G. Z., & Imamizu, H. (2001). The cerebellum coordinates eye and hand tracking movements. *Nature Neuroscience, 4,* 638–644.

Miall, R. C., & Wolpert, D. M. (1996). Forward models for physiological motor control. *Neural Networks, 9,* 1265–1279.

Miles, F. A., Braitman, D. J., & Dow, B. M. (1980). Long-term adaptive changes in primate vestibuloocular reflex. IV. Electrophysiological observations in flocculus of adapted monkeys. *Journal of Neurophysiology, 43,* 1477–1493.

Miles, F. A., Fuller, J. H., Braitman, D. J., & Dow, B. M. (1980). Long-term adaptive changes in primate vestibuloocular reflex. III. Electrophysiological observations in flocculus of normal monkeys. *Journal of Neurophysiology, 43,* 1437–1476.

Miles, F. A., & Lisberger, S. G. (1981). The "error" signals subserving adaptive gain control in the primate vestibulo-ocular reflex. *Annals of the New York Academy of Sciences, 374,* 513–525.

Miles, O. B., Cerminara, N. L., & Marple-Horvat, D. E. (2006). Purkinje cells in the lateral cerebellum of the cat encode visual events and target motion during visually guided reaching. *Journal of Physiology, 571,* 619–637.

Molinari, M., Chiricozzi, F. R., Clausi, S., Tedesco, A. M., De Lisa, M., & Leggio, M. G. (2008). Cerebellum and detection of sequences, from perception to cognition. *Cerebellum, 7,* 611–615.

Molinari, M., Leggio, M. G., Solida, A., Ciorra, R., Misciagna, S., Silveri, M. C., et al. (1997). Cerebellum and procedural learning: evidence from focal cerebellar lesions. *Brain, 120* (Pt 10), 1753–1762.

Morton, S. M., & Bastian, A. J. (2006). Cerebellar contributions to locomotor adaptations during splitbelt treadmill walking. *Journal of Neuroscience, 26,* 9107–9116.

Muller, F., & Dichgans, J. (1994). Impairments of precision grip in two patients with acute unilateral cerebellar lesions: a simple parametric test for clinical use. *Neuropsychologia, 32,* 265–269.

Najafi, F., Giovannucci, A., Wang, S. S., & Medina, J. F. (2014a). Coding of stimulus strength via analog calcium signals in Purkinje cell dendrites of awake mice. *Elife, 3,* e03663.

Najafi, F., Giovannucci, A., Wang, S. S., & Medina, J. F. (2014b). Sensory-driven enhancement of calcium signals in individual Purkinje cell dendrites of awake mice. *Cell Reports, 6,* 792–798.

Napper, R. M., & Harvey, R. J. (1988). Number of parallel fiber synapses on an individual Purkinje cell in the cerebellum of the rat. *Journal of Comparative Neurology, 274,* 168–177.

Nezafat, R., Shadmehr, R., & Holcomb, H. H. (2001). Long-term adaptation to dynamics of reaching movements: a PET study. *Experimental Brain Research, 140,* 66–76.

Nguyen-Vu, T. D., Kimpo, R. R., Rinaldi, J. M., Kohli, A., Zeng, H., Deisseroth, K., et al. (2013). Cerebellar Purkinje cell activity drives motor learning. *Nature Neuroscience, 16,* 1734–1736.

Nixon, P. D., & Passingham, R. E. (2000). The cerebellum and cognition: cerebellar lesions impair sequence learning but not conditional visuomotor learning in monkeys. *Neuropsychologia, 38,* 1054–1072.

Noda, H., & Suzuki, D. A. (1979). The role of the flocculus of the monkey in saccadic eye movements. *Journal of Physiology, 294,* 317–334.

Noto, C. T., & Robinson, F. R. (2001). Visual error is the stimulus for saccade gain adaptation. *Cognitive Brain Research, 12,* 301–305.

Nowak, D. A., Hermsdorfer, J., Rost, K., Timmann, D., & Topka, H. (2004). Predictive and reactive finger force control during catching in cerebellar degeneration. *Cerebellum, 3,* 227–235.

Ohmae, S., Uematsu, A., & Tanaka, M. (2013). Temporally specific sensory signals for the detection of stimulus omission in the primate deep cerebellar nuclei. *Journal of Neuroscience, 33*, 15432–15441.

Ojakangas, C. L., & Ebner, T. J. (1992). Purkinje cell complex and simple spike changes during a voluntary arm movement learning task in the monkey. *Journal of Neurophysiology, 68*, 2222–2236.

Ojakangas, C. L., & Ebner, T. J. (1994). Purkinje cell complex spike activity during voluntary motor learning: relationship to kinematics. *Journal of Neurophysiology, 72*, 2617–2630.

O'Reilly, J. X., Mesulam, M. M., & Nobre, A. C. (2008). The cerebellum predicts the timing of perceptual events. *Journal of Neuroscience, 28*, 2252–2260.

Paninski, L., Fellows, M. R., Hatsopoulos, N. G., & Donoghue, J. P. (2004). Spatiotemporal tuning of motor cortical neurons for hand position and velocity. *Journal of Neurophysiology, 91*, 515–532.

Pasalar, S., Roitman, A. V., Durfee, W. K., & Ebner, T. J. (2006). Force field effects on cerebellar Purkinje cell discharge with implications for internal models. *Nature Neuroscience, 9*, 1404–1411.

Person, A. L., & Raman, I. M. (2012). Purkinje neuron synchrony elicits time-locked spiking in the cerebellar nuclei. *Nature, 481*, 502–505.

Ploghaus, A., Tracey, I., Clare, S., Gati, J. S., Rawlins, J. N., & Matthews, P. M. (2000). Learning about pain: the neural substrate of the prediction error for aversive events. *Proceedings of the National Academy of Sciences of the United States of America, 97*, 9281–9286.

Popa. L.S. (2013). *Computational studies of cerebellar cortical circuitry.* (Ph.D. thesis). University of Minnesota.

Popa, L. S., Hewitt, A. L., & Ebner, T. J. (2012). Predictive and feedback performance errors are signaled in the simple spike discharge of individual Purkinje cells. *Journal of Neuroscience, 32*, 15345–15358.

Popa, L. S., Hewitt, A. L., & Ebner, T. J. (2014). The cerebellum for jocks and nerds alike. *Frontiers in Systems Neuroscience, 8*, 1–13.

Prsa, M., & Thier, P. (2011). The role of the cerebellum in saccadic adaptation as a window into neural mechanisms of motor learning. *European Journal of Neuroscience, 33*, 2114–2128.

Ramnani, N. (2006). The primate cortico-cerebellar system: anatomy and function. *Nature Reviews Neuroscience, 7*, 511–522.

Rasmussen, A., Jirenhed, D. A., Zucca, R., Johansson, F., Svensson, P., & Hesslow, G. (2013). Number of spikes in climbing fibers determines the direction of cerebellar learning. *Journal of Neuroscience, 33*, 13436–13440.

Requarth, T., & Sawtell, N. B. (2011). Neural mechanisms for filtering self-generated sensory signals in cerebellum-like circuits. *Current Opinion in Neurobiology, 21*, 602–608.

Robinson, D. A. (1975). Oculomotor control signals. In P. Bachyrita, & G. Lennerstrand (Eds.), *Basic mechanisms of ocular motility and their clinical implications* (pp. 337–374). Oxford, UK: Pergamon.

Roitman, A. V., Pasalar, S., & Ebner, T. J. (2009). Single trial coupling of Purkinje cell activity to speed and error signals during circular manual tracking. *Experimental Brain Research, 192*, 241–251.

Roitman, A. V., Pasalar, S., Johnson, M. T., & Ebner, T. J. (2005). Position, direction of movement, and speed tuning of cerebellar Purkinje cells during circular manual tracking in monkey. *Journal of Neuroscience, 25*, 9244–9257.

Rubia, F. J., & Kolb, F. P. (1978). Responses of cerebellar units to a passive movement in the decerebrate cat. *Experimental Brain Research, 31*, 387–401.

Sasaki, K., Bower, J. M., & Llinas, R. (1989). Multiple Purkinje cell recording in rodent cerebellar cortex. *European Journal of Neuroscience, 1*, 572–586.

Sawtell, N. B., & Bell, C. C. (2008). Adaptive processing in electrosensory systems: links to cerebellar plasticity and learning. *Journal of Physiology, Paris, 102*, 223–232.

Schlerf, J. E., Ivry, R. B., & Diedrichsen, J. (2012). Encoding of sensory prediction errors in the human cerebellum. *Journal of Neuroscience, 32*, 4913–4922.

Schmahmann, J. D. (2010). The role of the cerebellum in cognition and emotion: personal reflections since 1982 on the dysmetria of thought hypothesis, and its historical evolution from theory to therapy. *Neuropsychology Review, 20,* 236–260.

Serrien, D. J., & Wiesendanger, M. (2000). Temporal control of a bimanual task in patients with cerebellar dysfunction. *Neuropsychologia, 38,* 558–565.

Shadmehr, R., & Holcomb, H. H. (1997). Neural correlates of motor memory consolidation. *Science, 277,* 821–825.

Shadmehr, R., & Krakauer, J. W. (2008). A computational neuroanatomy for motor control. *Experimental Brain Research, 185,* 359–381.

Shadmehr, R., Smith, M. A., & Krakauer, J. W. (2010). Error correction, sensory prediction, and adaptation in motor control. *Annual Review of Neuroscience, 33,* 89–108.

Shidara, M., Kawano, K., Gomi, H., & Kawato, M. (1993). Inverse-dynamics model eye movement control by Purkinje cells in the cerebellum. *Nature, 365,* 50–52.

Smith, A. M. (1981). The coactivation of antagonist muscles. *Canadian Journal of Physiology and Pharmacology, 59,* 733–747.

Smith, M. A., & Shadmehr, R. (2005). Intact ability to learn internal models of arm dynamics in Huntington's disease but not cerebellar degeneration. *Journal of Neurophysiology, 93,* 2809–2821.

Soetedjo, R., & Fuchs, A. F. (2006). Complex spike activity of Purkinje cells in the oculomotor vermis during behavioral adaptation of monkey saccades. *Journal of Neuroscience, 26,* 7741–7755.

Soetedjo, R., Kojima, Y., & Fuchs, A. (2008). Complex spike activity signals the direction and size of dysmetric saccade errors. *Progress in Brain Research, 171,* 153–159.

Stocker, A. A., & Simoncelli, E. P. (2006). Noise characteristics and prior expectations in human visual speed perception. *Nature Neuroscience, 9,* 578–585.

Stone, L. S., & Lisberger, S. G. (1986). Detection of tracking errors by visual climbing fiber inputs to monkey cerebellar flocculus during pursuit eye movements. *Neuroscience Letters, 72,* 163–168.

Stone, L. S., & Lisberger, S. G. (1990). Visual responses of Purkinje cells in the cerebellar flocculus during smooth-pursuit eye movements in monkeys. I. Simple spikes. *Journal of Neurophysiology, 63,* 1241–1261.

Stoodley, C. J. (2012). The cerebellum and cognition: evidence from functional imaging studies. *Cerebellum, 11,* 352–365.

Taylor, J. A., & Ivry, R. B. (2012). The role of strategies in motor learning. *Annals of the New York Academy of Sciences, 1241,* 1–12.

Tesche, C. D., & Karhu, J. J. (2000). Anticipatory cerebellar responses during somatosensory omission in man. *Human Brain Mapping, 9,* 119–142.

Thach, W. T. (1968). Discharge of Purkinje and cerebellar nuclear neurons during rapidly alternating arm movements in the monkey. *Journal of Neurophysiology, 31,* 785–797.

Thach, W. T. (1970). Discharge of cerebellar neurons related to two maintained postures and two prompt movements. II. Purkinje cell output and input. *Journal of Neurophysiology, 33,* 537–547.

Thach, W. T. (2007). On the mechanism of cerebellar contributions to cognition. *Cerebellum, 6,* 163–167.

Thach, W. T., Goodkin, H. P., & Keating, J. G. (1992). The cerebellum and the adaptive coordination of movement. *Annual Review of Neuroscience, 15,* 403–442.

Thier, P., Dicke, P. W., Haas, R., & Barash, S. (2000). Encoding of movement time by populations of cerebellar Purkinje cells. *Nature, 405,* 72–76.

Timmann, D., Drepper, J., Frings, M., Maschke, M., Richter, S., Gerwig, M., et al. (2010). The human cerebellum contributes to motor, emotional and cognitive associative learning. A review. *Cortex, 46,* 845–857.

Todorov, E. (2004). Optimality principles in sensorimotor control. *Nature Neuroscience, 7,* 907–915.

Todorov, E., & Jordan, M. I. (2002). Optimal feedback control as a theory of motor coordination. *Nature Neuroscience, 5*, 1226–1235.

Tseng, Y. W., Diedrichsen, J., Krakauer, J. W., Shadmehr, R., & Bastian, A. J. (2007). Sensory prediction errors drive cerebellum-dependent adaptation of reaching. *Journal of Neurophysiology, 98*, 54–62.

Valle, M. S., Bosco, G., & Poppele, R. (2000). Information processing in the spinocerebellar system. *Neuroreport, 11*, 4075–4079.

Wagner, M. J., & Smith, M. A. (2008). Shared internal models for feedforward and feedback control. *Journal of Neuroscience, 28*, 10663–10673.

Wallman, J., & Fuchs, A. F. (1998). Saccadic gain modification: visual error drives motor adaptation. *Journal of Neurophysiology, 80*, 2405–2416.

Walter, J. T., & Khodakhah, K. (2006). The linear computational algorithm of cerebellar Purkinje cells. *Journal of Neuroscience, 26*, 12861–12872.

Walter, J. T., & Khodakhah, K. (2009). The advantages of linear information processing for cerebellar computation. *Proceedings of the National Academy of Sciences of the United States of America, 106*, 4471–4476.

Wang, J. J., Kim, J. H., & Ebner, T. J. (1987). Climbing fiber afferent modulation during a visually guided, multi-joint arm movement in the monkey. *Brain Research, 410*, 323–329.

Waterhouse, B. D., & Mcelligott, J. G. (1980). Simple spike activity of Purkinje cells in the posterior vermis of awake cats during spontaneous saccadic eye movements. *Brain Research Bulletin, 5*, 159–168.

Welsh, J. P., Lang, E. J., Suglhara, I., & Llinas, R. (1995). Dynamic organization of motor control within the olivocerebellar system. *Nature, 374*, 453–457.

Witter, L., Canto, C. B., Hoogland, T. M., de Gruijl, J. R., & De Zeeuw, C. I. (2013). Strength and timing of motor responses mediated by rebound firing in the cerebellar nuclei after Purkinje cell activation. *Frontiers in Neural Circuits, 7*, 133.

Wolpert, D. M., & Ghahramani, Z. (2000). Computational principles of movement neuroscience. *Nature Neuroscience*, 1212–1217.

Wolpert, D. M., Ghahramani, Z., & Jordan, M. I. (1995). An internal model for sensorimotor integration. *Science, 269*, 1880–1882.

Wolpert, D. M., Miall, R. C., & Kawato, M. (1998). Internal models in the cerebellum. *Trends in Cognitive Sciences, 2*, 338–347.

Xu-Wilson, M., Chen-Harris, H., Zee, D. S., & Shadmehr, R. (2009). Cerebellar contributions to adaptive control of saccades in humans. *Journal of Neuroscience, 29*, 12930–12939.

Yamamoto, K., Kawato, M., Kotosaka, S., & Kitazawa, S. (2007). Encoding of movement dynamics by Purkinje cell simple spike activity during fast arm movements under resistive and assistive force fields. *Journal of Neurophysiology, 97*, 1588–1599.

Yang, Y., & Lisberger, S. G. (2014). Purkinje-cell plasticity and cerebellar motor learning are graded by complex-spike duration. *Nature, 510*, 529–532.

2

Deep Cerebellar Nuclei Rebound Firing In Vivo: Much Ado About Almost Nothing?

Davide Reato, Esra Tara, Kamran Khodakhah

Dominick P. Purpura Department of Neuroscience, Albert Einstein College of Medicine, Bronx, NY, USA

INTRODUCTION

Broadly speaking, there are at least two excellent reasons to be enchanted by the cerebellum and to study it. The first is that, as the structure bestowed with the function of motor coordination (Armstrong & Edgley, 1984; Lisberger & Fuchs, 1978; Ojakangas & Ebner, 1992; Thach, 1968) (and maybe even elements of cognitive processing (Allen, Buxton, Wong, & Courchesne, 1997; Gao et al., 1996)), it is clearly important to delineate its computational principles (Albus, 1971; Eccles, 1973; Heck, De Zeeuw, Jaeger, Khodakhah, & Person, 2013; Ito, 1984; Wolpert, Miall, & Kawato, 1998). This is necessary not only for unraveling on how it performs its tasks, but also for obtaining the requisite knowledge needed to correct its dysfunction in cerebellar-related ataxia and cognitive disorders (Courchesne, Yeung-Courchesne, Press, Hesselink, & Jernigan, 1988; Jen, Kim, & Baloh, 2004; Levin et al., 2006; Mullen, Eicher, & Sidman, 1976; Walter, Alvina, Womack, Chevez, & Khodakhah, 2006). The second reason to be cerebellum-centric is that the cerebellum is most likely the structure that will lead us to an understanding of higher order brain function. This is because compared to other structures in the brain the cerebellum has the best understood circuitry, clear input–output pathways, and tractable behavioral paradigms that allow one to scrutinize its function. In short, as once eloquently put by David Linden "the cerebellum ... is the place where the 'holy grail' of neuroscience will first be found: a complete molecules-to-cells-to-circuits-to-behavior understanding" (Linden, 2003).

THE COMPUTATIONAL PRINCIPLES OF THE CEREBELLUM

Given the appeal of the cerebellum to neuroscientists, it is not surprising that it has attracted a diverse group of capable researchers, from theoreticians to synaptic physiologists, and from single-molecule biophysicists to system neurobiologists. The rich composition of scientists interested in cerebellar function in recent years has yielded brisk progress. However, because of their intense interest, many primary questions regarding cerebellar function and computation remain hotly debated. Perhaps one of the most fundamental of these debates is the question of how information is encoded and decoded by the cerebellar circuitry. For example, it remains to be determined whether cerebellar Purkinje cells, the principal computational element of the cerebellar cortex, encode information linearly in their firing rate (Allen, Azzena, & Ohno, 1974; Eccles, Sabah, Schmidt, & Taborikova, 1972; Thach, 1967; Walter & Khodakhah, 2006, 2009), in the duration of pauses in their activity (De Schutter & Steuber, 2009; Steuber et al., 2007), or in their activity pattern (Shin et al., 2007). Similarly, it is unclear how neurons of the deep cerebellar nuclei (DCN) integrate the information transmitted to them by Purkinje cells to provide the major output of the cerebellum (De Zeeuw et al., 2011; Gauck & Jaeger, 2000; Person & Raman, 2012). An intriguing related question, and the subject matter of this chapter, is whether DCN neurons use rebound firing to transform their inhibitory Purkinje cells inputs into excitatory signals.

THE DEEP CEREBELLAR NUCLEI: THE CEREBELLUM'S GATEWAY TO THE BRAIN

Like some other principal neurons of the basal ganglia, cerebellum, and thalamus that are involved in the control of movement, DCN neurons are spontaneously active (Rowland & Jaeger, 2005; Thach, 1968). In fact, in the absence of any synaptic input DCN neurons, similar to Purkinje cells (Nam & Hockberger, 1997; Raman & Bean, 1999), reliably fire action potentials with great regularity and precision such that the coefficient of variation of their interspike intervals is merely an astonishing 5% or so (Alvina & Khodakhah, 2008). Their firing rate in vivo, however, is dynamically modulated over a wide range of frequencies by GABAergic Purkinje cell inputs and by excitatory glutamatergic inputs formed mainly by mossy and climbing fiber collaterals (De Zeeuw et al., 2011). It is nowadays well established that DCN neurons, unlike a simple relay station, actively process information received from Purkinje cells to generate the output of the cerebellum.

REBOUND DEPOLARIZATION: A POTENTIAL FEATURE OF SPONTANEOUSLY ACTIVE NEURONS

An intriguing biophysical feature of any spontaneously active neuron is rebound excitation (Llinas & Sugimori, 1980). If the membrane potential of a spontaneously active neuron is hyperpolarized to a negative enough potential and for a long enough duration its membrane potential at the end of the hyperpolarization is likely to rebound to a more depolarized level compared to its baseline (Aizenman & Linden, 1999; Aizenman, Manis, & Linden, 1998). The reason for this rebound excitation is that during spontaneous activity not all voltage-gated sodium channels that inactivate with each action potential have the chance to recover from inactivation before the next spike. Thus, depending on the rate of its spontaneous activity, a neuron might be operating with only a small fraction of its sodium channels (Raman, Gustafson, & Padgett, 2000). A long and deep enough hyperpolarization will allow the bulk of sodium channels to recover from inactivation. In this case as the cell repolarizes after the hyperpolarizing episode the higher proportion of available sodium channels will yield a more depolarized membrane potential. This rebound excitation pursuant to an "anodal break" (as referred to by the old-timers) is in fact fairly common.

LOW-THRESHOLD T-TYPE CALCIUM CHANNELS AND REBOUND FIRING

In some cells rebound excitation, and by extension rebound firing, is augmented by the presence of low-threshold calcium channels (Aizenman & Linden, 1999; Alvina, Ellis-Davies, & Khodakhah, 2009; Boehme, Uebele, Renger, & Pedroarena, 2011; Llinas & Muhlethaler, 1988; Molineux et al., 2006; Pugh & Raman, 2006). Conductances such as T-type calcium channels have the property that they activate, and rapidly inactivate, at relatively hyperpolarized membrane potentials such as those experienced by a spontaneously active cell. Very much like those discussed for sodium channels earlier, periods of hyperpolarization facilitate recovery of these calcium channels from inactivation. The only difference in the contributions of these two conductances to rebound excitation is that low-threshold calcium channels generally inactivate much faster than sodium channels. The consequence of this difference is that when T-type calcium channels make a significant contribution to rebound excitation in a cell the rebound is more transient. In many cells a T-type-mediated rebound firing presents as a brief high-frequency burst, which lasts for only a few tens of milliseconds. This transient burst of high-frequency firing is an ideal coding mechanism with a very good signal-to-noise ratio (SNR) because the firing rate during the burst is typically an order of magnitude or so higher than that during the cell's "resting" activity. Moreover, the very brief and transient nature of the burst allows it to precisely mark the timing of an event (Kistler, van Hemmen, & De Zeeuw, 2000; Wetmore, Mukamel, & Schnitzer, 2008).

REBOUND FIRING: AN INTRIGUING AND EFFECTIVE CODING MECHANISM THAT CONVERTS INHIBITORY INPUTS TO EXCITATORY ONES

The more depolarized membrane potential during rebound excitation may result in a higher firing rate after the pause. This increase in the firing rate, termed rebound firing, is transient and lasts a few hundreds of milliseconds (Aizenman & Linden, 1999; Engbers et al., 2011; Jahnsen, 1986a; Llinas & Muhlethaler, 1988; Molineux et al., 2008; Pugh & Raman, 2006; Tadayonnejad, Mehaffey, Anderson, & Turner, 2009; Zheng & Raman, 2011). How high the firing rate goes during rebound firing depends on several factors, including the fraction of sodium channels that remain inactivated during normal pacemaking and the extent to which the hyperpolarization is successful in removing inactivation (Sangrey & Jaeger, 2010).

The transient period of increased activity during rebound firing can be an effective signaling mechanism and is one in which an inhibitory input is literally transformed into a pseudo-excitatory one (Eccles, 1973; Witter, Canto, Hoogland, de Gruijl, & De Zeeuw, 2013). Moreover, the magnitude of rebound firing can be a reliable indicator of the strength of the inhibitory input since the stronger the inhibition, the longer and (if the chloride reversal potential is not already reached) the more hyperpolarized the membrane potential would be (Sangrey & Jaeger, 2010). As discussed, longer and deeper hyperpolarizations translate into recovery of a larger fraction of sodium channels from inactivation and thus a greater rebound excitation (Aizenman & Linden, 1999; Raman et al., 2000).

REBOUND FIRING IN THE DEEP CEREBELLAR NUCLEI NEURONS: A PROMINENT BIOPHYSICAL FEATURE

Given that the information content of the computational circuitry of the cerebellar cortex is relayed to DCN neurons solely by inhibitory GABAergic inputs, whether DCN neurons encode information by rebound firing has been a long-standing question (Alvina, Walter, Kohn, Ellis-Davies, & Khodakhah, 2008; Bengtsson, Ekerot, & Jorntell, 2011; De Schutter & Steuber, 2009; De Zeeuw et al., 2011; Hoebeek, Witter, Ruigrok, & De Zeeuw, 2010; Wetmore et al., 2008). In fact, biophysically, DCN neurons satisfy all the requisites of a good "rebound burster." They operate with only a fraction of their total sodium channels (Raman et al., 2000), and most of them express a relatively high density of low-threshold T-type calcium channels (Gauck, Thomann, Jaeger, & Borst, 2001; Molineux et al., 2006; Muri & Knopfel, 1994; Volsen et al., 1995). Indeed, it is universally found that strong hyperpolarizations lead to significant rebound firing in the form of brief, transient high-frequency bursts. The primary conductance in DCN neurons that contributes to rebound firing appears to be T-type calcium channels, because blocking them with mibefradil or NNC 55-0396 completely abolishes rebound firing (Alvina et al., 2009). Given the ease with which rebound firing can be demonstrated in DCN neurons, and the attractiveness of a coding mechanism whereby the strength of the inhibitory Purkinje cell inputs can be converted to graded excitatory responses in DCN neurons (Witter et al., 2013), it is of little surprise that rebound firing has become the centerpiece of many theories of cerebellar function (De Schutter & Steuber, 2009; Jaeger, 2011; Kistler et al., 2000; Wetmore et al., 2008). In fact, many in the field have postulated that rebound firing may be the main, if not the sole, mechanism by which DCN neurons dynamically encode information relayed to them by Purkinje cells.

DEEP CEREBELLAR NUCLEI REBOUND FIRING: THE DEVIL IS IN THE DETAILS

Despite the robustness of rebound firing in DCN neurons under many experimental conditions in vitro, whether it is in fact the mechanism by which the cerebellum encodes information in vivo is a matter of some debate (Aksenov, Serdyukova, Irwin, & Bracha, 2004; Alvina et al., 2008; Bengtsson et al., 2011; Chaumont et al., 2013; Hoebeek et al., 2010; Holdefer, Houk, & Miller, 2005; Rowland & Jaeger, 2005). At the core of these debates is the question of how effective GABAergic Purkinje cell synaptic inputs are at hyperpolarizing DCN neurons. Do hyperpolarizations caused by physiologically relevant activity of Purkinje cells actually drive the membrane potential of DCN neurons to become negative enough and for long enough periods of time to yield meaningful rebound firing? Is rebound firing-like activity present during common behaviors?

How Effective are Purkinje Cell Inputs in Hyperpolarizing Deep Cerebellar Nuclei Neurons?

A theory on DCN rebound firing suggests that it is the activity of Purkinje cells that hyperpolarizes the membrane potential of DCN neurons to yield rebound firing. Evidence suggests that Purkinje cells' GABAergic inputs onto DCN neurons are not very effective at activating metabotropic GABAergic receptors (Billard, Vigot, & Batini, 1993). Instead, it is widely accepted that these inputs increase the membrane permeability of DCN neurons to chloride ions by activating GABA-gated chloride channels (De Zeeuw & Berrebi, 1995; Palkovits, Mezey, Hamori, & Szentagothai, 1977). Therefore, activation of Purkinje cell inputs can maximally hyperpolarize DCN neurons to their chloride reversal potential (E_{Cl}). The chloride reversal potential of DCN neurons has been measured in various preparations and species, all of which have yielded comparable values (Aizenman & Linden, 1999; Jahnsen, 1986b). Using gramicidin-perforated recordings in juvenile mice Zheng and Raman (2009) estimated the E_{Cl} to be around −75 mV. This is relatively shallow compared to membrane potentials as negative as −90 mV reported in studies in which rebound firing was examined by direct hyperpolarization of the membrane (Aizenman & Linden, 1999). Indeed, careful examination of the biophysical properties of T-type calcium channels in DCN neurons revealed that a membrane potential of −75 mV is not very effective at recovering T-type calcium channels from inactivation (McRory et al., 2001; Perez-Reyes, 2003). This suggests that for Purkinje cell synaptic inputs to produce T-type calcium channel-dependent rebound firing in DCN neurons either the duration of the synaptically induced hyperpolarization must be quite long or the chloride reversal potential in the cells must be made more negative (perhaps by an activity-dependent modification of the chloride transporters).

Rebound Firing Following Electrical or Optogenetic Stimulation In Vivo

There is no disagreement among any labs that with a strong hyperpolarization it is possible to generate strong and transient rebound firing in DCN neurons. Less clear are the conditions in vivo that are capable of generating strong and transient rebound firing.

In a previous study, when pauses in DCN activity were induced by stimulating Purkinje cells electrically in anesthetized mice, 90% of the cells were found to have comparable pre- and post-stimulus-induced-pause firing rates (Alvina et al., 2008) (Fig. 1). This result is in contrast to another study showing increased postpause firing rates (43%) in about half of the DCN neurons after electrical stimulation of the cerebellar cortex (Hoebeek et al., 2010). A possible explanation for the lack of rebound firing in Alvina et al.

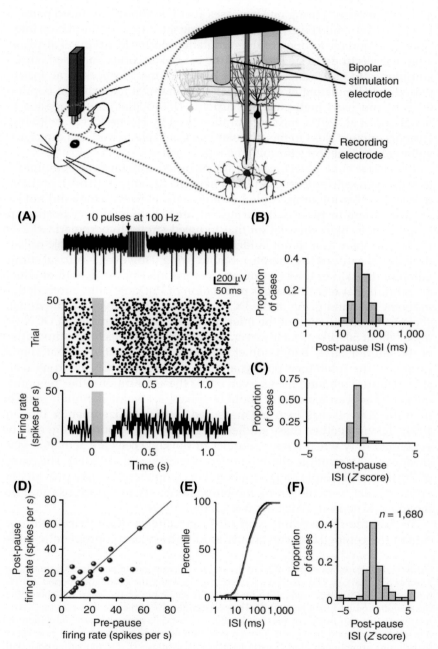

FIGURE 1 Rebound firing is not a common response in vivo. Single-unit activity of DCN neurons was monitored in vivo while the Purkinje cells overlaying them were electrically activated (10 electrical pulses at 100 Hz) to produce prominent pauses in DCN firing.

and the presence of firing rate increases after the stimulus-induced pause in Hoebeek et al. could be given by considering the different stimulation intensities used and the location of the stimulation electrode. Alvina et al. placed a bipolar electrode to simply touch the cerebellar cortex and used current amplitudes to just induce pauses of about 250 ms. Hoebeek et al. instead placed the stimulating electrode inside the brain, at a maximum depth of 0.5 mm, and used high-intensity currents (150–300 μA). As suggested by Bengtsson et al. (2011), the configuration used by Hoebeek et al., with high currents applied close to the granular layer, is likely to lead to a direct activation of DCN neurons through the mossy fibers.

Bengtsson et al. (2011), using cats, recorded spontaneous large inhibitory postsynaptic potentials in DCN neurons (usually 3–10 mV), probably due to coactivation of multiple Purkinje cells. However, they did not see any significant increase in the firing rate after these inhibitory postsynaptic potentials. Skin stimulation that induced strong hyperpolarization in DCN neurons was also not sufficient to activate enough Purkinje cells to drive DCN neurons to generate rebound firing. However, electrical stimulation of the skin or direct stimulation of the inferior olive, both of which are stimuli that recruit a larger population of Purkinje cells, succeeded in inducing rebound firing in the DCN. Hoebeek et al. have also previously shown that stimulation of the inferior olive leads to increases in DCN firing of about 50 spikes/s. However, even using direct electrical stimulation of the inferior olive, Bengtsson et al. found that only stimuli that almost saturated the inhibitory postsynaptic potentials in DCN neurons were able to induce rebound firing. Even under these conditions, the "rebound" measured was an increase of about 50 spikes/s, a value definitely smaller than the 200 spikes/s increase measured in slices (Aizenman & Linden, 1999). Taken together, these studies suggested that rebound firing may be generated only when a large number of Purkinje cells are activated synchronously by multiple climbing fibers (De Zeeuw et al., 2011). The pause of Purkinje cell simple spikes following a complex spike may provide the optimal relief from the strong inhibition necessary to induce rebound firing in DCN neurons (Aizenman & Linden, 1999).

To exclude the possibility of off-target effects of electrical stimulation of the cerebellar cortex, many studies have used optogenetic tools.

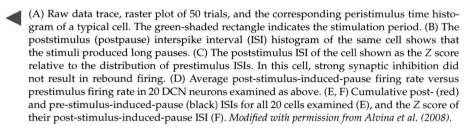

(A) Raw data trace, raster plot of 50 trials, and the corresponding peristimulus time histogram of a typical cell. The green-shaded rectangle indicates the stimulation period. (B) The poststimulus (postpause) interspike interval (ISI) histogram of the same cell shows that the stimuli produced long pauses. (C) The poststimulus ISI of the cell shown as the Z score relative to the distribution of prestimulus ISIs. In this cell, strong synaptic inhibition did not result in rebound firing. (D) Average post-stimulus-induced-pause firing rate versus prestimulus firing rate in 20 DCN neurons examined as above. (E, F) Cumulative post- (red) and pre-stimulus-induced-pause (black) ISIs for all 20 cells examined (E), and the Z score of their post-stimulus-induced-pause ISI (F). *Modified with permission from Alvina et al. (2008).*

Witter et al. (2013), using mice expressing channel rhodopsin-2 specifically in Purkinje cells, found that light stimulation led to the inhibition of DCN neuron firing and, in turn, precisely timed firing rate increases in 77% of the cells tested. The 50% increase in the firing rate of DCN neurons was induced by an increase of 50 spikes/s in Purkinje cells firing during light stimulation. In a separate study Lee et al. (2015) found that rebounds of 200 spikes/s could be induced if a number of Purkinje cells were strongly stimulated optogenetically (with their firing rates reaching 400 spikes/s). In both Lee et al. (2015) and Witter et al. (2013), the authors also showed that very strong stimulation of Purkinje cells was able to induce movement. Whether the movement requires or is caused by rebound firing in DCN is, however, not clear. In contrast to the studies of Witter et al. and Lee et al., Chaumont et al., using a similar optogenetic approach, did not report any rebound firing in DCN neurons after direct activation of Purkinje cells (Chaumont et al., 2013). In a following study, the same group reported that optogenetic stimulation of Purkinje cells affected some parameters of whisker movements in rats (Proville et al., 2014). The inhibition of DCN neurons caused by Purkinje cells induced a subsequent increase in the firing rate of only ~15 spikes/s.

In all the previously cited studies, DCN rebound firing was induced "artificially" and often using very strong stimulation. An obvious question is whether the conditions to generate rebound firing are present during physiological behaviors. Before tackling this issue, we must define what may constitute rebound firing.

What Constitutes Meaningful Rebound Firing?

The output of DCN neurons is thought to provide the signals required for the timing of specific tasks and thus mediate the temporal control of motor behaviors (Rowland & Jaeger, 2005). The finding that the physiological properties of DCN neurons allow for reliably triggering postinhibitory rebound bursts in vitro has led to the incorporation of this phenomenon into multiple theories of cerebellar function (Kistler et al., 2000; Mauk, Medina, Nores, & Ohyama, 2000; Wetmore et al., 2008).

While the ability of DCN neurons to mediate rebound firing has been well documented in vitro, the prevalence of rebound firing in vivo has been a topic of much debate. One reason for this is the lack of agreement on what constitutes meaningful rebound firing. The absence of an accepted threshold above which an increase in the firing rate of DCN neurons following a pause can be considered rebound has made the interpretation of experimental results highly dependent on the criteria set by the interpreter.

The number of criteria for rebound in the literature is so great that it is in fact challenging to find two papers that use the same definition. As such, post-stimulus-induced-pause increases in the firing rate as low as 6 spikes/s, as high as 435, and any number in between have been reported as rebound (Aizenman & Linden, 1999; Alvina et al., 2009, 2008; Jahnsen, 1986a; Kistler et al., 2000; Molineux et al., 2006, 2008; Uusisaari, Obata, & Knopfel, 2007). Alternatively, one can also find a number of thresholds above which an increase in the firing rate has been considered rebound, such as an increase in the poststimulus firing rate that is higher than 2 or 3 standard deviations of the firing rate within a certain length of time before the stimulus-induced pause (Tadayonnejad et al., 2009). Moreover, the definition of a threshold is not the only criterion that differs in the literature. The time following a stimulus-induced pause within which an increase in the firing rate of DCN neurons is considered rebound can be 1, 3, 5, 6, or more interspike intervals or anywhere from 100 ms to as high as 3 s (Aizenman & Linden, 1999; Alvina et al., 2009, 2008; Molineux et al., 2008; Uusisaari et al., 2007). There are also different opinions on what can be considered a meaningful "baseline" period before a pause and what is a physiologically relevant pause duration. It is in fact astonishing how many different definitions of rebound exist in the field. This may partially explain why much of the debate has been focused on whether rebound exists in vivo. However, before we can ask this question, we have to take a step back and decide what is a physiologically meaningful rebound firing.

Technically, one extra spike after the pause relative to baseline firing could count as rebound. A shortcoming of this, or any of the above thresholds, is that this is an arbitrary definition that does not take into account whether the downstream neurons have the ability to detect such "rebound input." In a system in which the intrinsic noise is zero, any increase in the postpause firing rate (even a single spike) would in fact result in an ideal SNR. However, the situation may be different in vivo, where there is substantial noise in the activity of DCN neurons. Because of noise, if the baseline firing rate is fluctuating by 10 spikes/s, then clearly an extra spike at the end of the pause cannot reliably encode information. Thus, a more physiologically meaningful threshold can be set by considering the reliability of the rebound signal, or its SNR calculated using

the equation $\text{SNR} = \dfrac{2\left(\mu_{\text{postpause}} - \mu_{\text{prepause}}\right)^2}{\sigma^2_{\text{postpause}} + \sigma^2_{\text{prepause}}}$, where μ_{prepause} and $\mu_{\text{postpause}}$

are the means and σ_{prepause} and $\sigma_{\text{postpause}}$ the standard deviations of the pre- and postpause firing rates. What is a good SNR for DCN neurons? We here provide an estimate based on realistic firing rate changes of

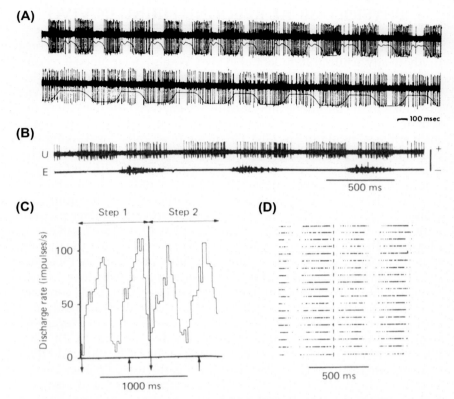

FIGURE 2   DCN neuron firing rate tracks movement dynamics. (A) Extracellular recordings of a monkey DCN neuron while moving the ipsilateral wrist (top) or the ipsilateral
shoulder. Movement dynamics is represented at the bottom of the extracellular traces. DCN
firing activity strongly correlates with movement. (B, C, D) Extracellular recordings of a cat
DCN neuron during locomotion. (B) Extracellular recordings from a DCN neuron and simultaneous electromyograph from the triceps during locomotion. (C) Firing rate during step
cycles. (D) Raster plot across trials of the spiking activity that is summarized in (C). DCN
neurons encode the movement in their firing rate fluctuations (rate code). *Panel (A) is reproduced with permission from Thach (1968), while (B, C, and D) are reproduced with permission from
Armstrong and Edgley (1984).*

DCN neurons during movement (Fig. 2). Based on our own data, we
assume an average firing rate of 30 spikes/s ($\mu_{prepause}$) and a coefficient
of variation (CV) of 0.5 (CV = $\sigma_{prepause}/\mu_{prepause}$), and we consider that a
movement can induce changes in firing rate on the order of 50 spikes/s
($\mu_{postpause} - \mu_{prepause}$) (Thach, 1968). We also assume a very ideal case in
which the standard deviation of the neuron during movement does not
change much ($\sigma_{prepause} = \sigma_{postpause}$). Under these conditions, the SNR is ~11.
While there are many assumptions in this calculation, it provides a reference for our following analysis using in vivo recordings.

PHYSIOLOGICAL REBOUND FIRING IN VIVO

Here we examined whether rebound firing occurs spontaneously (without any artificial stimulation) in vivo. We also determined if rebound firing could potentially provide extra information to a rate code.

To do so, we recorded 53 cells in the DCN extracellularly under various behavioral conditions. Specifically, we analyzed the activity of neurons in awake head-restrained mice ($n = 35$ cells) and in freely moving mice while standing ($n = 6$ cells), balancing ($n = 7$ cells), or walking ($n = 5$ cells) (Fig. 3(A)). Balancing and walking were chosen as behaviors characterized by high cerebellar activity. Firing rates, predominant firing rate (mode of the interspike interval (ISI)) and CV of the ISI are shown in Fig. 3(B1–B3). Consistent with previous studies, when the animal was walking, firing rates were more variable as shown by higher predominant firing rates and CV (Armstrong & Edgley, 1984). From spike trains of sorted single cells (example in Fig. 3(C1)), we calculated the distribution of ISIs. Fig. 3(C2) represents the probability of measuring ISIs longer than the duration denoted on the x axis. Consistent with previous studies (Thach, 1968), movements produced more brief and long ISIs compared to resting conditions. In general long ISIs occurred infrequently even during cerebellar intensive tasks such as balancing. On an average less than 1% of the ISIs were longer than 200 ms (inset in Fig. 3(C2)). These long ISIs may represent pauses in the firing of the DCN and could therefore precede rebound firing. In the following, the word "pauses" is used to indicate long ISIs, which were used to calculate pre- and postpause firing rates to look for rebound firing.

Because recovery from the inactivation of T-type calcium channels is voltage- and time-dependent, we performed the analysis considering different pause durations in case some were more effective at generating rebound firing than others. We did not consider pauses longer than 550 ms because fast and precise motor coordination (Mauk & Buonomano, 2004) must operate at short time scales. First, we estimated firing rates as the inverse of the average of five consecutive ISIs before and after the pause (Fig. 4(A)). We chose to use five ISIs to be consistent with previous studies but we additionally performed the same analysis considering two ISIs and found qualitatively similar results (see the following text). Fig. 4(B) shows the distribution of the difference in firing rates before and after the pause for representative cells from each behavioral condition. The difference between post- and prepause firing rates was small and symmetric for all the conditions and for all pause durations considered. In the example of cells shown, the vast majority of firing rate increases and decreases were less than 20 spikes/s. To explore whether these small changes in firing rates could be meaningful, we calculated the SNR. In Fig. 4(C) we show the estimated SNR for the same cells in Fig. 4(B). The distribution of the SNR was

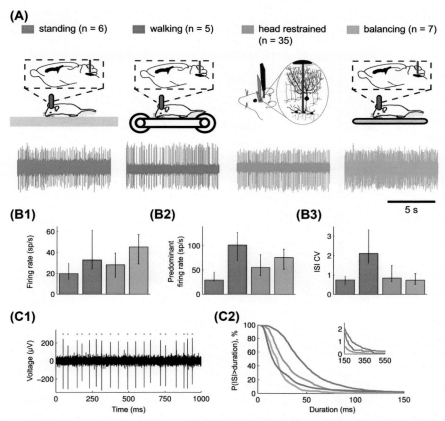

FIGURE 3   Extracellular recordings from awake mice were performed in vivo in accordance with the guidelines set by Albert Einstein College of Medicine. (A) Recordings of neurons in the DCN were taken under various behavioral conditions: while the animal was standing, walking on a treadmill, on a balance beam, or head restrained. Below the schematics of the experimental settings are representative voltage traces for each condition. (B1, 2, 3) Average firing rate, predominant firing rate (mode of the interspike interval (ISI) distribution), and CV of the ISI in the four different behavioral conditions. Error bars represent medians and interquartile range. (C1) Example of sorted extracellular recording of a neuron in the DCN. Spikes from extracellular recordings were sorted by thresholding and applying principal component analysis. (C2) Percentage probability of measuring ISIs longer than the duration reported on the x axis. The inset shows the same plot for a longer pause duration (>150 ms). Lines represent medians across cells for each behavioral condition.

symmetric and around zero. To generate this plot we denoted an increase in firing rate with a positive SNR and a decrease with a negative SNR. The average SNR for the increase in firing rate was around 0.1. In all cases, the values we measured were between 1 and 2 orders of magnitude smaller than what we estimated in the previous paragraph for DCN neurons during locomotion assuming a rate code (~11).

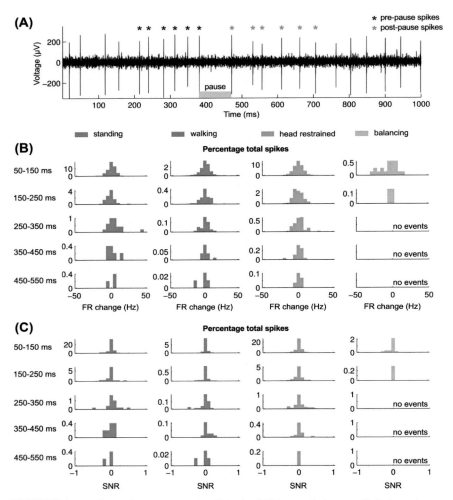

FIGURE 4   Analysis of representative cells in the DCN, recorded extracellularly as shown in Fig. 3. (A) Firing rates before and after pauses were estimated by considering five ISIs before and after the pause. (B) Distribution of firing rate changes for representative cells from each behavioral condition and for various pause durations (binned from 50 to 550 ms in steps of 100 ms). (C) Signal-to-noise ratio (SNR) distribution for the same cells as in (B). A positive SNR indicates a firing rate increase, while a negative one indicates a decrease. Both firing rate change and SNR were small and symmetric.

The representative results in Fig. 4 were confirmed by performing the same analysis on all the cells we recorded. As shown in Fig. 5(A), the pre- and postpause firing rates were very similar (the majority of points lay on the identity line) and symmetrical, with both increases and decreases in firing rates. Note that with increasing pause duration, the overall firing rate,

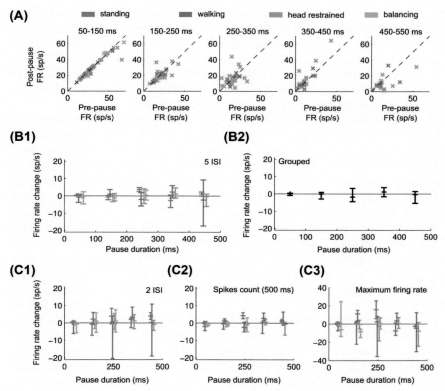

FIGURE 5 Firing rate changes as a function of pause duration for all the recorded cells in the DCN. (A) Pre- and postpause firing rate as a function of the pause duration under the four different experimental conditions (color coded). Each cross represents the average value for each cell. Pauses were binned from 50 to 550 ms in steps of 100 ms. Firing rates were estimated by considering the inverse of the first five ISIs before and after the pause. The identity line is dashed. Note that the firing before and after the pause was always very similar. This suggests that there was no rebound firing in DCN neurons. (B1) Differences between pre- and postpause firing rates for the various behavioral conditions. (B2) Same as in (B1) but grouping all the cells from all the conditions. (C1, 2, 3) Results using two ISIs instead of five to estimate firing rates (C1), considering the average firing rate in a 500-ms time window (C2), or considering the maximum instantaneous firing rate for five ISIs (C3). In (B1, 2) and (C1–3), error bars represent median and interquartile ranges.

both pre- and postpause, decreased. This suggests that the pause duration was simply determined by firing fluctuations, with longer pauses occurring during periods of low firing rate. Any increase in firing rate was always less than 20 spikes/s and on average less than 5 spikes/s for conditions and pause durations (Fig. 5(B1)). Fig. 5(B2) shows the same data but grouping together all the cells from all the various conditions. Again, the average change in the firing rate was never higher than a few spikes per second.

To check whether our results depend on the specific way in which we estimated firing rates, we performed the same analysis considering two ISIs instead of five to calculate firing rates (Fig. 5(C1)), average spike counts in a 500-ms window (Fig. 5(C2)), or maximum firing rates (Fig. 5(C3)) before and after the pause. Even if the use of two ISIs or the maximum to estimate firing rates obviously resulted in noisier estimations, we still found that the changes after the pause were small and symmetric.

To quantify the efficacy of firing rate changes to encode information, we quantified the SNR for all cells (Fig. 6(A1)). Rebound firing should lead to high values of the SNR. Instead, we found the SNR to be on average less than 0.1. SNRs of this order of magnitude are too low to transmit meaningful signals to downstream areas (see Conclusions). To check if the distribution of the SNR was skewed toward positive values, meaning that there were more increases than decreases in the firing rate, we estimated for each cell the skewness of the SNR distribution considering all the pauses. This analysis performed for each cell gave the results shown in Fig. 6(A2). The average skewness was always around zero, suggesting no biases toward positive increases in the postpause firing rate. On average, the SNR was less than 0.1 for all the conditions and all pause durations considered (Fig. 6(B1)). Moreover, as mentioned before, pauses longer than 200 ms occurred on average in less than 0.5% of all ISIs (Fig. 6(B2) and the inset). To further strengthen our analysis we estimated rebound events by setting an arbitrary threshold on the basis of the changes in firing rate, as done in some other studies (Sangrey & Jaeger, 2010). We considered rebound firing as every postpause event in which the first instantaneous firing rate (inverse of the first ISI) was more than two times the standard deviation of the firing rate before the pause. On average, the number of detections was 0.05% of all ISIs using this thresholding procedure. Finally, in our analysis we binned pauses equally for all the neurons. This was based on the assumption that the set of ionic channels necessary for rebound firing must be the same for all neurons in the DCN. However, there are different types of DCN neurons (Uusisaari & Knopfel, 2011; Uusisaari et al., 2007) characterized by different rebound properties (Najac & Raman, 2015; Uusisaari & Knopfel, 2011). In particular, large cells in the DCN exhibit large rebound firing compared to small cells (Najac & Raman, 2015). In our recordings we did not find any bimodal distribution of the effects. In any case, we also tried to bin pauses based on the specific ISI distribution of each neuron. Even in that case, we did not find any evidence for rebound firing and we measured even lower SNR (data not shown).

Hoebeek et al. (Hoebeek et al., 2010) showed that single electric pulses to the cerebellar cortex induced well-timed spiking activity in DCN neurons without changing the overall firing rate. We tested whether this effect was also present in our recordings. We aligned spike trains to the spike before the pause (Fig. 6(C)). We considered pauses binned as in all our

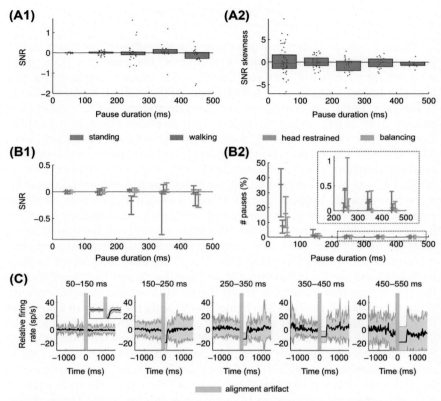

FIGURE 6 No clear evidence for rebound firing in DCN neurons. (A1) Signal-to-noise ratio (SNR) for all the cells considered. Each dot represents a cell and the rectangle the median and interquartile range computed across cells. The SNR values are very small, suggesting again the absence of significant rebound firing. (A2) Skewness of SNR distribution for each cell and medians and interquartile ranges across cells. The values around zero indicate that the distributions of the SNR were very symmetric, with no bias toward firing rate increases. (B1) SNR estimated for each behavioral condition and binned pause duration. (B2) Number of pauses for each time bin considered. In both (B1) and (B2), error bars represent medians and interquartile ranges. (C) Average firing rates after aligning all the spike trains with the last spike before a pause. Firing rates were estimated binning spike trains (20 ms) and the baselines were subtracted for each cell. Averages across trials for each cell were then averaged across cells. Black lines represent the mean values considering cells from all the conditions. Gray shading represents the standard deviation across cells.

previous analyses. On average, we did not see any clear increase in the alignment of spikes after the pause for any of the pause durations considered. In some cases, we found a gradual increase in the firing rate after the pause toward the baseline value. Note also that the standard deviation of the firing rate did not change significantly after the pause compared to that immediately before the pause, suggesting that our results were not an artifact of averaging across trials and neurons.

CONCLUSIONS

There is good evidence supporting the hypothesis that the cerebellum uses a rate code to encode movements. For example, there is an astonishing correlation between Purkinje cell instantaneous firing rate and eye movement (Medina & Lisberger, 2007; Shidara, Kawano, Gomi, & Kawato, 1993). An analogous case for rate coding in DCN neurons is provided by classic experiments showing in-phase firing rate modulation of DCN neurons during movement (Armstrong & Edgley, 1984; Thach, 1968). However, rebound firing of DCN neurons could provide additional information to a rate code (Kistler et al., 2000; Wetmore et al., 2008). DCN neurons contain all the prerequisites to generate rebound firing when strongly hyperpolarized. Here we sought to determine whether rebound firing occurs in vivo under physiological conditions, in particular in behaviors requiring intense cerebellar activity. We compared firing rates before and after naturally occurring pauses of varying durations and computed the SNR of the firing rate changes to also account for spiking variability during the behaviors. On average the change in firing rate after the pause was less than 5 Hz for all the conditions and symmetric, with both increases and decreases in firing. To evaluate the ability of a signal of this magnitude to transfer information considering the physiological firing variability, we then computed the SNR. On average, we found that the SNR was never higher than 0.1 for any pause duration. To put this SNR in context, we estimated the SNR of firing rate changes in DCN neurons during behaviors known to be encoded in their firing as a rate code, such as arm movement or locomotion (Armstrong & Edgley, 1984; Thach, 1968). On the basis of the firing rate changes seen during these movements and assuming a rate code, we estimated the SNR to be higher than 10. Therefore, at the single-cell level the information conveyed using rebound firing looks marginal compared to that using a rate code.

Could the SNR be improved by some extra mechanisms? If different neurons in the DCN increase their firing synchronously after a pause and send projections to the same neuron, their uncorrelated variation in firing rate could be averaged out postsynaptically. In other words, convergence of DCN neuron inputs to downstream areas, as a population, could improve the SNR. Based on previous studies (Shinoda, Futami, Mitoma, & Yokota, 1988; Toyama, Tsukahara, Kosaka, & Matsunami, 1970), Person and Raman (Person & Raman, 2012) indeed suggested that about 50 interpositus axons project to each neuron in the red nucleus. Therefore, the SNR could in theory be improved by synaptic convergence of DCN neurons. SNR, as we defined it here, scales linearly with the number of neurons. For the pause duration, for which we recorded the highest SNR, this value was on average 0.1. Therefore, the signal transmitted to red nucleus neurons could have an SNR of about $0.1 \times 50 = 5$, a value still smaller than that obtained using a simple rate code applied to a single neuron. However, whether pauses are indeed synchronized across DCN neurons, a key factor for improving the SNR, is still not known. In contrast, using a rate code the convergence of synaptic inputs would still lead to an increased SNR but without the strong constraint of the need for synchronous and precisely matched pauses.

Are the pauses that we used to estimate firing rates pre- and post-pause really meaningful? Using our data, we found that pause durations were simply determined by normal firing rate fluctuations, with briefer pauses occurring during high-frequency firing and longer ones when the neuron was firing less. Pause duration therefore may not add any extra information beyond a rate code. Notably, this is exactly what Cao, Maran, Dhamala, Jaeger, and Heck (2012), using awake mice, found for Purkinje cells. The simple spike pause durations correlated with behavior (licking and breathing). However these pauses occurred during the periods of low firing rates and indeed did not add any information beyond a rate code (Walter & Khodakhah, 2009). The use of pauses followed by rebounds in DCN neurons as a coding strategy also seems very unlikely for the cerebellar control of continuous movements. If any motor-related information was transmitted in this way, delays of hundreds of milliseconds would always be added (baseline plus pause plus rebound duration). For a structure known to coordinate fast motor behavior (Ivry, 1997; Mauk et al., 2000), this looks like a very deleterious strategy.

In summary, we did not find any evidence of rebound firing after a physiological pause. Our data do not support the hypothesis that rebound firing in DCN neurons may be a very common coding mechanism in the cerebellum. This raises a very important question. If rebound firing in DCN neurons does not occur "spontaneously" in vivo, why are DCN neurons such good "rebounders"? When could the rebound occur and why? Neurons in the DCN receive continuous GABAergic inputs from Purkinje cells but also glutamatergic signals from mossy and climbing fibers (De Zeeuw et al., 2011). Both Hoebeek et al. (2010) and Bengtsson et al. (2011) found that strong stimulation of the inferior olive in vivo induced rebound firing in DCN neurons. They conclude that only strong synchronous coactivation of a large number of Purkinje cells by many climbing fibers can lead to rebound firing. This finding is also consistent with studies using optogenetics to drive a large number of Purkinje cells (Lee et al., 2015; Witter et al., 2013). Perhaps it is the concerted activity of a number of climbing fibers that drives a large number of Purkinje cells physiologically. However, inferior olive activity is usually unchanged or inhibited during movement or movement initiation (Apps, Atkins, & Garwicz, 1997; Armstrong, Edgley, & Lidierth, 1988; Gellman, Gibson, & Houk, 1985; Gibson, Horn, & Pong, 2004; Harvey, Porter, & Rawson, 1977). Therefore, as suggested by Bengtsson et al. (2011), it is unlikely that the inferior olive causes rebound firing in DCN neurons during movement. The role of rebound firing thus may be of minor importance compared to a rate code for encoding movements. This conclusion is also supported by experimental studies showing firing rate modulation of DCN neurons, but no rebound firing, during vestibular stimulation or eye movement (Chubb & Fuchs, 1982; Gardner & Fuchs, 1975).

Nevertheless, it is still possible that rebound firing occurs in very specific situations. Considering that strong stimulation of the inferior olive leads to rebound firing in DCN neurons, it seems plausible that cerebellar learning (Kimpo, Rinaldi, Kim, Payne, & Raymond, 2014; Medina & Lisberger, 2008; Nguyen-Vu et al., 2013; Raymond & Lisberger, 1998; Raymond, Lisberger, & Mauk, 1996; Schonewille et al., 2011; Wulff et al., 2009; Yang & Lisberger, 2014) is potentially the most likely situation in which rebound firing may occur. To our knowledge, however, it remains to be shown that rebound firing in DCN occurs and is important for cerebellar learning.

References

Aizenman, C. D., & Linden, D. J. (1999). Regulation of the rebound depolarization and spontaneous firing patterns of deep nuclear neurons in slices of rat cerebellum. *Journal of Neurophysiology, 82*(4), 1697–1709.

Aizenman, C. D., Manis, P. B., & Linden, D. J. (1998). Polarity of long-term synaptic gain change is related to postsynaptic spike firing at a cerebellar inhibitory synapse. *Neuron, 21*(4), 827–835.

Aksenov, D., Serdyukova, N., Irwin, K., & Bracha, V. (2004). GABA neurotransmission in the cerebellar interposed nuclei: involvement in classically conditioned eyeblinks and neuronal activity. *Journal of Neurophysiology, 91*(2), 719–727. http://dx.doi.org/10.1152/jn.00859.2003.

Albus, J. S. (1971). A theory of cerebellar function. *Mathematical Biosciences*.

Allen, G. I., Azzena, G. B., & Ohno, T. (1974). Somatotopically organized inputs from fore- and hindlimb areas of sensorimotor cortex to cerebellar Purkyne cells. *Experimental Brain Research, 20*(3), 255–272.

Allen, G., Buxton, R. B., Wong, E. C., & Courchesne, E. (1997). Attentional activation of the cerebellum independent of motor involvement. *Science, 275*(5308), 1940–1943.

Alvina, K., Ellis-Davies, G., & Khodakhah, K. (2009). T-type calcium channels mediate rebound firing in intact deep cerebellar neurons. *Neuroscience, 158*(2), 635–641. http://dx.doi.org/10.1016/j.neuroscience.2008.09.052.

Alvina, K., & Khodakhah, K. (2008). Selective regulation of spontaneous activity of neurons of the deep cerebellar nuclei by N-type calcium channels in juvenile rats. *The Journal of Physiology, 586*(10), 2523–2538. http://dx.doi.org/10.1113/jphysiol.2007.148197.

Alvina, K., Walter, J. T., Kohn, A., Ellis-Davies, G., & Khodakhah, K. (2008). Questioning the role of rebound firing in the cerebellum. *Nature Neuroscience, 11*(11), 1256–1258. http://dx.doi.org/10.1038/nn.2195.

Apps, R., Atkins, M. J., & Garwicz, M. (1997). Gating of cutaneous input to cerebellar climbing fibres during a reaching task in the cat. *The Journal of Physiology, 502*(Pt 1), 203–214.

Armstrong, D. M., & Edgley, S. A. (1984). Discharges of nucleus interpositus neurones during locomotion in the cat. *The Journal of Physiology, 351*, 411–432.

Armstrong, D. M., Edgley, S. A., & Lidierth, M. (1988). Complex spikes in Purkinje cells of the paravermal part of the anterior lobe of the cat cerebellum during locomotion. *The Journal of Physiology, 400,* 405–414.

Bengtsson, F., Ekerot, C. F., & Jorntell, H. (2011). In vivo analysis of inhibitory synaptic inputs and rebounds in deep cerebellar nuclear neurons. *PLoS One, 6*(4), e18822. http://dx.doi.org/10.1371/journal.pone.0018822.

Billard, J. M., Vigot, R., & Batini, C. (1993). GABA, THIP and baclofen inhibition of Purkinje cells and cerebellar nuclei neurons. *Neuroscience Research, 16*(1), 65–69.

Boehme, R., Uebele, V. N., Renger, J. J., & Pedroarena, C. (2011). Rebound excitation triggered by synaptic inhibition in cerebellar nuclear neurons is suppressed by selective T-type calcium channel block. *Journal of Neurophysiology, 106*(5), 2653–2661. http://dx.doi.org/10.1152/jn.00612.2011.

Cao, Y., Maran, S. K., Dhamala, M., Jaeger, D., & Heck, D. H. (2012). Behavior-related pauses in simple-spike activity of mouse Purkinje cells are linked to spike rate modulation. *The Journal of Neuroscience, 32*(25), 8678–8685. http://dx.doi.org/10.1523/JNEUROSCI.4969-11.2012.

Chaumont, J., Guyon, N., Valera, A. M., Dugue, G. P., Popa, D., Marcaggi, P., & Isope, P. (2013). Clusters of cerebellar Purkinje cells control their afferent climbing fiber discharge. *Proceedings of the National Academy of Sciences of the United States of America, 110*(40), 16223–16228. http://dx.doi.org/10.1073/pnas.1302310110.

Chubb, M. C., & Fuchs, A. F. (1982). Contribution of y group of vestibular nuclei and dentate nucleus of cerebellum to generation of vertical smooth eye movements. *Journal of Neurophysiology, 48*(1), 75–99.

Courchesne, E., Yeung-Courchesne, R., Press, G. A., Hesselink, J. R., & Jernigan, T. L. (1988). Hypoplasia of cerebellar vermal lobules VI and VII in autism. *The New England Journal of Medicine, 318*(21), 1349–1354. http://dx.doi.org/10.1056/NEJM198805263182102.

De Schutter, E., & Steuber, V. (2009). Patterns and pauses in Purkinje cell simple spike trains: experiments, modeling and theory. *Neuroscience, 162*(3), 816–826. http://dx.doi.org/10.1016/j.neuroscience.2009.02.040.

De Zeeuw, C. I., & Berrebi, A. S. (1995). Postsynaptic targets of Purkinje cell terminals in the cerebellar and vestibular nuclei of the rat. *European Journal of Neuroscience, 7*(11), 2322–2333.

De Zeeuw, C. I., Hoebeek, F. E., Bosman, L. W., Schonewille, M., Witter, L., & Koekkoek, S. K. (2011). Spatiotemporal firing patterns in the cerebellum. *Nature Reviews Neuroscience, 12*(6), 327–344. http://dx.doi.org/10.1038/nrn3011.

Eccles, J. C. (1973). The cerebellum as a computer: patterns in space and time. *The Journal of Physiology, 229*(1), 1–32.

Eccles, J. C., Sabah, N. H., Schmidt, R. F., & Taborikova, H. (1972). Integration by Purkyne cells of mossy and climbing fiber inputs from cutaneous mechanoreceptors. *Experimental Brain Research, 15*(5), 498–520.

Engbers, J. D., Anderson, D., Tadayonnejad, R., Mehaffey, W. H., Molineux, M. L., & Turner, R. W. (2011). Distinct roles for I(T) and I(H) in controlling the frequency and timing of rebound spike responses. *The Journal of Physiology, 589*(Pt 22), 5391–5413. http://dx.doi.org/10.1113/jphysiol.2011.215632.

Gao, J. H., Parsons, L. M., Bower, J. M., Xiong, J., Li, J., & Fox, P. T. (1996). Cerebellum implicated in sensory acquisition and discrimination rather than motor control. *Science, 272*(5261), 545–547.

Gardner, E. P., & Fuchs, A. F. (1975). Single-unit responses to natural vestibular stimuli and eye movements in deep cerebellar nuclei of the alert rhesus monkey. *Journal of Neurophysiology, 38*(3), 627–649.

Gauck, V., & Jaeger, D. (2000). The control of rate and timing of spikes in the deep cerebellar nuclei by inhibition. *The Journal of Neuroscience, 20*(8), 3006–3016.

Gauck, V., Thomann, M., Jaeger, D., & Borst, A. (2001). Spatial distribution of low- and high-voltage-activated calcium currents in neurons of the deep cerebellar nuclei. *The Journal of Neuroscience, 21*(15), RC158.

Gellman, R., Gibson, A. R., & Houk, J. C. (1985). Inferior olivary neurons in the awake cat: detection of contact and passive body displacement. *Journal of Neurophysiology, 54*(1), 40–60.

Gibson, A. R., Horn, K. M., & Pong, M. (2004). Activation of climbing fibers. *Cerebellum, 3*(4), 212–221. http://dx.doi.org/10.1080/14734220410018995.

Harvey, R. J., Porter, R., & Rawson, J. A. (1977). The natural discharges of Purkinje cells in paravermal regions of lobules V and VI of the monkey's cerebellum. *The Journal of Physiology, 271*(2), 515–536.

Heck, D. H., De Zeeuw, C. I., Jaeger, D., Khodakhah, K., & Person, A. L. (2013). The neuronal code(s) of the cerebellum. *The Journal of Neuroscience, 33*(45), 17603–17609. http://dx.doi.org/10.1523/JNEUROSCI.2759-13.2013.

Hoebeek, F. E., Witter, L., Ruigrok, T. J., & De Zeeuw, C. I. (2010). Differential olivo-cerebellar cortical control of rebound activity in the cerebellar nuclei. *Proceedings of the National Academy of Sciences of the United States of America, 107*(18), 8410–8415. http://dx.doi.org/10.1073/pnas.0907118107.

Holdefer, R. N., Houk, J. C., & Miller, L. E. (2005). Movement-related discharge in the cerebellar nuclei persists after local injections of GABA(A) antagonists. *Journal of Neurophysiology, 93*(1), 35–43. http://dx.doi.org/10.1152/jn.00603.2004.

Ito, M. (1984). *Cerebellum and neural control*. New York: Raven Press.

Ivry, R. (1997). Cerebellar timing systems. *International Review of Neurobiology, 41*, 555–573.

Jaeger, D. (2011). Mini-review: synaptic integration in the cerebellar nuclei–perspectives from dynamic clamp and computer simulation studies. *Cerebellum, 10*(4), 659–666. http://dx.doi.org/10.1007/s12311-011-0248-3.

Jahnsen, H. (1986a). Electrophysiological characteristics of neurones in the guinea-pig deep cerebellar nuclei in vitro. *The Journal of Physiology, 372*, 129–147.

Jahnsen, H. (1986b). Extracellular activation and membrane conductances of neurones in the guinea-pig deep cerebellar nuclei in vitro. *The Journal of Physiology, 372*, 149–168.

Jen, J., Kim, G. W., & Baloh, R. W. (2004). Clinical spectrum of episodic ataxia type 2. *Neurology, 62*(1), 17–22.

Kimpo, R. R., Rinaldi, J. M., Kim, C. K., Payne, H. L., & Raymond, J. L. (2014). Gating of neural error signals during motor learning. *Elife, 3*, e02076. http://dx.doi.org/10.7554/eLife.02076.

Kistler, W. M., van Hemmen, J. L., & De Zeeuw, C. I. (2000). Time window control: a model for cerebellar function based on synchronization, reverberation, and time slicing. *Progress in Brain Research, 124*, 275–297. http://dx.doi.org/10.1016/S0079-6123(00)24023-5.

Lee, K. H., Mathews, P. J., Reeves, A. M., Choe, K. Y., Jami, S. A., Serrano, R. E., et al. (2015). Circuit mechanisms underlying motor memory formation in the cerebellum. *Neuron*. http://dx.doi.org/10.1016/j.neuron.2015.03.010.

Levin, S. I., Khaliq, Z. M., Aman, T. K., Grieco, T. M., Kearney, J. A., Raman, I. M., et al. (2006). Impaired motor function in mice with cell-specific knockout of sodium channel Scn8a (NaV1.6) in cerebellar purkinje neurons and granule cells. *Journal of Neurophysiology, 96*(2), 785–793. http://dx.doi.org/10.1152/jn.01193.2005.

Linden, D. J. (2003). Neuroscience. From molecules to memory in the cerebellum. *Science, 301*(5640), 1682–1685. http://dx.doi.org/10.1126/science.1090462.

Lisberger, S. G., & Fuchs, A. F. (1978). Role of primate flocculus during rapid behavioral modification of vestibuloocular reflex. II. Mossy fiber firing patterns during horizontal head rotation and eye movement. *Journal of Neurophysiology, 41*(3), 764–777.

Llinas, R., & Muhlethaler, M. (1988). Electrophysiology of guinea-pig cerebellar nuclear cells in the in vitro brain stem-cerebellar preparation. *The Journal of Physiology, 404*, 241–258.

Llinas, R., & Sugimori, M. (1980). Electrophysiological properties of in vitro Purkinje cell dendrites in mammalian cerebellar slices. *The Journal of Physiology, 305*, 197–213.

Mauk, M. D., & Buonomano, D. V. (2004). The neural basis of temporal processing. *Annual Review of Neuroscience*, *27*, 307–340. http://dx.doi.org/10.1146/annurev.neuro.27.070203.144247.

Mauk, M. D., Medina, J. F., Nores, W. L., & Ohyama, T. (2000). Cerebellar function: coordination, learning or timing? *Current Biology*, *10*(14), R522–R525.

McRory, J. E., Santi, C. M., Hamming, K. S., Mezeyova, J., Sutton, K. G., Baillie, D. L., & Snutch, T. P. (2001). Molecular and functional characterization of a family of rat brain T-type calcium channels. *The Journal of Biological Chemistry*, *276*(6), 3999–4011. http://dx.doi.org/10.1074/jbc.M008215200.

Medina, J. F., & Lisberger, S. G. (2007). Variation, signal, and noise in cerebellar sensory-motor processing for smooth-pursuit eye movements. *The Journal of Neuroscience*, *27*(25), 6832–6842. http://dx.doi.org/10.1523/JNEUROSCI.1323-07.2007.

Medina, J. F., & Lisberger, S. G. (2008). Links from complex spikes to local plasticity and motor learning in the cerebellum of awake-behaving monkeys. *Nature Neuroscience*, *11*(10), 1185–1192. http://dx.doi.org/10.1038/nn.2197.

Molineux, M. L., McRory, J. E., McKay, B. E., Hamid, J., Mehaffey, W. H., Rehak, R., & Turner, R. W. (2006). Specific T-type calcium channel isoforms are associated with distinct burst phenotypes in deep cerebellar nuclear neurons. *Proceedings of the National Academy of Sciences of the United States of America*, *103*(14), 5555–5560. http://dx.doi.org/10.1073/pnas.0601261103.

Molineux, M. L., Mehaffey, W. H., Tadayonnejad, R., Anderson, D., Tennent, A. F., & Turner, R. W. (2008). Ionic factors governing rebound burst phenotype in rat deep cerebellar neurons. *Journal of Neurophysiology*, *100*(5), 2684–2701. http://dx.doi.org/10.1152/jn.90427.2008.

Mullen, R. J., Eicher, E. M., & Sidman, R. L. (1976). Purkinje cell degeneration, a new neurological mutation in the mouse. *Proceedings of the National Academy of Sciences of the United States of America*, *73*(1), 208–212.

Muri, R., & Knopfel, T. (1994). Activity induced elevations of intracellular calcium concentration in neurons of the deep cerebellar nuclei. *Journal of Neurophysiology*, *71*(1), 420–428.

Najac, M., & Raman, I. M. (2015). Integration of Purkinje cell inhibition by cerebellar nucleo-olivary neurons. *The Journal of Neuroscience*, *35*(2), 544–549. http://dx.doi.org/10.1523/JNEUROSCI.3583-14.2015.

Nam, S. C., & Hockberger, P. E. (1997). Analysis of spontaneous electrical activity in cerebellar Purkinje cells acutely isolated from postnatal rats. *Journal of Neurobiology*, *33*(1), 18–32.

Nguyen-Vu, T. D., Kimpo, R. R., Rinaldi, J. M., Kohli, A., Zeng, H., Deisseroth, K., et al. (2013). Cerebellar Purkinje cell activity drives motor learning. *Nature Neuroscience*, *16*(12), 1734–1736. http://dx.doi.org/10.1038/nn.3576.

Ojakangas, C. L., & Ebner, T. J. (1992). Purkinje cell complex and simple spike changes during a voluntary arm movement learning task in the monkey. *Journal of Neurophysiology*, *68*(6), 2222–2236.

Palkovits, M., Mezey, E., Hamori, J., & Szentagothai, J. (1977). Quantitative histological analysis of the cerebellar nuclei in the cat. I. Numerical data on cells and on synapses. *Experimental Brain Research*, *28*(1–2), 189–209.

Perez-Reyes, E. (2003). Molecular physiology of low-voltage-activated t-type calcium channels. *Physiological Reviews*, *83*(1), 117–161. http://dx.doi.org/10.1152/physrev.00018.2002.

Person, A. L., & Raman, I. M. (2012). Purkinje neuron synchrony elicits time-locked spiking in the cerebellar nuclei. *Nature*, *481*(7382), 502–505. http://dx.doi.org/10.1038/nature10732.

Proville, R. D., Spolidoro, M., Guyon, N., Dugue, G. P., Selimi, F., Isope, P., & Lena, C. (2014). Cerebellum involvement in cortical sensorimotor circuits for the control of voluntary movements. *Nature Neuroscience*, *17*(9), 1233–1239. http://dx.doi.org/10.1038/nn.3773.

Pugh, J. R., & Raman, I. M. (2006). Potentiation of mossy fiber EPSCs in the cerebellar nuclei by NMDA receptor activation followed by postinhibitory rebound current. *Neuron*, *51*(1), 113–123. http://dx.doi.org/10.1016/j.neuron.2006.05.021.

Raman, I. M., & Bean, B. P. (1999). Ionic currents underlying spontaneous action potentials in isolated cerebellar Purkinje neurons. *The Journal of Neuroscience*, *19*(5), 1663–1674.

Raman, I. M., Gustafson, A. E., & Padgett, D. (2000). Ionic currents and spontaneous firing in neurons isolated from the cerebellar nuclei. *The Journal of Neuroscience, 20*(24), 9004–9016.

Raymond, J. L., & Lisberger, S. G. (1998). Neural learning rules for the vestibulo-ocular reflex. *The Journal of Neuroscience, 18*(21), 9112–9129.

Raymond, J. L., Lisberger, S. G., & Mauk, M. D. (1996). The cerebellum: a neuronal learning machine? *Science, 272*(5265), 1126–1131.

Rowland, N. C., & Jaeger, D. (2005). Coding of tactile response properties in the rat deep cerebellar nuclei. *Journal of Neurophysiology, 94*(2), 1236–1251. http://dx.doi.org/10.1152/jn.00285.2005.

Sangrey, T., & Jaeger, D. (2010). Analysis of distinct short and prolonged components in rebound spiking of deep cerebellar nucleus neurons. *European Journal of Neuroscience, 32*(10), 1646–1657. http://dx.doi.org/10.1111/j.1460-9568.2010.07408.x.

Schonewille, M., Gao, Z., Boele, H. J., Veloz, M. F., Amerika, W. E., Simek, A. A., & De Zeeuw, C. I. (2011). Reevaluating the role of LTD in cerebellar motor learning. *Neuron, 70*(1), 43–50. http://dx.doi.org/10.1016/j.neuron.2011.02.044.

Shidara, M., Kawano, K., Gomi, H., & Kawato, M. (1993). Inverse-dynamics model eye movement control by Purkinje cells in the cerebellum. *Nature, 365*(6441), 50–52. http://dx.doi.org/10.1038/365050a0.

Shin, S. L., Hoebeek, F. E., Schonewille, M., De Zeeuw, C. I., Aertsen, A., & De Schutter, E. (2007). Regular patterns in cerebellar Purkinje cell simple spike trains. *PLoS One, 2*(5), e485. http://dx.doi.org/10.1371/journal.pone.0000485.

Shinoda, Y., Futami, T., Mitoma, H., & Yokota, J. (1988). Morphology of single neurones in the cerebello-rubrospinal system. *Behavioural Brain Research, 28*(1–2), 59–64.

Steuber, V., Mittmann, W., Hoebeek, F. E., Silver, R. A., De Zeeuw, C. I., Hausser, M., et al. (2007). Cerebellar LTD and pattern recognition by Purkinje cells. *Neuron, 54*(1), 121–136. http://dx.doi.org/10.1016/j.neuron.2007.03.015.

Tadayonnejad, R., Mehaffey, W. H., Anderson, D., & Turner, R. W. (2009). Reliability of triggering postinhibitory rebound bursts in deep cerebellar neurons. *Channels (Austin), 3*(3), 149–155.

Thach, W. T. (1968). Discharge of Purkinje and cerebellar nuclear neurons during rapidly alternating arm movements in the monkey. *Journal of Neurophysiology, 31*(5), 785–797.

Thach, W. T., Jr. (1967). Somatosensory receptive fields of single units in cat cerebellar cortex. *Journal of Neurophysiology, 30*(4), 675–696.

Toyama, K., Tsukahara, N., Kosaka, K., & Matsunami, K. (1970). Synaptic excitation of red nucleus neurones by fibres from interpositus nucleus. *Experimental Brain Research, 11*(2), 187–198.

Uusisaari, M., & Knopfel, T. (2011). Functional classification of neurons in the mouse lateral cerebellar nuclei. *Cerebellum, 10*(4), 637–646. http://dx.doi.org/10.1007/s12311-010-0240-3.

Uusisaari, M., Obata, K., & Knopfel, T. (2007). Morphological and electrophysiological properties of GABAergic and non-GABAergic cells in the deep cerebellar nuclei. *Journal of Neurophysiology, 97*(1), 901–911. http://dx.doi.org/10.1152/jn.00974.2006.

Volsen, S. G., Day, N. C., McCormack, A. L., Smith, W., Craig, P. J., Beattie, R., et al. (1995). The expression of neuronal voltage-dependent calcium channels in human cerebellum. *Brain Research. Molecular Brain Research, 34*(2), 271–282.

Walter, J. T., Alvina, K., Womack, M. D., Chevez, C., & Khodakhah, K. (2006). Decreases in the precision of Purkinje cell pacemaking cause cerebellar dysfunction and ataxia. *Nature Neuroscience, 9*(3), 389–397. http://dx.doi.org/10.1038/nn1648.

Walter, J. T., & Khodakhah, K. (2006). The linear computational algorithm of cerebellar Purkinje cells. *The Journal of Neuroscience, 26*(50), 12861–12872. http://dx.doi.org/10.1523/JNEUROSCI.4507-05.2006.

Walter, J. T., & Khodakhah, K. (2009). The advantages of linear information processing for cerebellar computation. *Proceedings of the National Academy of Sciences of the United States of America, 106*(11), 4471–4476. http://dx.doi.org/10.1073/pnas.0812348106.

Wetmore, D. Z., Mukamel, E. A., & Schnitzer, M. J. (2008). Lock-and-key mechanisms of cerebellar memory recall based on rebound currents. *Journal of Neurophysiology, 100*(4), 2328–2347. http://dx.doi.org/10.1152/jn.00344.2007.

Witter, L., Canto, C. B., Hoogland, T. M., de Gruijl, J. R., & De Zeeuw, C. I. (2013). Strength and timing of motor responses mediated by rebound firing in the cerebellar nuclei after Purkinje cell activation. *Frontiers in Neural Circuits, 7,* 133. http://dx.doi.org/10.3389/fncir.2013.00133.

Wolpert, D. M., Miall, R. C., & Kawato, M. (1998). Internal models in the cerebellum. *Trends in Cognitive Sciences, 2*(9), 338–347.

Wulff, P., Schonewille, M., Renzi, M., Viltono, L., Sassoe-Pognetto, M., Badura, A., & De Zeeuw, C. I. (2009). Synaptic inhibition of Purkinje cells mediates consolidation of vestibulo-cerebellar motor learning. *Nature Neuroscience, 12*(8), 1042–1049. http://dx.doi.org/10.1038/nn.2348.

Yang, Y., & Lisberger, S. G. (2014). Purkinje-cell plasticity and cerebellar motor learning are graded by complex-spike duration. *Nature, 510*(7506), 529–532. http://dx.doi.org/10.1038/nature13282.

Zheng, N., & Raman, I. M. (2009). Ca currents activated by spontaneous firing and synaptic disinhibition in neurons of the cerebellar nuclei. *The Journal of Neuroscience, 29*(31), 9826–9838. http://dx.doi.org/10.1523/JNEUROSCI.2069-09.2009.

Zheng, N., & Raman, I. M. (2011). Prolonged postinhibitory rebound firing in the cerebellar nuclei mediated by group I metabotropic glutamate receptor potentiation of L-type calcium currents. *The Journal of Neuroscience, 31*(28), 10283–10292. http://dx.doi.org/10.1523/JNEUROSCI.1834-11.2011.

Classical Conditioning of Timed Motor Responses: Neural Coding in Cerebellar Cortex and Cerebellar Nuclei

H.J. Boele[1], M.M. ten Brinke[1], C.I. De Zeeuw[1,2]

[1]Department of Neuroscience, Erasmus MC, Rotterdam, The Netherlands;
[2]Netherlands Institute for Neuroscience, Royal Academy of Arts and
Sciences (KNAW), Amsterdam, The Netherlands

BEHAVIORAL ASPECTS OF EYEBLINK CONDITIONING

Soon after Pavlov's first description of classical conditioning of the salivation response at the beginning of the twentieth century (Pavlov, 1927), other scientists, also motivated to develop objective methods for studying learning and memory formation and the underlying neural mechanisms, extended the study of classical conditioning to other responses. In 1922 Cason showed that the eyelid response in humans could be successfully conditioned (Cason, 1922). The first eyeblink conditioning studies in animals were done by Hilgard and Marquis in the 1930s, first in dogs and later in monkeys (Hilgard & Marquis, 1935, 1936). In the 1960s Gormezano and co-workers started fundamental work on the behavioral aspects of eyeblink conditioning in rabbits, measuring the movements of the nictitating membrane instead of the eyelid responses directly (Gormezano, Schneiderman, Deaux, & Fuentes, 1962; Schneiderman & Gormezano, 1964). Today, also due to mouse transgenics, eyeblink conditioning is one of the most extensively studied forms of classical or Pavlovian conditioning. As a result the neuroanatomical circuits involved in eyeblink conditioning and the electrophysiological changes they exhibit are described at a relatively high level of detail.

In a typical eyeblink conditioning experiment, the conditional stimulus (CS) consists of an auditory or visual stimulus and the unconditional stimulus (US) of a periocular electrical stimulation or—in a more operant form of conditioning—a corneal air puff (for discussion of classical versus more operant forms of eyeblink conditioning, we refer to Longley & Yeo (2014). In a delay paradigm, the CS onset precedes the US onset usually by a couple hundreds of milliseconds, and CS and US coterminate. Repeated pairings of CS and US will gradually lead to an eyelid closure in response to the CS, which is called the conditioned response (CR). The behavioral similarities between nictitating membrane CRs and eyelid CRs allow the use of a common term for both: eyeblink CR. Although the eyelid response is extremely simple compared to, for instance, complex limb movements, it can be identified as a motor response. Since the fundamental features of a motor response, such as timing and strength, can be measured relatively easily and reliably in the nictitating membrane eyelid response, eyeblink conditioning has become a popular model to investigate not only associative learning but also motor learning.

Conditional Stimulus–Unconditional Stimulus Interval

The length of the interval between the CS and US onset in an eyeblink conditioning delay paradigm greatly affects the rate of acquisition of eyeblink CRs. In rabbits, there is hardly any eyeblink conditioning possible when using CS–US intervals below 100ms or above 4000ms, and the best learning, in terms of the percentage of trials showing CRs, occurs with a CS–US interval between 250 and 500ms (Schneiderman, 1966; Schneiderman & Gormezano, 1964; Smith, 1968). The same pattern has been reported for other species. Apart from some exceptions (for humans, see Bolbecker et al., 2011; Kimble, 1947; Woodruff-Pak & Finkbiner, 1995), the overall trend seems to be that at intervals between 150 and 1000ms, the duration of the CS–US interval is negatively correlated with the rate of eyeblink CR acquisition, that is, the longer the CS–US interval, the lower the rate of acquisition (for humans, see Boneau, 1958; McAllister, 1953; Steinmetz et al., 2011; for rabbits, see Schneiderman, 1966; Schneiderman & Gormezano, 1964; Smith, 1968; Solomon, Blanchard, Levine, Velazquez, & Groccia-Ellison, 1991; Vogel, Amundson, Lindquist, & Steinmetz, 2009; for mice, see Chettih, McDougle, Ruffolo, & Medina, 2011)

Conditioned Response Amplitude

Eyeblink CRs are not all-or-nothing responses in the sense that they suddenly pop up during the conditioning process. Instead, they seem to be acquired gradually. Although there is substantial variability between subjects and between trials in one subject, one can observe in averaged data a clear rise in the amplitude of eyeblink CRs over training, starting with small "hesitating" eyeblink CRs at the beginning and ending with full eyelid closures after training (Garcia, Mauk, Weidemann, & Kehoe, 2003; Gormezano & Kehoe, 1975; Mauk & Ruiz, 1992; Smith, 1968; Gallistel, Fairhurst, & Balsam, 2004; Kehoe, Ludvig, Dudeney, Neufeld, & Sutton, 2008).

Latency to Conditioned Response Peak

Eyeblink CRs are perfectly timed responses of which the peak coincides with the time point at which the US is about to be delivered. For instance, when training occurs with a CS–US interval of 250 ms the eyeblink CR will reach its maximum amplitude at about 250 ms after the CS onset. If a 500-ms CS–US interval were used instead, the CR would peak at 500 ms after the CS onset (Fig. 1) (Boneau, 1958; Chettih et al., 2011; Ebel & Prokasy, 1963; Garcia et al., 2003; Kehoe et al., 2008; Koekkoek et al., 2003; Mauk & Ruiz, 1992; Schneiderman & Gormezano, 1964; Smith, 1968; Vogel et al., 2009; Vogel, Brandon, & Wagner, 2003; Welsh et al., 2005). After the peak around the US, the eyelid will open quickly again. This way, an eyeblink CR provides optimal protection against the aversive US and vision is disrupted for the shortest possible period. In contrast to the CR amplitude, the latency to CR peak seems to be relatively constant during training. Although some initial studies report a slow migration of the (median) latency to a CR peak toward either earlier (Schneiderman & Gormezano, 1964) or later portions of the CS–US interval (Boneau, 1958) during training, more recent work shows only very minimal migration within the CS–US interval. Both day-by-day analysis, in which each data point is computed by averaging all mean values for a particular day or session (Garcia et al., 2003; Kehoe et al., 2008; Mauk & Ruiz, 1992; Vogel et al., 2003), and trial-by-trial analysis, in which each data point is computed by averaging together all individual traces for a specific trial (Kehoe et al., 2008), show that the CR peak seems to be timed properly with respect to the US from the first moment they appear, that is, from the moment they surpass a preset threshold (in rabbits, 0.2 or 0.5 mm movement of the nictitating membrane). In line with this "nonmigration phenomenon" is the finding that a sudden change in the CS–US interval during training does not lead to a gradual migration of the CR peak from the old US onset toward the new US onset but rather to a selective extinction of the CR for the old interval together with an acquisition of CRs to the new interval (Boneau, 1958; Kehoe & Joscelyne, 2005; Yeo, Lobo, & Baum, 1997). Previous studies reporting a gradual shift of the CR peak amplitude as a result of a switch in the CS–US interval could be explained by the type of analysis, in which CRs with bimodal

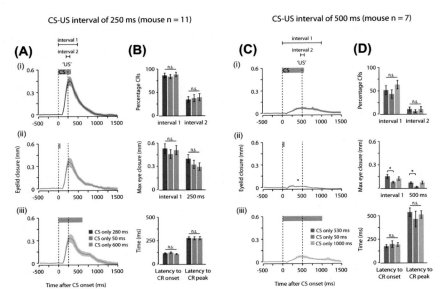

FIGURE 1 **Eyeblink CRs in CS-only trials with various CS durations.** (A) Averaged eyelid response traces (±SEM) of mice in a probe session consisting of paired CS–US trials (not depicted) intermingled with three types of CS-only trials: (i) normal-CS-only trials with a duration of 280 ms (dark green), (ii) short-CS-only trials with a duration of 50 ms (light green), and (iii) long-CS-only trials with a duration of 600 ms (blue). Prior to this probe session, the mice were trained in 10 consecutive daily acquisition sessions, each consisting of 100 paired CS–US trails with CS-US interval of 250 ms. (B) Between eyeblink CRs in the three types of CS-only trial no significant differences were found for CR percentage (calculated for interval 1 (0–500 m after the CS onset) and interval 2 (200–300 m after the CS onset)), maximum eyelid closure in interval 1, maximum eyelid closure at the expected US onset at 250 ms after the CS onset, latency to CR onset, or latency to CR peak. (C) Averaged eyelid response traces (±SEM) of mice in a probe session consisting of paired CS–US trials (not depicted) intermingled with three types of CS-only trials: (i) normal-CS-only trials with a duration of 530 ms (dark orange), (ii) short-CS-only trials with a duration of 50 ms (orange), and (iii) long-CS-only trials with a duration of 1000 ms (light orange). Prior to this probe session, the mice were trained in 10 consecutive daily acquisition sessions, each consisting of 100 paired CS–US trails with CS-US interval of 500 ms. (D) No significant difference could be established between CR percentage (calculated for interval 1 (0–1000 m after CS onset) and interval 2 (450–550 m after CS onset)), latency to CR onset, and latency to CR peak. Instead, maximum eyelid closure in interval 1 and maximum eyelid closure at expected US onset at 500 ms after CS onset were significantly smaller in trials with a short CS compared to eyelid responses in trials with a normal and long CS.

distributions were averaged over successive sessions (for humans, Ebel & Prokasy, 1963; Leonard & Theios, 1967; Prokasy, Ebel, & Thompson, 1963; for rabbits, Coleman & Gormezano, 1971; Prokasy & Papsdorf, 1965; Salafia, Martino, Cloutman, & Romano, 1979; for rats, Welsh et al., 2005 (report that "the peak of the CRs shifted to a longer latency")).

Latency to the Conditioned Response Onset

Interestingly, the same absence of migration can be observed in the latency to CR onset during training. In rabbits, early reports again suggest a gradual migration of the latency to CR onset from just before the US onset to earlier parts of the CS–US interval (Gormezano, Kehoe, & Marshall, 1983). Although at first glance some later studies suggest a similar trend, this migration to earlier portions of the CS–US interval appeared to be nonsignificant (Garcia et al., 2003; Kehoe et al., 2008). In rabbits, cats, ferrets, and humans the latency to CR onset is determined by the CS–US interval used, that is, the longer the CS–US interval the longer the latency to CR onset (Mauk & Ruiz, 1992). However, in rats and mice it seems that the latency to CR onset is rather independent of the CS–US interval used (Chettih et al., 2011; Welsh et al., 2005). In mice, it has been reported that regardless of the CS–US interval used, the latency to CR onset seems to be about 100 ms after the CS onset (but compare this finding with Fig. 1(B) and (D)). Interestingly, in rabbits and ferrets the latency to CR onset may be changed by alterations in the CS: CS intensities higher than the one used during acquisition training sessions appears to decrease the latency to CR onset (Frey, 1969; Svensson, Ivarsson, & Hesslow, 1997; Svensson, Jirenhed, Bengtsson, & Hesslow, 2010). In mice this phenomenon has not been demonstrated so far, probably because mice exhibit, when using higher (auditory) CS intensities, more startle responses and short-latency fear responses, which precede and easily mask eyeblink CR onsets (Boele, Koekkoek, & De Zeeuw, 2010; Chettih et al., 2011).

Varying Conditional Stimulus Duration after Acquisition

Interestingly, the duration of the CS seems to be rather dissociated from the kinetic profile of the eyeblink CR. It has been shown that the presentation of CS-only trials, in which the duration of the CS either extends beyond the used CS–US interval (Kehoe & Joscelyne, 2005) or is much shorter than the CS–US interval during training (Svensson & Ivarsson, 1999), results in normal eyeblink CRs. However, particularly for the short CS, it remains to be elucidated whether this result also holds for longer CS–US intervals and for more natural CSs instead of direct mossy fiber stimulation. We therefore trained 11 mice (C57Bl/6, male, aged 15–20 weeks) in 10 daily acquisition sessions (100 paired CS–US trials per daily session) in a delay paradigm with a CS–US interval of 250 ms (CS duration of 280 ms and US duration of 30 ms). After this training protocol we presented in a probe session (session 11) the same 100 paired CS–US trials, but now intermingled with three different types of CS-only trials: 10 normal-CS-only trials with a duration of 280 ms, 10 short-CS-only trials with a duration of 50 ms, and 10 long-CS-only trials with a duration of 600 ms. For a second group of seven mice (C57Bl/6, male, aged 15–20 weeks) we used the same training procedures except that these mice were trained with a CS–US interval of 500 ms (CS duration of 530 ms and US duration of 30 ms), and the probe session consisted of 100 paired CS–US trials intermingled with three different types of CS-only trials, 10 of which were normal-CS-only trials with a duration of 530 ms, 10 short-CS-only trials with a duration of 50 ms, and 10 long-CS-only trials with a duration of 1000 ms. For both groups the CS was a green LED light placed at ±7 cm in front of the animal and the US a weak air puff applied to the cornea, which elicited a reflexive full eyelid closure. Animals were head restrained but able to walk freely on a foam cylinder and eyelid movements were recorded with MDMT (for further details on the experimental setup, MDMT, and training procedures, see Chettih et al., 2011; Koekkoek, Den Ouden, Perry, Highstein, & De Zeeuw, 2002). For the CS–US interval of 250 ms, eyelid responses were considered significant if the (1) CR amplitude was >5% of full eyelid closure (UR = 100%), (2) latency to CR onset was between 50 and 250 ms, and (3) the latency to CR peak amplitude was between 100 and 500 ms (interval 1) or 200 and 300 ms (interval 2; so-called "perfectly timed eyeblink CRs"). For the CS–US interval of 500 ms, eyelid responses were considered significant if the (1) CR amplitude was >5% of full eyelid closure (UR = 100%), (2) latency to CR onset was between 50 and 500 ms, and (3) latency to CR peak was between 100 and 1000 ms (interval 1) or 450 and 550 ms (interval 2).

When first comparing mice that were trained with a 250-ms CS–US interval versus mice trained with a 500-ms CS–US interval, we found that the averaged CR percentage and CR amplitude were both higher for animals trained with the shorter interval, which is in line with previous mouse work (Chettih et al., 2011) (CR percentage interval 1, $F(1, 16) = 13.604$, $p = 0.002$; averaged eye closure in interval 1, $F(1, 16) = 23.309$, $p < 0.001$; values were calculated in normal-CS-only trials) (Fig. 1). In addition, we found a significant difference in the timing of eyeblink CRs: both the latency to CR onset and the latency to CR peak time were shorter for animals that were trained with a 250-ms CS–US interval (latency to CR onset, $F(1, 16) = 18.973$, $p < 0.001$; latency to CR peak time, $F(1, 16) = 33.555$, $p < 0.001$; the values calculated in normal-CS-only trials). This shorter latency to CR onset in mice trained with a 250-ms CS–US interval is in agreement with previous rabbit work (e.g., Mauk & Ruiz, 1992) but seems to be in contrast to the mouse work reported by Chettih et al. (2011). It can be explained by the fact that the longest CS–US interval used in the Chettih study was only 400 ms.

Second, for mice trained with a 250-ms CS–US interval, eyeblink CRs in all the three types of CS-only trials were indistinguishable (Fig. 1(A) and (B)). No differences could be established between the averaged CR percentage (interval 1, $F(2, 30) = 0.244$, $p = 0.785$; interval 2, $F(2, 30) = 0.103$, $p = 0.903$), averaged eyelid closure in interval 1 ($F(2, 30) = 0.406$, $p = 0.670$), averaged eyelid closure at 250 ms after CS onset ($F(2, 30) = 0.592$, $p = 0.559$), latency to CR onset $F(2, 30) = 1.761$, $p = 0.189$), or latency to CR peak amplitude ($F(2, 30) = 0.010$, $p = 0.990$). However, for mice that were trained with a 500-ms CS–US interval, things appear to be quite different. Although no significant differences were found between averaged CR percentage (interval 1, $F(2, 18) = 1.223$, $p = 0.318$; interval 2, $F(2, 18) = 0.300$, $p = 0.744$), latency to CR onset ($F(2, 17) = 0.242$, $p = 0.788$), or latency to CR peak ($F(2, 17) = 0.421$, $p = 0.663$), averaged eyelid closures in interval 1 and at the expected US onset were undeniably smaller in the short 50-ms CS-only trials than in trials with a normal 500-ms CS or 1000-ms CS (interval 1, $F(2, 18) = 4.493$, $p = 0.026$; Bonferroni post hoc, 50 vs. 500, $p = 0.025$, 50 vs. 1000, $p = 0.22$; eyelid closure at 500 ms after CS onset, $F(2, 18) = 6.192$, $p = 0.009$; Bonferroni post hoc, 50 vs. 500, $p = 0.023$, 50 vs. 1000, $p = 0.019$) (Fig. 1(C) and (D)). The almost complete absence of eyeblink CRs in the short 50-ms CS-only trials might explain why the latency to CR peak was not significantly different from those in the normal 500-ms CS-only trials.

In short, a very brief CS does not seem to affect the kinetic profile of the eyeblink CRs when training occurs with a CS–US interval of 250 ms. Instead, for a 500-ms interval, the short CS seems to be insufficient to elicit proper CRs. In addition, a long CS that extends beyond the time point at which the US would be delivered does not significantly change the CR profile for either the 250-ms or the 500-ms CS–US interval.

NEURAL CIRCUITS ENGAGED DURING EYEBLINK CONDITIONING

Where in the brain is the memory formed during eyeblink conditioning? Theoretically, such a brain locus should (1) receive converging inputs from CS and US, (2) innervate the eyelid premotoneurons, and (3) be able to undergo plasticity as a result of CS–US pairings. Early lesion experiments aimed at defining the minimal brain tissue sufficient for normal conditioning revealed that lesions of the cerebral hemispheres, hippocampus, or diencephalon could not prevent the acquisition and expression of eyeblink CRs (Norman, Buchwald, & Villablanca, 1977; Norman, Villablanca, Brown, Schwafel, & Buchwald, 1974; Oakley & Russell, 1972, 1975, 1976, 1977; Schmaltz & Theios, 1972), suggesting that the memory formation takes place at "lower" levels of the brain stem and/or cerebellum.

Lesions of the Cerebellar Nuclei

In the early 1980s Desmond and Moore found that lesions of the superior cerebellar peduncle prevented both CR acquisition and CR expression without affecting the URs (Desmond & Moore, 1982). Around the same time McCormick and Thompson reported that lesions of the cerebellar nuclei permanently abolished eyeblink CRs (McCormick et al., 1981, 1982), which was a little later confined by Yeo et al. to the anterior interposed nucleus (AIN) (Yeo, Hardiman, & Glickstein, 1985a). To date, many groups have replicated these initial findings in different species. In addition to a permanent eyeblink CR abolishment as a result of electrolytic or aspiration lesions of the AIN, eyeblink CRs could also be reversibly abolished by cooling, lidocaine or muscimol infusion in the AIN (Aksenov, Serdyukova, Irwin, & Bracha, 2004; Bracha, Webster, Winters, Irwin, & Bloedel, 1994; Bracha, Zhao, Irwin, & Bloedel, 2001; Chapman, Steinmetz, Sears, & Thompson, 1990; Clark, Zhang, & Lavond, 1992; Freeman, Halverson, & Poremba, 2005; Garcia & Mauk, 1998; Hardiman, Ramnani, & Yeo, 1996; Krupa, Thompson, & Thompson, 1993; Nordholm, Thompson, Dersarkissian, & Thompson, 1993). In addition, Delgado-Garcia and colleagues targeted the posterior interposed nucleus (PIN), instead of the AIN, as one of the main cerebellar nuclei involved in eyeblink conditioning in cats, serving a modulatory role (Delgado-Garcia & Gruart, 2006; Jimenez-Diaz, Gruart, Minano, & Delgado-Garcia, 2002; Jimenez-Diaz, Navarro-Lopez Jde, Gruart, Delgado-Garcia, 2004). Koekkoek and colleagues (Koekkoek et al., 2003, 2005) found that lesions of the AIN in mice affected their eyeblink responses in the CS–US interval in an incomplete fashion (see also Boele et al., 2010).

Lesions of the Cerebellar Cortex

Yeo et al. (1985b) demonstrated that unilateral electrolytic lesions of the cerebellar cortical lobule HVI, sparing the cerebellar nuclei, *completely* abolished CRs. Lesions of other parts of the cerebellar cortex did not affect CRs (Yeo et al., 1985b). Attwell, Rahman, and Yeo (2001) and Attwell, Ivarsson, Millar, and Yeo (2002) replicated these findings, showing that blocking Purkinje cell input to the AIN by infusions with PTX (picrotoxin; a $GABA_A$ chloride channel blocker) or gabazine (a $GABA_A$ receptor antagonist) completely abolished CRs; no remnant CRs with short latency to onset and peak were observed, neither in the nictitating membrane response nor in the eyelid response (Attwell et al., 2001, 2002). Mostofi et al. showed in rabbits that extremely small infusions of CNQX (6-cyano-7-nitroquinoxaline-2,3-dione; a non-NMDA ionotropic glutamate receptor antagonist) in the D0 zone of lobule HVI, the eyeblink-controlling microzone, were sufficient to completely abolish eyeblink CRs (Mostofi, Holtzman, Grout, Yeo, & Edgley, 2010). Other groups, however, initially reported that lesions of the cerebellar cortex would have *no effect* on eyeblink CRs (Clark, McCormick, Lavond, & Thompson, 1984; McCormick, Clark, Lavond, & Thompson, 1982; McCormick et al., 1981; McCormick & Thompson, 1984), which might be explained by the fact that the lesioned areas in these studies spared the eyeblink-controlling microzone. Instead, Lavond and colleagues found that both the amplitude and timing of eyeblink CRs would be affected following lesions of the eyeblink-controlling microzone, albeit in an incomplete fashion (Lavond & Steinmetz, 1989; Lavond, Steinmetz, Yokaitis, & Thompson, 1987). In line with this finding, Mauk and co-workers reported that both permanent lesions of the cerebellar cortex and reversible disconnections of the AIN from the cerebellar cortex by PTX infusions in the AIN or muscimol infusions in the cerebellar cortex mainly disrupted the learning-dependent timing of eyeblink CRs: after cortical inputs were removed from the AIN, rabbits still showed CRs, but these residual CRs had an extremely short latency to onset and latency to peak and therefore are called short-latency responses (SLRs) (Bao, Chen, Kim, & Thompson, 2002; Garcia & Mauk, 1998; Medina, Garcia, & Mauk, 2001; Ohyama, Nores, & Mauk, 2003; Ohyama, Nores, Medina, Riusech, Mauk, 2006; Perrett, Ruiz, & Mauk, 1993). In short, inactivation of the interposed nucleus generally severely affects eyeblink CRs, whereas inactivation of the cerebellar cortex leads to more conflicting results, with some groups reporting a full abolishment of eyeblink CRs and others reporting residual SLRs.

Unconditional Stimulus and Unconditioned Response Pathway

Sensory stimulation of the cornea, conjunctiva, or periocular regions will normally elicit a reflexive eyeblink. This eyeblink consists of a rapid contraction of the external eyelids together with, in some animals, a passive lateral sweep of the nictitating membrane or the third eyelid due to retraction of the eyeball in the orbita. The sensory information is relayed via the ophthalmic division of the trigeminal nerve to the trigeminal nucleus (N. V), which in turn innervates the oculomotor nucleus (N. III), the (accessory) abducens nucleus (N. VI), and the orbicularis oculi motor neurons of the facial nucleus (N. VII) (Fig. 2) (van Ham & Yeo, 1996a,b; Holstege, van Ham, & Tan, 1986; Pellegrini, Horn, & Evinger, 1995). The eyeblink is a result of the simultaneous action of these three motor nuclei: the facial nucleus activates the orbicularis oculi muscle, the oculomotor nucleus deactivates the levator palpebrae muscle, and the oculomotor and abducens nuclei together retract the eyeball (Delgado-Garcia, Gruart, & Munera, 2002; Delgado-Garcia, Gruart, & Trigo, 2003; van Ham & Yeo, 1996a,b; Trigo, Gruart, & Delgado-Garcia, 1999).

In addition to these eyeblink motoneurons, the trigeminal neurons also project to the medial part of the dorsal accessory inferior olive and dorsomedial group of the principal olive (De Zeeuw et al., 1996). These olivary regions provide the climbing fiber input via the inferior cerebellar peduncle to the eyeblink-controlling microzones in the cerebellar cortex (Fig. 2). In cats, Hesslow identified four of these cortical microzones in the C1 and C3

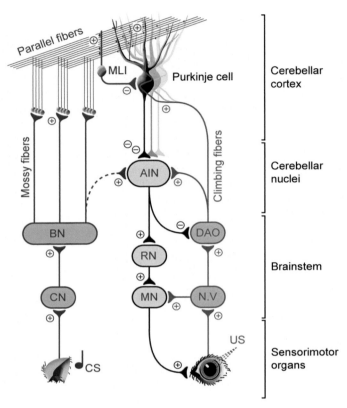

FIGURE 2   **Neural circuits engaged during eyeblink conditioning.** Purkinje cells in eyeblink-controlling microzones receive the climbing fiber input from the dorsal accessory olive, which relays sensory information from the periorbital facial region (US pathway in red). Additionally, the same Purkinje cells receive a continuous stream of virtually all sensory information from some 200,000 parallel fibers, originating from mossy fibers from various brain-stem nuclei including the basilar pontine nuclei (CS pathway in green). The Purkinje cells project to the AIN, which in turn innervates, via the red nucleus, the motor neurons that control the eyeblink (CR pathway in gray). Abbreviations: AIN, anterior interposed nucleus; BN, brain-stem nuclei (e.g., basilar pontine nuclei, nucleus reticularis tegmentis pontis, lateral reticular nucleus); CN, cochlear nucleus; DAO, dorsal accessory olive; MLI, molecular layer interneuron; MN, motor neurons innervating the eyeblink muscles (oculomotor nucleus (III), accessory nucleus (VI), and facial nucleus (VII)); N. V, trigeminal nucleus; RN, red nucleus.

zones of lobules VI and VII, which showed complex spike responses with a short latency of about 10 ms on ipsilateral periorbital stimulation. Stimulation of these areas can produce eyeblink responses, and microstimulation of these areas during the CS–US interval in conditioned animals can completely abolish eyeblink CRs (Hesslow, 1994). The directly adjacent C2 regions also showed complex spikes on periorbital stimulation, but these complex spikes can be elicited by both ipsi- and contralateral stimulation and have longer latencies (ipsilateral ± 15 ms; contralateral ± 20 ms) (Hesslow, 1994). Since microstimulation of these adjacent C2 areas does not produce an eyeblink response, they may not directly control the eyeblink CR. Hesslow's finding of multiple eyeblink-controlling microzones is in agreement with the hypothesis that microzones themselves are part of an entity of so-called multizonal microcomplexes (Apps & Hawkes, 2009). In ferrets, a more or less similar cortical pattern of eyeblink-controlling microzones can be found (Hesslow & Ivarsson, 1994). For rabbits an eyeblink-controlling microzone has been found in the zebrin-negative D0 zone, which, according to Sugihara's terminology, represents zebrin band P5– (Mostofi et al., 2010; Sugihara & Shinoda, 2004; Voogd, 2003; Voogd & Ruigrok, 2004). For other species such as rats and mice, evidence is now accumulating that this microzone in the depth of lobule VI also controls eyeblink responses (Heiney, Kim, Augustine, & Medina, 2014; Steinmetz & Freeman, 2014; Van Der Giessen et al., 2008).

Climbing fibers originating from the medial part of the dorsal accessory inferior olive and the dorsomedial group of the principal olive do not only innervate Purkinje cells in the cerebellar cortex but also give off collaterals to the cerebellar nuclei, predominantly to the lateral AIN and its dorsolateral hump (DLH) (Pijpers, Voogd, & Ruigrok, 2005), which are the nuclear parts of the eyeblink-controlling module. These climbing fiber collaterals are excitatory and seem to innervate particularly inhibitory glutamic acid decarboxylase 67 (GAD67)-positive cerebellar nuclei neurons (Uusisaari & Knopfel, 2011), but also GAD67-negative projection neurons (Fig. 3) (Hoebeek, Witter, Ruigrok, & De Zeeuw, 2010; McCrea, Bishop, & Kitai, 1978).

As proposed by Marr (1969) and Albus (1971), climbing fibers indeed seem to transmit US or error information (Marr, 1969; Albus, 1971). Electrical stimulation of the inferior olive or climbing fibers directly can serve as an effective US during eyeblink conditioning and has been demonstrated to result in normal eyeblink CR acquisition (Jirenhed, Bengtsson, & Hesslow, 2007; Mauk, Steinmetz, & Thompson, 1986; Rasmussen et al., 2013; Steinmetz, Lavond, & Thompson, 1989; Yeo & Hardiman, 1992; Yeo, Hardiman, & Glickstein, 1985c). Interestingly, only a train of several stimulus pulses can cause acquisition; a single climbing fiber pulse even causes extinction (Rasmussen et al., 2013). This finding is in line with behavioral work using a periocular US, which shows that a stronger US induces faster acquisition, and a very weak US indeed leads to extinction of eyeblink CRs (Freeman, Spencer, Skelton, & Stanton, 1993; Kehoe & White, 2002; Najafi & Medina, 2013; Passey, 1948; Smith, 1968; Spence, 1953).

Lesions of the inferior olive severely impair CR acquisition (Welsh & Harvey, 1998), although data are less consistent on this point. Intuitively, one would expect that lesions of the inferior olive after CR acquisition cause an extinction-like behavior during normal paired CS–US training.

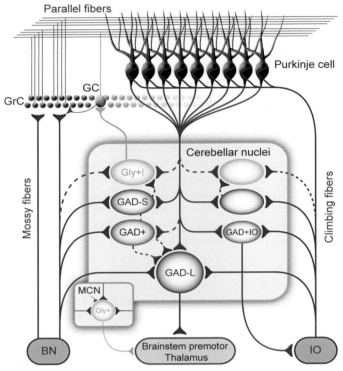

FIGURE 3   **The cerebellar nuclei contain various cell types and form the final integra-tive processing unit in the cerebellum.** In the cerebellar nuclei one can categorize at least six neuronal types based on electrophysiological properties and activity of the glutamic acid decarboxylase (GAD67) and glycine transporter (GlyT2) promoters. The cerebellar nuclei contain at least two glutamatergic neuron types, namely large GAD67-negative projec-tion (GAD-L) neurons and small GAD67-negative interneurons (GAD-S); two GABAergic neuron types, namely GAD67-positive projection neurons (GAD+IO, IO stands for inferior olive) and GAD67-positive interneurons (GAD+); and two glycinergic neuron types, namely GlyT2-positive projection neurons in the MCN (Gly+) and GlyT2 neurons (Gly+I, I stands for inactive), which project back to the Golgi cells and Purkinje cells in the cerebellar cortex. In contrast to other cerebellar nuclei neurons, Gly+I neurons are not spontaneously active. Dashed lines denote connections of uncertain strength. Gray projections are GABAergic, purple are glutamatergic, and orange are glycinergic or mixed glycinergic/GABAergic. (Figure based on Ankri et al., 2015; Uusisaari & Knopfel, 2011). Since the focus of this figure is on the cerebellar nuclei neurons we did not depict all cortical neurons and projections. Abbreviations: BN, brain-stem nuclei; IO, inferior olive; MCN, medial cerebellar nucleus.

Since the US cannot be transmitted to the Purkinje cell, paired CS–US may be seen by the Purkinje cell as "CS-only" trials. Such extinction-like behav-ior has indeed been reported (McCormick, Steinmetz, & Thompson, 1985; Welsh & Harvey, 1998). On the other hand, removal of climbing fiber input from the Purkinje cells is also known to increase simple spike firing of Purkinje cells within several minutes to exceptionally high levels, and sustained climbing fiber inactivation (30 min–5 h) will even lead to simple spike oscillations with high-frequency bursts (up to 150 Hz) with in-between periods of complete spiking silence (Cerminara & Rawson, 2004; Colin, Manil, & Desclin, 1980; Montarolo, Palestini, & Strata, 1982). More in line with these robust changes in Purkinje cell physiology, other groups report an immediate abolishment of CRs after removal of climbing fiber inputs (Yeo, Hardiman, & Glickstein, 1986; Zbarska, Bloedel, & Bracha, 2008; Zbarska, Holland, Bloedel, & Bracha, 2007). Thus specific parts in the inferior olive receive periorbital sensory information and these olivary parts innervate with their climbing fibers Purkinje cells in specific eyeblink-controlling zones in the cerebellar cortex and, by means of collaterals, neurons in the eyeblink-controlling zones in the cerebellar nuclei. These climbing fibers transmit error information or, in classical conditioning terminology, the US, which elicits a short-latency complex spike in the Purkinje cells.

Conditional Stimulus Pathway

Mossy fibers transmit sensory information from many modalities, including auditory and visual, to the cerebellar cortex (Altman, Bechterev, Radionova, Shmigidina, & Syka, 1976; Buchtel, Iosif, Marchesi, Provini, & Strata, 1972; Freeman & Duffel, 2008; Freeman, Halverson, & Hubbard, 2007; Halverson & Freeman, 2009, 2010; Halverson, Poremba, & Freeman, 2008; Leergaard & Bjaalie, 2007; Steinmetz et al., 1987). These mossy fibers originate from various brain-stem nuclei, including the basilar pontine nuclei. The basilar pontine nuclei receive a massive amount of sensory information from cortical and subcortical areas (Glickstein, Cohen, Dixon, Gibson, Hollins, Labossiere, et al., 1980; Glickstein, Stein, & King, 1972; Kosinski, Azizi, & Mihailoff, 1988; Legg, Mercier, & Glickstein, 1989; Mihailoff, Kosinski, Azizi, & Border, 1989; Mihailoff, Lee, Watt, & Yates, 1985; Mower, Gibson, Robinson, Stein, & Glickstein, 1980; Wells, Hardiman, & Yeo, 1989). Mossy fibers innervate granule cells, which in turn, with their massive parallel fiber projection, supply input to the Purkinje cells, including those in the eyeblink-controlling microzone. In unconditioned animals, mossy fibers originating from the basilar pontine nuclei sparsely give off collaterals to the lateral cerebellar nuclei but do not project to the eyeblink-controlling regions of the cerebellar nuclei, which would be the lateral AIN and the DLH (Boele, Koekkoek, De Zeeuw, & Ruigrok, 2013; Brodal, Dietrichs, & Walberg, 1986; Cicirata et al., 2005; Dietrichs, Bjaalie, & Brodal, 1983; Parenti, Zappala, Serapide, Panto, & Cicirata, 2002). For other mossy fiber sources, such as the nucleus reticularis tegmentis pontis, the innervation of the AIN and DLH is probably slightly more pronounced. The sparse mossy fiber collaterals, which are, just like climbing fiber collaterals, excitatory, innervate mainly the large GAD67-negative projection neurons (Fig. 3) (Uusisaari & Knopfel, 2011).

Electrical stimulation of mossy fiber origins such as the basilar pontine nuclei (Freeman, Rabinak, & Campolattaro, 2005; Steinmetz, Rosen, Chapman, Lavond, & Thompson, 1986; Tracy & Steinmetz, 1998), but also of mossy fibers directly in the middle cerebellar peduncle (Hesslow, Svensson, & Ivarsson, 1999; Steinmetz et al., 1986; Svensson et al., 1997), can serve as a CS and can result in robust conditioning. In addition, lesioning of the middle cerebellar peduncle prevents both CR acquisition and CR expression (Lewis, Lo Turco, & Solomon, 1987). Thus, mossy fibers seem to transmit multimodal conditional or contextual information, in classical conditioning terminology the CS, via the granule cell–parallel fiber system to the Purkinje cells, including those in the eyeblink-controlling microzone.

Conditioned Response Pathway

Purkinje cells in cortical eyeblink-controlling microzones form the ultimate point of convergence of CS and US information transmitted by mossy and climbing fibers, respectively. Temporal silencing of these Purkinje cells' simple spike firing by optogenetic stimulation of molecular layer interneurons can produce eyeblink responses (Heiney et al., 2014). In addition, electrical microstimulation of these areas during the CS–US interval in conditioned animals can completely abolish eyeblink CRs (Hesslow, 1994). Purkinje cells in eyeblink-controlling microzones project to the lateral part of the AIN, including its DLH (Rosenfield & Moore, 1995). The cerebellar nuclei should not be treated as a simple relay nucleus with little neuronal diversity (Uusisaari & Knopfel, 2011). Evidence is accumulating that these nuclei act as the final, integrative processing unit in the cerebellar circuitry. In the cerebellar nuclei one can categorize at least six neuronal types based on electrophysiological properties and activity of the GAD67 and glycine transporter (GlyT2) promoters, which are often used as markers for γ-aminobutyric acid (GABA)-ergic and glycinergic neurons, respectively. The cerebellar nuclei contain at least two excitatory neuron types, namely large GAD67-negative projection neurons and small GAD67-negative interneurons, and four inhibitory neuron types, namely GAD67-positive projection neurons and interneurons, and GlyT2-positive projection neurons and interneurons (Fig. 3) (for monkeys, see Chan-Palay, 1977; for cat, Palkovits, Mezey, Hamori, & Szentagothai, 1977; for rats, see Aizenman, Huang, & Linden, 2003; Bagnall et al., 2009; Knopfel & Uusisaari, 2008; Uusisaari & Knopfel, 2011). Purkinje cells have a strong inhibitory effect on both types of excitatory cerebellar nuclei neurons (large and small GAD67-negative neurons) and at least one type of inhibitory cerebellar nuclei neuron (GAD67-positive neurons) (Uusisaari & Knopfel, 2011). As mentioned above, the AIN also receives excitatory inputs from climbing fiber collaterals transmitting the same US information, but in untrained animals mossy fiber collaterals are, depending on their source and thus the CS modality, extremely sparse (Boele et al., 2013; Brodal et al., 1986; Cicirata et al., 2005; Dietrichs et al., 1983; Parenti et al., 2002).

Retrograde transsynaptic tracing experiments using (pseudo)rabies virus showed that the orbicularis oculi muscle is mainly innervated by the ipsilateral AIN, including its dorsolateral hump, and lobule HVI (Gonzalez-Joekes & Schreurs, 2012; Morcuende, Delgado-Garcia, & Ugolini, 2002). Indeed, electrical stimulation of this AIN region can produce an eyelid closure (Freeman & Nicholson, 2000; Halverson, Lee, & Freeman, 2010; McCormick & Thompson, 1984). In addition, stimulation of the "downstream" magnocellular division of the red nucleus can induce eyeblink responses (Nowak, Marshall-Goodell, Kehoe, & Gormezano, 1997), whereas lesions of the red nucleus completely abolish eyeblink CRs (Ohyama et al., 2006; Rosenfield & Moore, 1983, 1985). Thus, the CR pathway contains AIN projections to the magnocellular division of the red nucleus, which projects to the motor nuclei that innervate the eyelid muscles, including N. VII to activate the orbicularis oculi muscle, N. III to deactivate the levator palpebrae muscle, and N. III and N. VI together ensuring retraction of the eyeball (Delgado-Garcia et al., 2002, 2003; van Ham & Yeo, 1996b; Trigo et al., 1999). It is important to note at this point that the reflexive eyeblink (unconditioned response; UR) and the conditioned eyeblink (CR) differ from each other in kinematics because of differences in their neural control. For URs the eyeblink motor neurons (III, VI, VII) receive their main input from N. V, whereas for CRs they receive their main input from the red nucleus. As a result, the temporal profile of the UR is determined by the US: a stronger stimulation leads to a bigger and faster eyeblink. The temporal profile of the CR instead is governed by the CS–US interval: the CR peaks just before the onset of the US.

Apart from the excitatory projection to the premotor neurons in the red nucleus provided by large glutamatergic projection neurons (large GAD67-negative), the cerebellar nuclei have an inhibitory projection back to the inferior olive, provided by small GAD67-positive neurons (De Zeeuw, Holstege, Calkoen, Ruigrok, & Voogd, 1988; De Zeeuw, Holstege, Ruigrok, & Voogd, 1989; Ruigrok & Voogd, 1990; Fredette & Mugnaini, 1991). In this GABAergic feedback loop, the cerebellar zonal arrangement is again preserved (Courville, Faraco-Cantin, & Legendre, 1983; De Zeeuw et al., 1989; Dietrichs & Walberg, 1981, 1986; Ruigrok, 2011) and thus the lateral AIN and DLH regions project back to the medial part of the dorsal accessory inferior olive and the dorsomedial group of the principal olive.

Since Purkinje cells innervate both excitatory and inhibitory neurons in the cerebellar nuclei, the excitatory cerebellar output system and the inhibitory feedback to the inferior olive are most probably controlled simultaneously (De Zeeuw & Berrebi, 1995; Teune, van der Burg, de Zeeuw, Voogd, & Ruigrok, 1998; Uusisaari & Knopfel, 2011). Indeed, cerebellar nuclear recordings show that, during acquisition, inputs from the inferior olive are being suppressed, suggesting that the inferior olive becomes functionally inhibited by the cerebellum during the generation of an eyeblink CR (Andersson, Garwicz, & Hesslow, 1988; Hesslow & Ivarsson, 1996; Kim, Krupa, & Thompson, 1998; Medina, Nores, & Mauk, 2002), resulting in a decreased complex spike frequency within the CS–US interval (Rasmussen & Hesslow, 2014; Rasmussen, Jirenhed, & Hesslow, 2008; Rasmussen, Jirenhed, Wetmore, & Hesslow, 2014). Interestingly, early recordings from Purkinje cells during eyeblink conditioning seem to suggest the opposite: some cells would show an increase in complex spikes within the CS–US interval in conditioned animals (Berthier & Moore, 1986). These intuitively conflicting results might partly be explained by differences in experimental design and data analysis. First, Rasmussen and coworkers conditioned their animals for several hours and looked particularly at the changes in the complex spike frequency in the last 100 ms of the CS (CS and US coterminate), whereas Berthier and Moore performed a longer training for several days and reported increased complex spike frequencies for some Purkinje cells in the first 100 ms of the CS. Second, Rasmussen et al. recorded specifically from Purkinje cells in the eyeblink-controlling microzone, whereas Berthier and Moore had a more global approach. Instead, manipulation of the nucleo-olivary pathway has provided more consistent results. Whereas blockade of nucleo-olivary feedback after acquisition prevents extinction of conditioned eyelid responses, blocking excitatory inputs to the inferior olive or stimulation of the nucleo-olivary feedback loop just before US presentation in a trained animal leads to extinction of eyeblink CRs (Bengtsson, Jirenhed, Svensson, & Hesslow, 2007; Medina et al., 2002).

Contribution of Extracerebellar Structures

Numerous studies have focused on the contribution of extracerebellar structures such as (medial) prefrontal cortex, hippocampus, thalamus, and amygdala to memory formation relating to delayed eyeblink conditioning (mPFC, Leal-Campanario, Fairen, Delgado-Garcia, & Gruart, 2007; Plakke, Freeman, & Poremba, 2009; Wu et al., 2012; hippocampus, Berger & Thompson, 1978; Blankenship, Huckfeldt, Steinmetz, & Steinmetz, 2005; Hoehler & Thompson, 1980; Lee & Kim, 2004; Wu et al., 2013; thalamus, Halverson & Freeman, 2009, 2010; Halverson, Hubbard, & Freeman, 2009; Halverson et al., 2010; Halverson et al., 2008; Ng & Freeman, 2012; Steinmetz, Buss, & Freeman, 2013; amygdala, Blankenship et al., 2005;

Boele et al., 2010; Lee & Kim, 2004; Neufeld & Mintz, 2001; Ng & Freeman, 2013). Especially amygdala inactivation seems to have major effects on the acquisition of eyeblink CR, and we have suggested that in mice particularly the amygdala contributes to the potentiation of startle and short-latency fear responses in the eyeblink trace (Boele et al., 2010). Since this chapter focuses on cerebellar coding, and since the role of extracerebellar structures seems to be mainly limited to either a modulation of CS inputs to the cerebellum or the potentiation of fear components in the eyeblink trace, they will not be further discussed here.

NEURAL PLASTICITY IN THE CEREBELLAR CORTEX AND CEREBELLAR NUCLEI

Learning versus Performance

As mentioned above, inactivation of the AIN can abolish eyeblink CRs. From the very beginning this finding was challenged by the argument that lesions of the AIN would produce a *performance* deficit rather than an impairment of *learning*. The first argument against the cerebellar learning hypothesis came from studies, suggesting that AIN lesions simply block the expression but not the learning of eyeblink CRs (Bracha et al., 1994; Llinas & Welsh, 1993; Welsh, 1992; Welsh & Harvey, 1989, 1991). This issue has to a large extent been tackled in several temporal (or reversible) inactivation studies using the local anesthetic lidocaine or the GABA agonist muscimol, with the rationale that inactivation of a brain region where memory formation takes place should result in no CRs during training and no CRs once the inactivation has been removed. In contrast, inactivation of a brain area that is not involved in memory storage but only in the expression of learning should result in no CRs during the inactivation, but CRs should be expressed once the inactivation has been removed. Lidocaine or muscimol infusions in the eyeblink-controlling parts of the cerebellar cortex and AIN prevent learning, reflected by the absence of CRs both during inactivation and after the removal of the inactivation (Aksenov et al., 2004; Attwell et al., 2001; Bracha et al., 1994, 2001; Hardiman et al., 1996; Krupa et al., 1993; Nordholm et al., 1993). In contrast, inactivation of cerebellar premotor efferents, such as the red nucleus, by the same drugs prevents the expression of CRs during the inactivation, but does not prevent learning, in that after the washout of the drug CRs are present (Krupa & Thompson, 1995; Krupa, Weng, & Thompson, 1996; Ohyama et al., 2006). Thus, learning takes place upstream from the red nucleus in the CR pathway, which is the cerebellum.

A second argument against the cerebellar learning hypothesis came from recording studies reporting that neurons in the interposed nucleus start firing about 20ms after the onset of the eyeblink CR, suggesting that the interposed nuclei cannot initiate/generate the eyeblink CR (Delgado-Garcia & Gruart, 2002, 2005, 2006; Gruart, Blazquez, & Delgado-Garcia, 1995; Gruart & Delgado-Garcia, 1994; Gruart, Guillazo-Blanch, Fernandez-Mas, Jimenez-Diaz, & Delgado-Garcia, 2000; Sanchez-Campusano, Gruart, & Delgado-Garcia, 2011). Also according to this work, the cerebellum is not involved in memory storage but rather in the timing of eyeblink CRs and dampening oscillations in the eyeblink. However, most of these recordings were made in the PIN, which is an area of the cerebellar nuclei that does not seem to be directly involved in the control of eyelid muscles as there are no major projections to the red nucleus (Teune, van der Burg, van der Moer, Voogd, & Ruigrok, 2000). In contrast, electrophysiological recordings from neurons in the AIN do exhibit a firing profile, which precedes the onset of the eyeblink CRs and is observed only in trials wherein a CR is present and its activity models the timing and amplitude of these CRs (Berthier & Moore, 1990; Choi & Moore, 2003; Freeman & Nicholson, 2000; Gould & Steinmetz, 1996; Green & Arenos, 2007; Halverson et al., 2010; McCormick et al., 1982; McCormick & Thompson, 1984; Nicholson & Freeman, 2002). Together, these recordings suggest that the AIN is causally related to eyeblink CRs by driving the premotor neurons that innervate the eyelid muscles, and that the PIN might contribute to the motion trajectory of CRs once they start.

Cerebellar Cortex versus Cerebellar Nuclei

It appeared to be much more challenging to tease apart the relative contributions of the cerebellar cortex and the cerebellar nuclei. Is the abolishment of CRs after AIN inactivation a result of disruption of the memory that is formed in the AIN itself or simply the effect of blocking the output of the memory that is formed "upstream" in the Purkinje cells? In other words, is the essential memory formed in the cerebellar nuclei or in the cerebellar cortex? Or maybe in both?

Learning in the Cerebellar Cortex

According to Marr's and Albus's theoretical work the essential learning of timed motor responses would take place in the cerebellar cortex (Albus, 1971; Marr, 1969). They hypothesize that simultaneous activation of a set of parallel fibers with a climber fiber results in a change in the synaptic strength of this set of parallel fiber–Purkinje cell synapses. According to Albus this process should be regarded as a form of classical conditioning: *"It is now hypothesized that the inactivation response pause [after a complex spike] in Purkinje spike rate is an unconditioned response (UR) in a classical learning sense caused by the unconditioned stimulus (US) of a climbing fiber burst. It is further hypothesized that the mossy fiber activity pattern ongoing at the time of the climbing fiber burst is the conditioned stimulus (CS). If this is true, the effect of learning should be that eventually the particular mossy fiber pattern (CS) should elicit a pause (CR) in Purkinje cell activity similar to the inactivation response (UR) that previously had been elicited only by the climbing fiber burst (US)"* (Albus, 1971). Thus, cerebellar learning requires context or conditional (CS) information from mossy fibers and an error or teaching signal (US) from climbing fibers. As a result of pairing the CS with the US, Purkinje cells in the cerebellar cortex eventually should pause their simple spike firing. Since Purkinje cells have a tonic inhibitory effect on the cerebellar nuclei, this simple spike suppression will disinhibit the cerebellar nuclei, which in turn should ultimately result in an increase in cerebellar output.

Thus, Purkinje cells in a cerebellar microzone receive on the one hand a large amount of sensory information from many modalities (CS) and on the other hand sensory information from a very specific receptive field (US). Therefore, they appear well suited to associative learning (Harvey & Napper, 1991). The best evidence that Purkinje cells in the cerebellar cortex indeed can acquire pauses in their simple spike firing during eyeblink conditioning comes from Hesslow's lab. Their exact identification of eyeblink-controlling microzones in the C1 and C3 regions and their decerebrated preparation make it possible to study changes in Purkinje cell activity as they might occur during eyeblink conditioning. In a training paradigm, using peripheral forelimb or direct mossy fiber stimulation as CS paired with a periocular or direct climbing fiber stimulation as US, they observed a gradual acquisition of a suppression and even complete silencing of Purkinje cell simple spike firing. This Purkinje cell pause or Purkinje cell CR is adaptively timed in that the response latency varies with the interval used between CS and US and the suppression is maximal just before the onset of the US (Fig. 4(A–C)) (Jirenhed et al., 2007; Jirenhed & Hesslow, 2011b; Rasmussen et al., 2008; Svensson et al., 2010). Moreover, many other known behavioral phenomena such as extinction and rapid reacquisition (Fig. 4(D–I)) (Jirenhed et al., 2007), adaptation of the timing of CRs after changing the CS–US interval (Jirenhed & Hesslow, 2011b), a minimal effective CS–US interval of about 100 ms (Wetmore et al., 2014), faster conditioning by increasing US intensity (Rasmussen et al., 2013), and an earlier CR onset after increasing the CS intensity (Svensson et al., 2010), can also be observed in the single Purkinje cell. Together, these findings strongly suggest that the essential learning takes place in these Purkinje cells in the eyeblink-controlling microzone. However, it is still unclear whether this Purkinje cell simple spike pause alone is sufficient to generate eyeblink CRs. First, in Hesslow's approach in the decerebrated ferret training occurs within a couple of hours and from behavioral experiments we know that, with a few exceptions, it is impossible to train an animal within this time window, even if the animal is used to spending long times in the experimental setup (observations by H.J. Boele, data not shown). Second, because of their preparation they do not record simultaneously

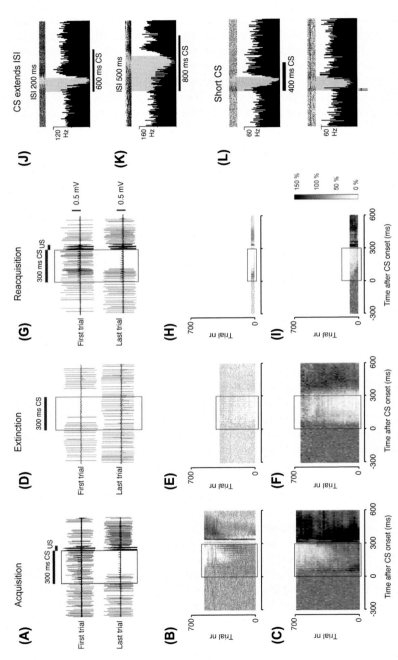

FIGURE 4 Extracellular Purkinje cell recordings during eyeblink conditioning. (A–C) Acquisition of Purkinje cell CR. (A) Two sample records from a Purkinje cell exposed to paired CS–US presentations (bars above graph), from trial 1 (top) and 640 trials later (bottom). The acquired Purkinje cell response had a latency relative to CS onset of ±60 ms. (B) Raster plot of the simple spike activity recorded from the same cell during 640 trials of paired CS–US presentations. (C) Average raster response during the CS period (framed) gradually developed as training progressed. The inhibitory response during the

plot based on 11 Purkinje cell records during acquisition. The plot is built up of squares, the shadings of which indicate the average firing rate across all cells. The light area that gradually appears represents the Purkinje cell CR, that is, an inhibitory response with a firing rate below background level (100%). The darker areas indicate increased simple spike activity. (D–F) Purkinje cell activity during extinction. (D) Two example records from a Purkinje cell exposed to unpaired CS–US stimulation (bar above graph indicates the 300-ms CS period), from trial 1 (top) and 440 trials later (bottom). The Purkinje cell CR had a latency relative to the CS onset of 60 ms and a duration of 300 ms. (E) Raster plot of simple spike activity recorded from the same cell as above during 440 trials of unpaired CS–US stimulation. The inhibitory response during the CS period (framed) was gradually extinguished as training progressed. (F) Average raster plot of simple spikes recorded from nine Purkinje cells during paired CS–US stimulation. (G–I) Purkinje cell activity during reacquisition. (G) Two example records from a Purkinje cell reexposed to paired CS–US stimulation (bars above graph) after extinction of the CR. Trial 1 (top) and 40 trials later (bottom) are shown. (H) Raster plot of simple spike activity (recorded from the same cell as above) during 40 trials of reintroduced pairing of CS–US stimulation. Notice the savings in the rate of reacquisition compared with acquisition. After only four trials, the CR was reacquired. (I) Average raster plot based on five Purkinje cell records during paired CS–US stimulation. (J, K) Conditioned Purkinje cell responses on a CS that extends the CS–US interval. (J) Example raster plot and histogram of responses from a cell conditioned to a 200-ms CS–US interval (gray shading), using a CS of 600 ms duration (black bar above graph). (K) Example raster plot and histogram of responses from a cell conditioned to a 500-ms CS–US interval (gray shading), using a CS of 800 ms duration (black bar below graph). (L) Conditioned Purkinje cell response on a short CS displayed as raster plot and histogram. Top shows the average response to CS-alone stimulation after conditioning with a 200-ms CS–US interval (gray shading) using a 400-ms duration CS (black bar below graph); the CS consisted of a 400-ms pulse train (50 Hz) to the mossy fibers. Bottom shows CRs from the same cell elicited with a short CS of only two pulses; each CS pulse is indicated by an arrow (interval between stimuli was 20 ms). For J, K, and L, each graph is based on 40 trials. The duration is 1.5 s. *Figure and legend used with permission from Jirenhed et al. (2007), Jirenhed & Hesslow (2011a,b).*

from Purkinje cells and the conditioned external eyelids. However, other studies, which do perform simultaneous recordings, show that indeed a subpopulation of Purkinje cells can show a learning-related inhibitory response of which the temporal profile corresponds with that of the eyelid CR (Hesslow & Ivarsson, 1994; Kotani, Kawahara, & Kirino, 2006). In addition, some Purkinje cells would instead increase their firing in the CS–US interval during conditioning (Berthier & Moore, 1986; Green & Steinmetz, 2005; Kotani, Kawahara, & Kirino, 2003; Kotani et al., 2006). However, these cells do not seem to control the eyeblink CR directly, since their firing profile does not seem to be correlated with the temporal profile of the eyeblink CR (Kotani et al., 2006). So far, a conclusive and quantitative study on the exact role and contributions of Purkinje cells controlling the overt eyeblink CR at different stages during the learning process is still lacking.

Plasticity Mechanisms in the Cerebellar Cortex

What is the neural mechanism underlying this adaptively timed simple spike suppression of a Purkinje cell? Albus proposed that the main underlying mechanism would be a synaptic weakening of the parallel fiber–Purkinje cell synapse (pf–PC synapse) (Albus, 1971). A few years later Masao Ito provided the first experimental support for this learning mechanism by showing that Purkinje cells (in the flocculus) indeed showed a clear suppression in excitability upon mossy fiber stimulation after it had been paired with conjunctive climbing fiber stimulation (Ito, Sakurai, & Tongroach, 1982). This suppression lasted for about an hour and was therefore called long-term depression (LTD). LTD was later confirmed in many other studies (Ekerot & Kano, 1985; Linden & Connor, 1991; Linden, Dickinson, Smeyne, & Connor, 1991). Further strengthened by reports that LTD-deficient mouse mutants showed impaired eyeblink conditioning, LTD was increasingly considered as the main learning mechanism underlying eyeblink conditioning (De Zeeuw et al., 1998; De Zeeuw & Yeo, 2005; Freeman & Steinmetz, 2011; Hansel & Linden, 2000; Hansel, Linden, & D'Angelo, 2001; Mauk & Buonomano, 2004; Mauk, Garcia, Medina, & Steele, 1998; Yamazaki & Tanaka, 2009; Yeo, 2004). For instance, LTD and eyeblink conditioning is impaired in (1) mutants lacking the metabotropic glutamate receptor mGluR1 in Purkinje cells (Aiba et al., 1994; Ichise et al., 2000; Kishimoto et al., 2002), (2) mutants lacking the glutamate receptor subunit δ2 (Kishimoto et al., 2001), (3) mutants lacking glial fibrillary acidic protein (Shibuki et al., 1996), and (4) Purkinje-cell specific mutants overexpressing protein kinase C (PKC) inhibitor (Koekkoek et al., 2003).

However, experimental and theoretical work has thrown some doubt on the essential role that pf–PC LTD would play in motor learning. First, Welsh et al. (2005) reported that application of T-588, which blocks LTD by acutely reducing calcium release from intracellular stores, does not prevent the adaptation of eyeblink CR timing to a new CS–US interval (Welsh et al., 2005). Second, Schonewille et al. (2010) demonstrated that in three different types of mutant mice (PICK1 KO, GluRD7 KI, and GluRK882A KI) that selectively lack expression of cerebellar LTD, eyeblink conditioning was not affected (Schonewille et al., 2011). In these mutants, the expression of pf–PC LTD is specifically targeted by modifications downstream of the molecular cytosolic pathways at the level of the intermediary PICK1 between PKC activation and AMPA receptor internalization or even at the level of the cell membrane (GluR2Δ7 KI and GluR2K882A KI). In contrast, in previous mutants, not only pf–PC LTD but also other forms of cerebellar plasticity are affected (Gao, van Beugen, & De Zeeuw, 2012). For example, inhibition of PKC may affect the efficacy of $GABA_A$ receptors at the molecular layer interneuron-to-Purkinje cell synapse by influencing their surface density and sensitivity to positive allosteric modulators and/or by modifying chloride conductance (Song & Messing, 2005). Similarly, Purkinje cells also display intrinsic plasticity (Zhang, & Linden, 2003), and protein kinases may well be required for persistent use-dependent modulation of one or more of the ion channels involved. Finally, the kinases might also play a role in presynaptic plasticity at the Purkinje cell-to-cerebellar nuclei neuron synapse (Belmeguenai et al., 2010) and/or postsynaptic plasticity at the mossy fiber or climbing fiber collateral-to-cerebellar nuclei neuron synapse (Pugh & Raman, 2008; Zhang & Linden, 2006). These more global effects might explain why in previous mutants with enzymatic deficits eyeblink conditioning was impaired and why in these improved and newer mutants with receptor-linked subtle deficits eyeblink conditioning is normal. Third, LTD of the pf–PC synapse seems to be insufficient to explain the millisecond precise timing of eyeblink CRs. The LTD hypothesis assumes that a specific CS will activate different sets of granule cells, which in response will fire with different latencies and durations. LTD then would occur specifically at those pf–PC synapses, whose burst activity coincides with the climbing fiber input provided by the US. As a result of LTD, simple spike firing would be suppressed in the CS–US interval and thus the eyelid will close in the CS–US interval. If this hypothesis were true, then one would expect that the duration of the relevant parallel fiber input is strongly tied to that of the resultant simple spike suppression and the eyeblink CR. In other words, the CS duration would determine the length of the CR. However, it has been shown in Purkinje cell CRs and eyeblink CRs that a long CS, which extends beyond the CS–US interval used, results in normally shaped CRs (Figs 1 and 4(J, K)) (Jirenhed & Hesslow, 2011b). Thus, even if the CS outlasts the CS–US interval used by several hundreds of milliseconds, the CR is perfectly timed, with its peak just at the point at which the US is about to be delivered. Interestingly, after training with a CS–US interval of 250 ms, a very brief CS of only tens of milliseconds is also sufficient to elicit normal Purkinje cell and eyeblink CRs (Figs 1(A, B) and 4(L)) (Jirenhed & Hesslow,

2011a; Svensson et al., 2010), but when training occurs with a longer CS–US interval of 500 ms, the brief CS seems to be insufficient to elicit proper CRs (Fig. 1(C) and (D)). Together, these data strongly suggest that the CR seems to be rather uncoupled from the CS duration and that for short CS–US intervals of about 250 ms, especially the first tens of milliseconds contain crucial information for the Purkinje cell to suppress its firing. This, in our view, cannot be merely explained by pf–PC LTD. At this point it is still unclear whether parallel fibers transmit a natural CS, an auditory tone for instance, during the full duration of the CS to the Purkinje cell, as in the approach with the mossy fiber stimulation as described above (cf. van Beugen, Gao, Boele, Hoebeek, & De Zeeuw, 2013; Jorntell & Ekerot, 2006; Ruigrok, Hensbroek, & Simpson, 2011). Fourth, it appeared that LTD of the pf–PC synapse cannot even be established after eyeblink conditioning (Jirenhed & Hesslow, 2011a). In an approach where animals were first trained with a CS consisting of direct mossy fiber stimulation for a duration of 800 ms and a US of direct climbing fiber stimulation for 20 ms, and starting at 200 ms after CS onset, the authors looked after training at the simple spike probability following single mossy fiber pulses in CS-alone trials at various time points in the 800-ms CS period. They argue that, if LTD would take place, then one would expect a lower simple spike probability at each time point in the 800-ms CS period, and thus a coupling of CS length and simple spike suppression. However, in conditioned Purkinje cells they could establish only a decreased simple spike probability within the CS–US interval and not in the 600-ms period wherein the CS outlasts the US, suggesting that LTD of the parallel fiber–Purkinje cell synapse has not taken place (Hesslow, Jirenhed, Rasmussen, & Johansson, 2013; Jirenhed & Hesslow, 2011a).

For further arguments against LTD as being the sole essential form of plasticity underlying eyeblink conditioning, we refer to Hesslow et al. (2013) and Gao et al. (2012). Hesslow et al. (2013) argue that the conditions under which LTD is induced in vitro do not match those of behavioral eyeblink conditioning experiments. In the slice preparation LTD can be induced within minutes and optimal LTD is obtained when the delay between "CS" and "US" would be close to zero milliseconds, whereas during behavioral experiments, the acquisition of eyeblink CRs takes several hundreds of paired trials, and the minimum interval to get proper conditioning between CS and US is about 100 ms. In contrast, Hansel and co-workers argue that LTD can also be successfully induced at longer intervals of hundreds of milliseconds (Piochon, Kruskal, Maclean, & Hansel, 2012; Titley & Hansel, 2015). Further, since Purkinje cells have an intrinsic spike-generating mechanism (Raman & Bean, 1997, 1999), removal of excitatory inputs from the Purkinje cell by the application of CNQX has only minor effects on the simple spike firing rate (Cerminara & Rawson, 2004; Zhou et al., 2014), and granule cells are mostly silent to begin with (Isope & Barbour, 2002), LTD of the parallel fiber–Purkinje cell synapse alone cannot easily explain the complete silencing of Purkinje cell simple spike firing for hundreds of milliseconds. In other words, removal of excitation seems unable to induce a complete pause in simple spike firing.

Which alternative plasticity mechanisms could potentially explain or contribute to timed simple spike pauses during eyeblink conditioning? First, Johansson, Jirenhed, Rasmussen, Zucca, and Hesslow (2014) have demonstrated that Purkinje cells can be successfully conditioned by direct stimulation of parallel fibers as CS and direct climbing fiber stimulation as US up to CS–US intervals of 300 ms. Moreover, application of the GABA antagonist gabazine seems to have no effect on acquired simple spike pauses (Johansson et al., 2014). Although the role of molecular layer interneurons can probably not be excluded completely because of the ephaptic inhibitory effects they have on Purkinje cells (Blot & Barbour, 2014), these data strongly suggest the existence of a cellular mechanism within the Purkinje cell that may suppress its simple spike firing for the duration of the CS–US interval (i.e., several hundreds of milliseconds). In other words, Purkinje cells seem to "convert" increases in parallel fiber input (by the CS) to decreased output. The exact nature of these cellular mechanisms remains to be elucidated, but group II and III metabotropic glutamate receptors are likely to play a role (Dutar, Vu, & Perkel, 1999; Johansson et al., 2014). Second, it should be noted that stellate and basket cells make strong inhibitory chemical but possibly also electrical synapses with Purkinje cells, as shown in lower vertebrates (Sotelo & Llinas, 1972). As a result their activity may contribute long simple spike pauses (Heiney et al., 2014; Korn & Axelrad, 1980; Mittmann, Koch, & Hausser, 2005) and thereby contribute to the CRs. However, how these cells contribute to the exact timing of CRs is unclear. Third, from a Purkinje cell's perspective, it seems unwise to decrease input strengths of relevant sets of parallel fibers transmitting CS information. If Purkinje cells indeed have an intrinsic mechanism to convert increases in parallel fiber input, caused by the CS, to a decreased output, then pf–PC long-term potentiation (LTP) would be an effective mechanism to enhance the input strength of specific parallel fiber inputs transmitting CS. This pf–PC LTP might enable the Purkinje cell to "pick up" the relevant CS information more easily. This optimization of input strength might explain why after conditioning a minimum of CS information, for instance, a very brief CS, can be sufficient to elicit perfectly timed CRs (Figs 1(A, B) and 4(L)) (Jirenhed & Hesslow, 2011a; Svensson et al., 2010). The importance of pf–PC LTP is further supported by the finding that eyeblink conditioning is severely impaired in L7-PP2B mice, which have a Purkinje cell-specific impairment in pf–PC LTP and cannot increase their intrinsic excitability (Belmeguenai & Hansel, 2005; Schonewille et al., 2010).

Plasticity in Cerebellar Nuclei

One of the main arguments for plasticity in the cerebellar nuclei during eyeblink conditioning comes from studies that show inactivation of cortical eyeblink-controlling zones could not completely abolish eyeblink CRs: after removal of cortical inputs from the AIN, animals would still display residual CRs with an extremely short latency to onset and latency to peak, therefore called SLRs (Bao et al., 2002; Garcia & Mauk, 1998; Medina et al., 2001; Ohyama et al., 2003, 2006; Perrett et al., 1993). Since other groups do not find these SLRs, they have been a matter of big dispute (Attwell et al., 2001, 2002; Yeo et al., 1985b). These conflicting results have been addressed extensively by Bracha and co-workers. Initially, they reported that PTX infusions in the AIN did not have any effect on eyeblink CRs and should even increase the amplitude of the eyelid responses (Bracha et al., 2001). However, later they showed that the effects of PTX and gabazine injection in the AIN are at least partly determined by the dosage used: a low dose of gabazine or PTX results in SLRs, whereas higher dosages result in a complete abolishment of CRs (Aksenov et al., 2004; Parker, Zbarska, Carrel, & Bracha, 2009). In addition, they also report that the effects of the low-dose PTX in similar AIN injections are surprisingly variable: some rabbits do show SLRs, whereas others do not. Importantly, before and after injection they also performed extracellular recordings from AIN neurons, which are categorized into three groups based on resting firing frequency before injection of PTX. The main effect of low-dose infusions (0.5 μl per side) of PTX in the AIN is an increased baseline firing frequency and diminished modulation during the CS–US interval in all three categories of AIN neurons (mainly lateral parts of the AIN). A consecutive second injection (again 0.5 μl per side) further increases the baseline firing frequency and almost completely abolishes modulation during the CS–US interval. No SLRs could be observed in the firing profile of AIN neurons (Fig. 5). The behavioral results of PTX injections comprise increased tonic eyelid closures and increased UR amplitudes. According to the same group, blocking climbing and mossy fiber collateral input with DGG (γ-D-glutamylglycine; glutamate receptor antagonist) does not abolish CRs but has only minor effects on CR latency (increase) and CR incidence (decrease) (Aksenov, Serdyukova, Bloedel, & Bracha, 2005), a finding that is in line with Attwell and co-workers (Attwell et al., 2001, 2002), suggesting that plasticity in the cerebellar nuclei plays only an accessory role in the expression of CRs.

Since, to our knowledge, SLRs have never been described for the firing profile of AIN neurons, this raises the question whether these SLRs indeed form the behavioral correlate of memory that has been formed in the cerebellar nuclei. Inactivation of the cerebellar cortex results in a tonic disinhibition of the cerebellar nuclei, which in turn results in an increased excitation of premotor areas innervating the eyelid motoneuron (N. III, VI, VII). As a result, sensory input from the trigeminal nucleus to these motoneurons might result in a stronger output. Indeed, it has been shown that the removal of cortical inputs to the AIN results in stronger and bigger reflexive eyelid closures (Parker et al., 2009; Yeo & Hardiman, 1992).

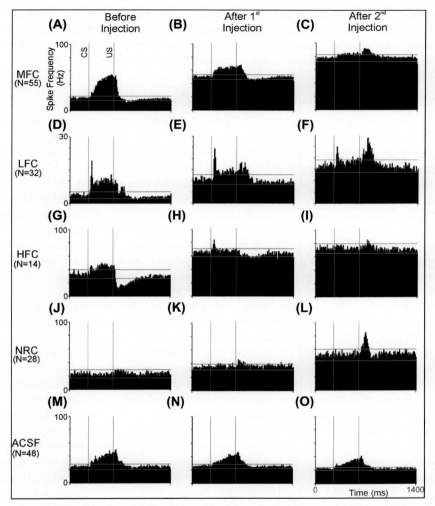

FIGURE 5   **Extracellular recordings from cerebellar nuclei neurons during eyeblink conditioning.** Effects of picrotoxin (PTX) and artificial cerebrospinal fluid (ACSF) injections on recorded populations of cells. Averaged peristimulus histograms are arranged in rows corresponding to cell type and in columns representing the activity before injection, after the first PTX injection, and after the second PTX injection. (A–C) Medium-frequency cells (MFC). (D–F) Low-frequency cells (LFC). (G–I) High-frequency cells (HFC). (J–L) Nonresponding cells (NRC). (M–O) Cells recorded during control injections of vehicle, ACSF. Note that the first injection of PTX increased baseline firing frequency and diminished the relative size of firing modulation in all cell types. The second injection further increased baseline activity and further reduced the depth of firing modulation. Also note the emerging response to the US in MFC, LFC, and NRC that becomes the most prominent response following the second PTX injection. Bin width, 10 ms. Horizontal lines in each histogram represent tolerance limits, which were computed based on the statistical assumption that 99% of observations should not exceed this limit with a probability of 0.95. Abbreviations: CS, conditioned stimulus onset; US, unconditioned stimulus onset. *Figure and legend used with permission from Aksenov et al. (2004).*

Similarly, the effects of other brain structures that (in)directly innervate the eyelid motoneurons might become more evident after lesions of the cerebellar cortex. Therefore, we propose that it cannot be excluded that SLRs in rabbits are also a result of extracerebellar learning.

Plasticity Mechanisms in the Cerebellar Nuclei

Plasticity in the AIN during eyeblink conditioning assumes convergence of CS and US at this site by mossy fibers and climbing fibers, respectively. But, as mentioned already, in untrained animals there is hardly any convergence of CS and US in the AIN. For climbing fibers it is clear that they give off collaterals to the cerebellar nuclei (Pijpers et al., 2005), thus US signals are also sent to the AIN. However, in unconditioned animals mossy fiber projections from the basilar pontine nuclei to the cerebellar nuclei are sparse and mainly restricted to the lateral cerebellar nuclei. For other sources of mossy fibers, such as the nucleus reticularis tegmentis pontis, projections to the cerebellar nuclei seem to be more predominantly present, but are also mainly restricted to the lateral cerebellar nuclei (Boele et al., 2013; Brodal et al., 1986; Cicirata et al., 2005; Dietrichs et al., 1983; Parenti et al., 2002). Thus, there seems to be an asymmetry in climbing fiber and mossy fiber projections to the AIN and the main neuronal pathway that would enable memory formation in the cerebellar nuclei, that is, the projection from the basilar pontine nuclei to AIN, appears to be virtually absent following standard tracing experiments in naïve animals. Therefore, we tested the hypothesis that during eyeblink conditioning mossy fiber collaterals can grow to specific eyeblink-controlling parts of the cerebellar nuclei, thus enabling the CS also to terminate in the AIN, and that as a consequence memory formation in the cerebellar nuclei can take place (Boele et al., 2013). Such reorganization of neuronal circuits by axonal growth and synaptogenesis has been recognized as a plausible mechanism for learning and memory formation for many decades (Holt, 1931), since it could robustly increase the memory storage capacity of the brain (Wen, Stepanyants, Elston, Grosberg, & Chklovskii, 2009). Yet, evidence for this learning mechanism still was missing. We demonstrated first that in untrained mice mossy fiber collaterals originating from the lateral parts of the basilar pontine nuclei, which are considered to convey auditory information to the cerebellum, are sparse and limited to the lateral cerebellar nucleus and caudolateral PIN, which is in perfect agreement with previous findings obtained in other species (Brodal et al., 1986; Cicirata et al., 2005; Dietrichs et al., 1983; Parenti et al., 2002). Second, we demonstrated that these mossy fiber collaterals to the cerebellar nuclei could expand considerably following Pavlovian eyeblink conditioning to a tone, whereas no changes are observed following pseudo-conditioning to this tone (Fig. 6(A–C)). Because pseudo-conditioned animals show

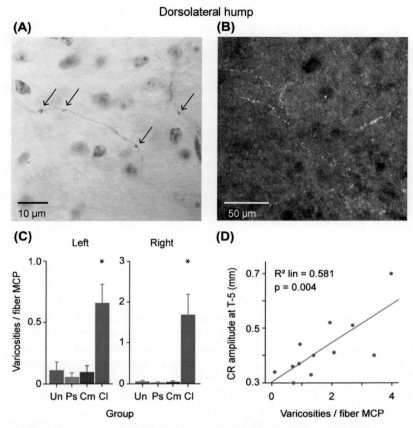

FIGURE 6 **Labeled mossy fiber collaterals and varicosities in the dorsolateral hump (DLH) for each group.** (A) Light microscopic image of a biotinylated dextran amine (BDA) -labeled mossy fiber collateral with varicosities in the DLH region of a conditioned animal. Bar, 10 μm. Arrows indicate labeled varicosities. (B) Dark-field microscopic image of BDA-labeled mossy fiber collaterals with varicosities in the DLH region of a conditioned animal. Bar, 50 μm. (C) Total number of synapses in the DLH per labeled fiber in the middle cerebellar peduncle (MCP) for all four groups. Conditioned animals with BDA injection in lateral right basilar pontine nuclei (BPN) show a significant increase in their number of varicosities per MCP fiber. (D) Mean number of labeled varicosities in the DLH per labeled MCP mossy fiber plotted against the mean CR amplitude (mm) at the last training session for conditioned animals with BDA injected in the lateral BPN. In conditioned animals the number of labeled varicosities in the DLH per MCP fiber correlates positively with the amplitude of the eyelid CRs in the last training sessions. Abbreviations: Cl, conditioned with BDA injection in lateral right BPN; Cm, conditioned with BDA injection in medial right BPN; Ps, pseudo-conditioned with BDA injected in lateral right BPN; Un, untrained with BDA injected in lateral right BPN. *Figure and legend used with permission from Boele et al. (2013).*

similar patterns of labeling compared to untrained animals, the data strongly suggest that the changed distribution and increased density of terminal labeling in the conditioned animals are specifically due to the paired presentation of CS and US rather than to the less specific aspects of the learning task, such as habituation or sensitization to the CS and US. Third, no changes are observed in conditioned animals after labeling non-auditory mossy fibers from the medial part of the basilar pontine nuclei. Therefore, we conclude that the observed conditioning-induced neuronal outgrowth specifically involves basilar pontine nuclei neurons that transmit the tone CS to the cerebellar nuclei. Fourth, and this last observation maybe gives the most important clue to the role of these mossy fiber collaterals, we established a positive correlation between the amplitude of the eyeblink CRs after training and the amount of mossy fiber collaterals in the DLH region (Fig. 6(D)), which is the part of the AIN in mice receiving input from Purkinje cells known to be involved in controlling eyelid movements (Gonzalez-Joekes & Schreurs, 2012; Morcuende et al., 2002; Mostofi et al., 2010). We could not establish any correlations between the CR timing and the amount of mossy fiber collaterals in this DLH region. We propose that this new excitatory input to the DLH and adjacent lateral AIN interacts with the well-timed Purkinje cell disinhibition of the same DLH neurons and results in a stronger output to the eyelid muscles than would happen with changes in the Purkinje cell input alone. In addition, it has been shown that excitatory mossy fiber input followed by inhibitory Purkinje cell input could induce LTP at the mossy fiber–cerebellar nuclei neuron synapse (Pugh & Raman, 2008; Zhang & Linden, 2006). On the other hand, the direct mossy and climbing fiber inputs to the AIN do not seem to be the major driver of the eyeblink CRs, since blockade of these inputs to the AIN with CNQX or DGG has only very minor effects on CRs in trained animals (Aksenov et al., 2004; Attwell et al., 2001, 2002).

CONCLUSIONS

Starting from the elegant models and work by Marr, Albus, and Ito, psychologists and cerebellar scientists have come a long way in understanding classical Pavlovian eyeblink conditioning. Even though the original concept of an interaction between the two main afferent pathways, that is, the mossy fiber and the climbing fiber systems, still stands, it has become increasingly clear that there is not a single essential form of plasticity in any part of the cerebellum that is doing the job by itself under normal physiological circumstances. Instead the picture is emerging that the cerebellar cortex directly and constantly interacts with the cerebellar nuclei and inferior olive to facilitate the learning process and that the cellular processes within all of these areas entail not only synaptic depression or potentiation but also hardwired plasticity. Indeed, one could state that the olivocerebellar system has evolved as a wonderful and diverse learning machine that can resist most mutations a single process that takes part in its computations required for memory formation.

CONFLICT OF INTEREST

Authors declare no competing financial interest.

Acknowledgments

We kindly thank A.C. IJpelaar for her technical assistance on eyeblink conditioning experiments. This work was financially supported by the Netherlands Organization for Health Research and Development (ZonMw) and Fundamental Science (NWO-ALW), ERC Advanced, CEREBNET, and C7 programs of the European Community.

References

Aiba, A., Kano, M., Chen, C., Stanton, M. E., Fox, G. D., Herrup, K., et al. (1994). Deficient cerebellar long-term depression and impaired motor learning in mGluR1 mutant mice. *Cell, 79*, 377–388.

Aizenman, C. D., Huang, E. J., & Linden, D. J. (2003). Morphological correlates of intrinsic electrical excitability in neurons of the deep cerebellar nuclei. *Journal of Neurophysiology, 89*, 1738–1747.

Aksenov, D. P., Serdyukova, N. A., Bloedel, J. R., & Bracha, V. (2005). Glutamate neurotransmission in the cerebellar interposed nuclei: involvement in classically conditioned eyeblinks and neuronal activity. *Journal of Neurophysiology, 93*, 44–52.

Aksenov, D., Serdyukova, N., Irwin, K., & Bracha, V. (2004). GABA neurotransmission in the cerebellar interposed nuclei: involvement in classically conditioned eyeblinks and neuronal activity. *Journal of Neurophysiology, 91*, 719–727.

Albus, J. S. (1971). *A theory of cerebellar function*.

Altman, J. A., Bechterev, N. N., Radionova, E. A., Shmigidina, G. N., & Syka, J. (1976). Electrical responses of the auditory area of the cerebellar cortex to acoustic stimulation. *Experimental Brain Research, 26*, 285–298.

Andersson, G., Garwicz, M., & Hesslow, G. (1988). Evidence for a GABA-mediated cerebellar inhibition of the inferior olive in the cat. *Experimental Brain Research, 72*, 450–456.

Ankri, L., Husson, Z., Pietrajtis, K., Proville, R., Lena, C., Yarom, Y., et al. (2015). A novel inhibitory nucleo-cortical circuit controls cerebellar Golgi cell activity. *eLife, 4*.

Apps, R., & Hawkes, R. (2009). Cerebellar cortical organization: a one-map hypothesis. *Nature Reviews Neuroscience, 10*, 670–681.

Attwell, P. J., Ivarsson, M., Millar, L., & Yeo, C. H. (2002). Cerebellar mechanisms in eyeblink conditioning. *Annals of the New York Academy of Sciences, 978*, 79–92.

Attwell, P. J., Rahman, S., & Yeo, C. H. (2001). Acquisition of eyeblink conditioning is critically dependent on normal function in cerebellar cortical lobule HVI. *Journal of Neurophysiology, 21*, 5715–5722.

Bagnall, M. W., Zingg, B., Sakatos, A., Moghadam, S. H., Zeilhofer, H. U., & du Lac, S. (2009). Glycinergic projection neurons of the cerebellum. *Journal of Neurophysiology, 29*, 10104–10110.

Bao, S., Chen, L., Kim, J. J., & Thompson, R. F. (2002). Cerebellar cortical inhibition and classical eyeblink conditioning. *Proceedings of the National Academy of Sciences of the United States of America, 99*, 1592–1597.

Belmeguenai, A., & Hansel, C. (2005). A role for protein phosphatases 1, 2A, and 2B in cerebellar long-term potentiation. *The Journal of Neuroscience, 25*, 10768–10772.

Belmeguenai, A., Hosy, E., Bengtsson, F., Pedroarena, C. M., Piochon, C., Teuling, E., et al. (2010). Intrinsic plasticity complements long-term potentiation in parallel fiber input gain control in cerebellar Purkinje cells. *The Journal of Neuroscience, 30*, 13630–13643.

Bengtsson, F., Jirenhed, D. A., Svensson, P., & Hesslow, G. (2007). Extinction of conditioned blink responses by cerebello-olivary pathway stimulation. *Neuroreport, 18*, 1479–1482.

Berger, T. W., & Thompson, R. F. (1978). Neuronal plasticity in the limbic system during classical conditioning of the rabbit nictitating membrane response. I. The hippocampus. *Brain Research, 145*, 323–346.

Berthier, N. E., & Moore, J. W. (1986). Cerebellar Purkinje cell activity related to the classically conditioned nictitating membrane response. *Experimental Brain Research, 63*, 341–350.

Berthier, N. E., & Moore, J. W. (1990). Activity of deep cerebellar nuclear cells during classical conditioning of nictitating membrane extension in rabbits. *Experimental Brain Research, 83*, 44–54.

van Beugen, B. J., Gao, Z., Boele, H. J., Hoebeek, F., & De Zeeuw, C. I. (2013). High frequency burst firing of granule cells ensures transmission at the parallel fiber to purkinje cell synapse at the cost of temporal coding. *Frontiers in Neural Circuits, 7*, 95.

Blankenship, M. R., Huckfeldt, R., Steinmetz, J. J., & Steinmetz, J. E. (2005). The effects of amygdala lesions on hippocampal activity and classical eyeblink conditioning in rats. *Brain Research, 1035*, 120–130.

Blot, A., & Barbour, B. (2014). Ultra-rapid axon-axon ephaptic inhibition of cerebellar Purkinje cells by the pinceau. *Nature Neuroscience, 17*, 289–295.

Boele, H. J., Koekkoek, S. K., & De Zeeuw, C. I. (2010). Cerebellar and extracerebellar involvement in mouse eyeblink conditioning: the ACDC model. *Frontiers in Cellular Neuroscience, 3*, 19.

Boele, H. J., Koekkoek, S. K., De Zeeuw, C. I., & Ruigrok, T. J. (2013). Axonal sprouting and formation of terminals in the adult cerebellum during associative motor learning. *The Journal of Neuroscience, 33*, 17897–17907.

Bolbecker, A. R., Steinmetz, A. B., Mehta, C. S., Forsyth, J. K., Klaunig, M. J., Lazar, E. K., et al. (2011). Exploration of cerebellar-dependent associative learning in schizophrenia: effects of varying and shifting interstimulus interval on eyeblink conditioning. *Behavioral Neuroscience, 125*, 687–698.

Boneau, C. A. (1958). The interstimulus interval and the latency of the conditioned eyelid response. *Journal of Experimental Psychology, 56*, 464–471.

Bracha, V., Webster, M. L., Winters, N. K., Irwin, K. B., & Bloedel, J. R. (1994). Effects of muscimol inactivation of the cerebellar interposed-dentate nuclear complex on the performance of the nictitating membrane response in the rabbit. *Experimental Brain Research, 100*, 453–468.

Bracha, V., Zhao, L., Irwin, K., & Bloedel, J. R. (2001). Intermediate cerebellum and conditioned eyeblinks. Parallel involvement in eyeblinks and tonic eyelid closure. *Experimental Brain Research, 136*, 41–49.

Brodal, P., Dietrichs, E., & Walberg, F. (1986). Do pontocerebellar mossy fibres give off collaterals to the cerebellar nuclei? an experimental study in the cat with implantation of crystalline HRP-WGA. *Neuroscience Research, 4*, 12–24.

Buchtel, H. A., Iosif, G., Marchesi, G. F., Provini, L., & Strata, P. (1972). Analysis of the activity evoked in the cerebellar cortex by stimulation of the visual pathways. *Experimental Brain Research, 15*, 278–288.

Cason, H. (1922). The conditioned eyelid reaction. *Journal of Experimental Psychology, 5*, 153–198.

Cerminara, N. L., & Rawson, J. A. (2004). Evidence that climbing fibers control an intrinsic spike generator in cerebellar Purkinje cells. *The Journal of Neuroscience, 24*, 4510–4517.

Chan-Palay, V. (1977). *Cerebellar dentate nucleus: Organization, cytology and transmitters.* Berlin: Springer-Verlag.

Chapman, P. F., Steinmetz, J. E., Sears, L. L., & Thompson, R. F. (1990). Effects of lidocaine injection in the interpositus nucleus and red nucleus on conditioned behavioral and neuronal responses. *Brain Research, 537,* 149–156.

Chettih, S. N., McDougle, S. D., Ruffolo, L. I., & Medina, J. F. (2011). Adaptive timing of motor output in the mouse: the role of movement oscillations in eyelid conditioning. *Frontiers in Integrative Neuroscience, 5,* 72.

Choi, J. S., & Moore, J. W. (2003). Cerebellar neuronal activity expresses the complex topography of conditioned eyeblink responses. *Behavioral Neuroscience, 117,* 1211–1219.

Cicirata, F., Zappala, A., Serapide, M. F., Parenti, R., Panto, M. R., & Paz, C. (2005). Different pontine projections to the two sides of the cerebellum. *Brain Research. Brain Research Reviews, 49,* 280–294.

Clark, G. A., McCormick, D. A., Lavond, D. G., & Thompson, R. F. (1984). Effects of lesions of cerebellar nuclei on conditioned behavioral and hippocampal neuronal responses. *Brain Research, 291,* 125–136.

Clark, R. E., Zhang, A. A., & Lavond, D. G. (1992). Reversible lesions of the cerebellar interpositus nucleus during acquisition and retention of a classically conditioned behavior. *Behavioral Neuroscience, 106,* 879–888.

Coleman, S. R., & Gormezano, I. (1971). Classical conditioning of the rabbit's (*Oryctolagus cuniculus*) nictitating membrane response under symmetrical CS-US interval shifts. *Journal of Comparative and Physiological Psychology, 77,* 447–455.

Colin, F., Manil, J., & Desclin, J. C. (1980). The olivocerebellar system. I. Delayed and slow inhibitory effects: an overlooked salient feature of cerebellar climbing fibers. *Brain Research, 187,* 3–27.

Courville, J., Faraco-Cantin, F., & Legendre, A. (1983). Detailed organization of cerebello-olivary projections in the cat. An autoradiographic study. *Archives italiennes de biologie, 121,* 219–236.

De Zeeuw, C. I., & Berrebi, A. S. (1995). Postsynaptic targets of Purkinje cell terminals in the cerebellar and vestibular nuclei of the rat. *The European Journal of Neuroscience, 7,* 2322–2333.

De Zeeuw, C. I., Hansel, C., Bian, F., Koekkoek, S. K., van Alphen, A. M., Linden, D. J., et al. (1998). Expression of a protein kinase C inhibitor in Purkinje cells blocks cerebellar LTD and adaptation of the vestibulo-ocular reflex. *Neuron, 20,* 495–508.

De Zeeuw, C. I., Holstege, J. C., Calkoen, F., Ruigrok, T. J., & Voogd, J. (1988). A new combination of WGA-HRP anterograde tracing and GABA immunocytochemistry applied to afferents of the cat inferior olive at the ultrastructural level. *Brain Research, 447,* 369–375.

De Zeeuw, C. I., Holstege, J. C., Ruigrok, T. J., & Voogd, J. (1989). Ultrastructural study of the GABAergic, cerebellar, and mesodiencephalic innervation of the cat medial accessory olive: anterograde tracing combined with immunocytochemistry. *Journal of Comparative Neurology, 284,* 12–35.

De Zeeuw, C. I., Lang, E. J., Sugihara, I., Ruigrok, T. J., Eisenman, L. M., Mugnaini, E., et al. (1996). Morphological correlates of bilateral synchrony in the rat cerebellar cortex. *The Journal of Neuroscience, 16,* 3412–3426.

De Zeeuw, C. I., & Yeo, C. H. (2005). Time and tide in cerebellar memory formation. *Current Opinion in Neurobiology, 15,* 667–674.

Delgado-Garcia, J. M., & Gruart, A. (2002). The role of interpositus nucleus in eyelid conditioned responses. *Cerebellum, 1,* 289–308.

Delgado-Garcia, J. M., & Gruart, A. (2005). Firing activities of identified posterior interpositus nucleus neurons during associative learning in behaving cats. *Brain Research. Brain Research Reviews, 49,* 367–376.

Delgado-Garcia, J. M., & Gruart, A. (2006). Building new motor responses: eyelid conditioning revisited. *Trends in Neurosciences, 29,* 330–338.

Delgado-Garcia, J. M., Gruart, A., & Munera, A. (2002). Neural organization of eyelid responses. *Movement Disorders, 17*(Suppl. 2), S33–S36.

Delgado-Garcia, J. M., Gruart, A., & Trigo, J. A. (2003). Physiology of the eyelid motor system. *Annals of the New York Academy of Sciences, 1004*, 1–9.

Desmond, J. E., & Moore, J. W. (1982). A brain stem region essential for the classically conditioned but not unconditioned nictitating membrane response. *Physiology & Behavior, 28*, 1029–1033.

Dietrichs, E., Bjaalie, J. G., & Brodal, P. (1983). Do pontocerebellar fibers send collaterals to the cerebellar nuclei? *Brain Research, 259*, 127–131.

Dietrichs, E., & Walberg, F. (1981). The cerebellar nucleo-olivary projection in the cat. *Anatomy and Embryology, 162*, 51–67.

Dietrichs, E., & Walberg, F. (1986). The cerebellar nucleo-olivary and olivocerebellar nuclear projections in the cat as studied with anterograde and retrograde transport in the same animal after implantation of crystalline WGA-HRP. III. The interposed nuclei. *Brain Research, 373*, 373–383.

Dutar, P., Vu, H. M., & Perkel, D. J. (1999). Pharmacological characterization of an unusual mGluR-evoked neuronal hyperpolarization mediated by activation of GIRK channels. *Neuropharmacology, 38*, 467–475.

Ebel, H. C., & Prokasy, W. F. (1963). Classical eyelid conditioning as a function of sustained and shifted interstimulus intervals. *Journal of Experimental Psychology, 65*, 52–58.

Ekerot, C. F., & Kano, M. (1985). Long-term depression of parallel fibre synapses following stimulation of climbing fibres. *Brain Research, 342*, 357–360.

Fredette, B. J., & Mugnaini, E. (1991). The GABAergic cerebello-olivary projection in the rat. *Anatomy and Embryology, 184*, 225–243.

Freeman, J. H., & Duffel, J. W. (2008). Eyeblink conditioning using cochlear nucleus stimulation as a conditioned stimulus in developing rats. *Developmental Psychobiology, 50*, 640–646.

Freeman, J. H., Halverson, H. E., & Hubbard, E. M. (2007). Inferior colliculus lesions impair eyeblink conditioning in rats. *Learning & Memory, 14*, 842–846.

Freeman, J. H., Jr., Halverson, H. E., & Poremba, A. (2005). Differential effects of cerebellar inactivation on eyeblink conditioned excitation and inhibition. *The Journal of Neuroscience, 25*, 889–895.

Freeman, J. H., Jr., & Nicholson, D. A. (2000). Developmental changes in eye-blink conditioning and neuronal activity in the cerebellar interpositus nucleus. *The Journal of Neuroscience, 20*, 813–819.

Freeman, J. H., Jr., Rabinak, C. A., & Campolattaro, M. M. (2005). Pontine stimulation overcomes developmental limitations in the neural mechanisms of eyeblink conditioning. *Learning & Memory, 12*, 255–259.

Freeman, J. H., Spencer, C. O., Skelton, R. W., & Stanton, M. E. (1993). Ontogeny of eyeblink conditioning in the rat: effects of US intensity and interstimulus interval on delay conditioning. *Psychobiology, 21*, 233–242.

Freeman, J. H., & Steinmetz, A. B. (2011). Neural circuitry and plasticity mechanisms underlying delay eyeblink conditioning. *Learning & Memory, 18*, 666–677.

Frey, W. P. (1969). Within and between session CS intensity performance effects in rabbit eyelid conditioning. *Psychonomic Science, 17*, 1–2.

Gallistel, C. R., Fairhurst, S., & Balsam, P. (2004). The learning curve: implications of a quantitative analysis. *Proceedings of the National Academy of Sciences of the United States of America, 101*, 13124–13131.

Gao, Z., van Beugen, B. J., & De Zeeuw, C. I. (2012). Distributed synergistic plasticity and cerebellar learning. *Nature Reviews Neuroscience, 13*, 619–635.

Garcia, K. S., & Mauk, M. D. (1998). Pharmacological analysis of cerebellar contributions to the timing and expression of conditioned eyelid responses. *Neuropharmacology, 37*, 471–480.

Garcia, K. S., Mauk, M. D., Weidemann, G., & Kehoe, E. J. (2003). Covariation of alternative measures of responding in rabbit (*Oryctolagus cuniculus*) eyeblink conditioning during acquisition training and tone generalization. *Behavioral Neuroscience, 117*, 292–303.

Glickstein, M., Cohen, J. L., Dixon, B., Gibson, A., Hollins, M., Labossiere, E., et al. (1980). Corticopontine visual projections in macaque monkeys. *Journal of Comparative Neurology, 190*, 209–229.

Glickstein, M., Stein, J., & King, R. A. (1972). Visual input to the pontine nuclei. *Science, 178*, 1110–1111.

Gonzalez-Joekes, J., & Schreurs, B. G. (2012). Anatomical characterization of a rabbit cerebellar eyeblink premotor pathway using pseudorabies and identification of a local modulatory network in anterior interpositus. *The Journal of Neuroscience, 32*, 12472–12487.

Gormezano, I., & Kehoe, E. J. (1975). Classical conditioning: some methodical-conceptual issues. In W. K. Estes (Ed.), *Handbook of learning and cognitive processes* (pp. 143–179). Hillsdale: Lawrence Erlbaum.

Gormezano, I., Kehoe, E. J., & Marshall, B. S. (1983). *Twenty years of classical conditioning research with the rabbit*. New York: Academic Press.

Gormezano, I., Schneiderman, N., Deaux, E., & Fuentes, I. (1962). Nictitating membrane: classical conditioning and extinction in the albino rabbit. *Science, 138*, 33–34.

Gould, T. J., & Steinmetz, J. E. (1996). Changes in rabbit cerebellar cortical and interpositus nucleus activity during acquisition, extinction, and backward classical eyelid conditioning. *Neurobiology of Learning and Memory, 65*, 17–34.

Green, J. T., & Arenos, J. D. (2007). Hippocampal and cerebellar single-unit activity during delay and trace eyeblink conditioning in the rat. *Neurobiology of Learning and Memory, 87*, 269–284.

Green, J. T., & Steinmetz, J. E. (2005). Purkinje cell activity in the cerebellar anterior lobe after rabbit eyeblink conditioning. *Learning & Memory, 12*, 260–269.

Gruart, A., Blazquez, P., & Delgado-Garcia, J. M. (1995). Kinematics of spontaneous, reflex, and conditioned eyelid movements in the alert cat. *Journal of Neurophysiology, 74*, 226–248.

Gruart, A., & Delgado-Garcia, J. M. (1994). Discharge of identified deep cerebellar nuclei neurons related to eye blinks in the alert cat. *Neuroscience, 61*, 665–681.

Gruart, A., Guillazo-Blanch, G., Fernandez-Mas, R., Jimenez-Diaz, L., & Delgado-Garcia, J. M. (2000). Cerebellar posterior interpositus nucleus as an enhancer of classically conditioned eyelid responses in alert cats. *Journal of Neurophysiology, 84*, 2680–2690.

Halverson, H. E., & Freeman, J. H. (2009). Medial auditory thalamic input to the lateral pontine nuclei is necessary for auditory eyeblink conditioning. *Neurobiology of Learning and Memory*.

Halverson, H. E., & Freeman, J. H. (2010). Ventral lateral geniculate input to the medial pons is necessary for visual eyeblink conditioning in rats. *Learning & Memory, 17*, 80–85.

Halverson, H. E., Hubbard, E. M., & Freeman, J. H. (2009). Stimulation of the lateral geniculate, superior colliculus, or visual cortex is sufficient for eyeblink conditioning in rats. *Learning & Memory, 16*, 300–307.

Halverson, H. E., Lee, I., & Freeman, J. H. (2010). Associative plasticity in the medial auditory thalamus and cerebellar interpositus nucleus during eyeblink conditioning. *The Journal of Neuroscience, 30*, 8787–8796.

Halverson, H. E., Poremba, A., & Freeman, J. H. (2008). Medial auditory thalamus inactivation prevents acquisition and retention of eyeblink conditioning. *Learning & Memory, 15*, 532–538.

van Ham, J. J., & Yeo, C. H. (1996a). The central distribution of primary afferents from the external eyelids, conjunctiva, and cornea in the rabbit, studied using WGA-HRP and B-HRP as transganglionic tracers. *Experimental Neurology, 142*, 217–225.

van Ham, J. J., & Yeo, C. H. (1996b). Trigeminal inputs to eyeblink motoneurons in the rabbit. *Experimental Neurology, 142*, 244–257.

Hansel, C., & Linden, D. J. (2000). Long-term depression of the cerebellar climbing fiber–Purkinje neuron synapse. *Neuron, 26*, 473–482.

Hansel, C., Linden, D. J., & D'Angelo, E. (2001). Beyond parallel fiber LTD: the diversity of synaptic and non-synaptic plasticity in the cerebellum. *Nature Neuroscience, 4*, 467–475.

Hardiman, M. J., Ramnani, N., & Yeo, C. H. (1996). Reversible inactivations of the cerebellum with muscimol prevent the acquisition and extinction of conditioned nictitating membrane responses in the rabbit. *Experimental Brain Research, 110*, 235–247.

Harvey, R. J., & Napper, R. M. (1991). Quantitative studies on the mammalian cerebellum. *Progress in Neurobiology, 36*, 437–463.

Heiney, S. A., Kim, J., Augustine, G. J., & Medina, J. F. (2014). Precise control of movement kinematics by optogenetic inhibition of Purkinje cell activity. *The Journal of Neuroscience, 34*, 2321–2330.

Hesslow, G. (1994). Correspondence between climbing fibre input and motor output in eyeblink-related areas in cat cerebellar cortex. *The Journal of Physiology, 476*, 229–244.

Hesslow, G., & Ivarsson, M. (1994). Suppression of cerebellar Purkinje cells during conditioned responses in ferrets. *Neuroreport, 5*, 649–652.

Hesslow, G., & Ivarsson, M. (1996). Inhibition of the inferior olive during conditioned responses in the decerebrate ferret. *Experimental Brain Research, 110*, 36–46.

Hesslow, G., Jirenhed, D. A., Rasmussen, A., & Johansson, F. (2013). Classical conditioning of motor responses: what is the learning mechanism? *Neural Networks: The Official Journal of the International Neural Network Society, 47*, 81–87.

Hesslow, G., Svensson, P., & Ivarsson, M. (1999). Learned movements elicited by direct stimulation of cerebellar mossy fiber afferents. *Neuron, 24*, 179–185.

Hilgard, E. R., & Marquis, D. G. (1935). Acquisition, extinction, and retention of conditioned lid responses to light in dogs. *Journal of Comparative Psychology, 19*, 29–58.

Hilgard, E. R., & Marquis, D. G. (1936). Conditioned eyelid responses in monkeys, with a comparison of dog, monkey, and man. *Phychological Monographs, 47*, 187–198.

Hoebeek, F. E., Witter, L., Ruigrok, T. J., & De Zeeuw, C. I. (2010). Differential olivo-cerebellar cortical control of rebound activity in the cerebellar nuclei. *Proceedings of the National Academy of Sciences of the United States of America, 107*, 8410–8415.

Hoehler, F. K., & Thompson, R. F. (1980). Effect of the interstimulus (CS-UCS) interval on hippocampal unit activity during classical conditioning of the nictitating membrane response of the rabbit (*Oryctolagus cuniculus*). *Journal of Comparative and Physiological Psychology, 94*, 201–215.

Holstege, G., van Ham, J. J., & Tan, J. (1986). Afferent projections to the orbicularis oculi motoneuronal cell group. An autoradiographical tracing study in the cat. *Brain Research, 374*, 306–320.

Holt, E. B. (1931). *Animal drive and the learning process* New York.

Ichise, T., Kano, M., Hashimoto, K., Yanagihara, D., Nakao, K., Shigemoto, R., et al. (2000). mGluR1 in cerebellar Purkinje cells essential for long-term depression, synapse elimination, and motor coordination. *Science, 288*, 1832–1835.

Isope, P., & Barbour, B. (2002). Properties of unitary granule cell-->Purkinje cell synapses in adult rat cerebellar slices. *The Journal of Neuroscience, 22*, 9668–9678.

Ito, M., Sakurai, M., & Tongroach, P. (1982). Climbing fibre induced depression of both mossy fibre responsiveness and glutamate sensitivity of cerebellar Purkinje cells. *The Journal of Physiology, 324*, 113–134.

Jimenez-Diaz, L., Gruart, A., Minano, F. J., & Delgado-Garcia, J. M. (2002). An experimental study of posterior interpositus involvement in the genesis and control of conditioned eyelid responses. *Annals of the New York Academy of Sciences, 978*, 106–118.

Jimenez-Diaz, L., Navarro-Lopez Jde, D., Gruart, A., & Delgado-Garcia, J. M. (2004). Role of cerebellar interpositus nucleus in the genesis and control of reflex and conditioned eyelid responses. *The Journal of Neuroscience, 24*, 9138–9145.

Jirenhed, D. A., Bengtsson, F., & Hesslow, G. (2007). Acquisition, extinction, and reacquisition of a cerebellar cortical memory trace. *The Journal of Neuroscience, 27*, 2493–2502.

Jirenhed, D. A., & Hesslow, G. (2011a). Time course of classically conditioned Purkinje cell response is determined by initial part of conditioned stimulus. *The Journal of Neuroscience, 31,* 9070–9074.

Jirenhed, D. A., & Hesslow, G. (2011b). Learning stimulus intervals–adaptive timing of conditioned purkinje cell responses. *Cerebellum, 10,* 523–535.

Johansson, F., Jirenhed, D. A., Rasmussen, A., Zucca, R., & Hesslow, G. (2014). Memory trace and timing mechanism localized to cerebellar Purkinje cells. *Proceedings of the National Academy of Sciences of the United States of America, 111,* 14930–14934.

Jorntell, H., & Ekerot, C. F. (2006). Properties of somatosensory synaptic integration in cerebellar granule cells in vivo. *The Journal of Neuroscience, 26,* 11786–11797.

Kehoe, E. J., & Joscelyne, A. (2005). Temporally specific extinction of conditioned responses in the rabbit (*Oryctolagus cuniculus*) nictitating membrane preparation. *Behavioral Neuroscience, 119,* 1011–1022.

Kehoe, E. J., Ludvig, E. A., Dudeney, J. E., Neufeld, J., & Sutton, R. S. (2008). Magnitude and timing of nictitating membrane movements during classical conditioning of the rabbit (*Oryctolagus cuniculus*). *Behavioral Neuroscience, 122,* 471–476.

Kehoe, E. J., & White, N. E. (2002). Extinction revisited: similarities between extinction and reductions in US intensity in classical conditioning of the rabbit's nictitating membrane response. *Animal Learning & Behavior, 30,* 96–111.

Kimble, G. A. (1947). Conditioning as a function of the time between conditioned and unconditioned stimuli. *Journal of Experimental Psychology, 37,* 1–15.

Kim, J. J., Krupa, D. J., & Thompson, R. F. (1998). Inhibitory cerebello-olivary projections and blocking effect in classical conditioning. *Science, 279,* 570–573.

Kishimoto, Y., Fujimichi, R., Araishi, K., Kawahara, S., Kano, M., Aiba, A., et al. (2002). mGluR1 in cerebellar Purkinje cells is required for normal association of temporally contiguous stimuli in classical conditioning. *The European Journal of Neuroscience, 16,* 2416–2424.

Kishimoto, Y., Kawahara, S., Fujimichi, R., Mori, H., Mishina, M., & Kirino, Y. (2001). Impairment of eyeblink conditioning in GluRdelta2-mutant mice depends on the temporal overlap between conditioned and unconditioned stimuli. *The European Journal of Neuroscience, 14,* 1515–1521.

Knopfel, T., & Uusisaari, M. (2008). Modulation of excitation by metabotropic glutamate receptors. *Results and Problems in Cell Differentiation, 44,* 163–175.

Koekkoek, S. K. E., Den Ouden, W. L., Perry, G., Highstein, S. M., & De Zeeuw, C. I. (2002). Monitoring kinetic and frequency-domain properties of eyelid responses in mice with magnetic distance measurement technique. *Journal of Neurophysiology, 88,* 2124–2133.

Koekkoek, S. K., et al. (2005). Deletion of FMR1 in Purkinje cells enhances parallel fiber LTD, enlarges spines, and attenuates cerebellar eyelid conditioning in Fragile X syndrome. *Neuron, 47,* 339–352.

Koekkoek, S. K., Hulscher, H. C., Dortland, B. R., Hensbroek, R. A., Elgersma, Y., Ruigrok, T. J., et al. (2003). Cerebellar LTD and learning-dependent timing of conditioned eyelid responses. *Science, 301,* 1736–1739.

Korn, H., & Axelrad, H. (1980). Electrical inhibition of Purkinje cells in the cerebellum of the rat. *Proceedings of the National Academy of Sciences of the United States of America, 77,* 6244–6247.

Kosinski, R. J., Azizi, S. A., & Mihailoff, G. A. (1988). Convergence of cortico- and cuneopontine projections onto components of the pontocerebellar system in the rat: an anatomical and electrophysiological study. *Experimental Brain Research, 71,* 541–556.

Kotani, S., Kawahara, S., & Kirino, Y. (2003). Purkinje cell activity during learning a new timing in classical eyeblink conditioning. *Brain Research, 994,* 193–202.

Kotani, S., Kawahara, S., & Kirino, Y. (2006). Purkinje cell activity during classical eyeblink conditioning in decerebrate guinea pigs. *Brain Research, 1068,* 70–81.

Krupa, D. J., & Thompson, R. F. (1995). Inactivation of the superior cerebellar peduncle blocks expression but not acquisition of the rabbit's classically conditioned eye-blink response. *Proceedings of the National Academy of Sciences of the United States of America, 92*, 5097–5101.

Krupa, D. J., Thompson, J. K., & Thompson, R. F. (1993). Localization of a memory trace in the mammalian brain. *Science, 260*, 989–991.

Krupa, D. J., Weng, J., & Thompson, R. F. (1996). Inactivation of brainstem motor nuclei blocks expression but not acquisition of the rabbit's classically conditioned eyeblink response. *Behavioral Neuroscience, 110*, 219–227.

Lavond, D. G., & Steinmetz, J. E. (1989). Acquisition of classical conditioning without cerebellar cortex. *Behavioural Brain Research, 33*, 113–164.

Lavond, D. G., Steinmetz, J. E., Yokaitis, M. H., & Thompson, R. F. (1987). Reacquisition of classical conditioning after removal of cerebellar cortex. *Experimental Brain Research, 67*, 569–593.

Leal-Campanario, R., Fairen, A., Delgado-Garcia, J. M., & Gruart, A. (2007). Electrical stimulation of the rostral medial prefrontal cortex in rabbits inhibits the expression of conditioned eyelid responses but not their acquisition. *Proceedings of the National Academy of Sciences of the United States of America, 104*, 11459–11464.

Lee, T., & Kim, J. J. (2004). Differential effects of cerebellar, amygdalar, and hippocampal lesions on classical eyeblink conditioning in rats. *The Journal of Neuroscience, 24*, 3242–3250.

Leergaard, T. B., & Bjaalie, J. G. (2007). Topography of the complete corticopontine projection: from experiments to principal maps. *Frontiers in Neuroscience, 1*, 211–223.

Legg, C. R., Mercier, B., & Glickstein, M. (1989). Corticopontine projection in the rat: the distribution of labelled cortical cells after large injections of horseradish peroxidase in the pontine nuclei. *Journal of Comparative Neurology, 286*, 427–441.

Leonard, D. W., & Theios, J. (1967). Effect of CS-US interval shift on classical conditioning of the nictitating membrane in the rabbit. *Journal of Comparative and Physiological Psychology, 63*, 355–358.

Lewis, J. L., Lo Turco, J. J., & Solomon, P. R. (1987). Lesions of the middle cerebellar peduncle disrupt acquisition and retention of the rabbit's classically conditioned nictitating membrane response. *Behavioral Neuroscience, 101*, 151–157.

Linden, D. J., & Connor, J. A. (1991). Participation of postsynaptic PKC in cerebellar long-term depression in culture. *Science, 254*, 1656–1659.

Linden, D. J., Dickinson, M. H., Smeyne, M., & Connor, J. A. (1991). A long-term depression of AMPA currents in cultured cerebellar Purkinje neurons. *Neuron, 7*, 81–89.

Llinas, R., & Welsh, J. P. (1993). On the cerebellum and motor learning. *Current Opinion in Neurobiology, 3*, 958–965.

Longley, M., & Yeo, C. H. (2014). Distribution of neural plasticity in cerebellum-dependent motor learning. *Progress in Brain Research, 210*, 79–101.

Marr, D. (1969). A theory of cerebellar cortex. *The Journal of Physiology, 202*, 437–470.

Mauk, M. D., & Buonomano, D. V. (2004). The neural basis of temporal processing. *Annual Review of Neuroscience, 27*, 307–340.

Mauk, M. D., Garcia, K. S., Medina, J. F., & Steele, P. M. (1998). Does cerebellar LTD mediate motor learning? Toward a resolution without a smoking gun. *Neuron, 20*, 359–362.

Mauk, M. D., & Ruiz, B. P. (1992). Learning-dependent timing of Pavlovian eyelid responses: differential conditioning using multiple interstimulus intervals. *Behavioral Neuroscience, 106*, 666–681.

Mauk, M. D., Steinmetz, J. E., & Thompson, R. F. (1986). Classical conditioning using stimulation of the inferior olive as the unconditioned stimulus. *Proceedings of the National Academy of Sciences of the United States of America, 83*, 5349–5353.

McAllister, W. R. (1953). Eyelid conditioning as a function of the CS-US interval. *Journal of Experimental Psychology, 45*, 417–422.

McCormick, D. A., Clark, G. A., Lavond, D. G., & Thompson, R. F. (1982). Initial localization of the memory trace for a basic form of learning. *Proceedings of the National Academy of Sciences of the United States of America, 79*, 2731–2735.

McCormick, D. A., Lavond, D. G., Clark, G. A., Kettner, R. E., Rising, C. E., & Thompson, R. F. (1981). The engram found? Role of the cerebellum in classical conditioning of nictitating membrane and eyelid responses. *Bulletin of the Psychonomic Society, 18*, 103–105.

McCormick, D. A., Steinmetz, J. E., & Thompson, R. F. (1985). Lesions of the inferior olivary complex cause extinction of the classically conditioned eyeblink response. *Brain Research, 359*, 120–130.

McCormick, D. A., & Thompson, R. F. (1984). Cerebellum: essential involvement in the classically conditioned eyelid response. *Science, 223*, 296–299.

McCrea, R. A., Bishop, G. A., & Kitai, S. T. (1978). Morphological and electrophysiological characteristics of projection neurons in the nucleus interpositus of the cat cerebellum. *Journal of Comparative Neurology, 181*, 397–419.

Medina, J. F., Garcia, K. S., & Mauk, M. D. (2001). A mechanism for savings in the cerebellum. *The Journal of Neuroscience, 21*, 4081–4089.

Medina, J. F., Nores, W. L., & Mauk, M. D. (2002). Inhibition of climbing fibres is a signal for the extinction of conditioned eyelid responses. *Nature, 416*, 330–333.

Mihailoff, G. A., Kosinski, R. J., Azizi, S. A., & Border, B. G. (1989). Survey of noncortical afferent projections to the basilar pontine nuclei: a retrograde tracing study in the rat. *Journal of Comparative Neurology, 282*, 617–643.

Mihailoff, G. A., Lee, H., Watt, C. B., & Yates, R. (1985). Projections to the basilar pontine nuclei from face sensory and motor regions of the cerebral cortex in the rat. *Journal of Comparative Neurology, 237*, 251–263.

Mittmann, W., Koch, U., & Hausser, M. (2005). Feed-forward inhibition shapes the spike output of cerebellar Purkinje cells. *The Journal of Physiology, 563*, 369–378.

Montarolo, P. G., Palestini, M., & Strata, P. (1982). The inhibitory effect of the olivocerebellar input on the cerebellar Purkinje cells in the rat. *The Journal of Physiology, 332*, 187–202.

Morcuende, S., Delgado-Garcia, J. M., & Ugolini, G. (2002). Neuronal premotor networks involved in eyelid responses: retrograde transneuronal tracing with rabies virus from the orbicularis oculi muscle in the rat. *The Journal of Neuroscience, 22*, 8808–8818.

Mostofi, A., Holtzman, T., Grout, A. S., Yeo, C. H., & Edgley, S. A. (2010). Electrophysiological localization of eyeblink-related microzones in rabbit cerebellar cortex. *The Journal of Neuroscience, 30*, 8920–8934.

Mower, G., Gibson, A., Robinson, F., Stein, J., & Glickstein, M. (1980). Visual pontocerebellar projections in the cat. *Journal of Neurophysiology, 43*, 355–366.

Najafi, F., & Medina, J. F. (2013). Beyond "all-or-nothing" climbing fibers: graded representation of teaching signals in Purkinje cells. *Frontiers in Neural Circuits, 7*, 115.

Neufeld, M., & Mintz, M. (2001). Involvement of the amygdala in classical conditioning of eyeblink response in the rat. *Brain Research, 889*, 112–117.

Ng, K. H., & Freeman, J. H. (2012). Developmental changes in medial auditory thalamic contributions to associative motor learning. *The Journal of Neuroscience, 32*, 6841–6850.

Ng, K. H., & Freeman, J. H. (2013). Amygdala inactivation impairs eyeblink conditioning in developing rats. *Developmental Psychobiology*.

Nicholson, D. A., & Freeman, J. H., Jr. (2002). Neuronal correlates of conditioned inhibition of the eyeblink response in the anterior interpositus nucleus. *Behavioral Neuroscience, 116*, 22–36.

Nordholm, A. F., Thompson, J. K., Dersarkissian, C., & Thompson, R. F. (1993). Lidocaine infusion in a critical region of cerebellum completely prevents learning of the conditioned eyeblink response. *Behavioral Neuroscience, 107*, 882–886.

Norman, R. J., Buchwald, J. S., & Villablanca, J. R. (1977). Classical conditioning with auditory discrimination of the eye blink in decerebrate cats. *Science, 196*, 551–553.

Norman, R. J., Villablanca, J. R., Brown, K. A., Schwafel, J. A., & Buchwald, J. S. (1974). Classical eyeblink conditioning in the bilaterally hemispherectomized cat. *Experimental Neurology, 44*, 363–380.

Nowak, A. J., Marshall-Goodell, B., Kehoe, E. J., & Gormezano, I. (1997). Elicitation, modification, and conditioning of the rabbit nictitating membrane response by electrical stimulation in the spinal trigeminal nucleus, inferior olive, interpositus nucleus, and red nucleus. *Behavioral Neuroscience, 111*, 1041–1055.

Oakley, D. A., & Russell, I. S. (1972). Neocortical lesions and Pavlovian conditioning. *Physiology & Behavior, 8*, 915–926.

Oakley, D. A., & Russell, I. S. (1975). Role of cortex in Pavlovian discrimination learning. *Physiology & Behavior, 15*, 315–321.

Oakley, D. A., & Russell, I. S. (1976). Subcortical nature of Pavlovian differentiation in the rabbit. *Physiology & Behavior, 17*, 947–954.

Oakley, D. A., & Russell, I. S. (1977). Subcortical storage of Pavlovian conditioning in the rabbit. *Physiology & Behavior, 18*, 931–937.

Ohyama, T., Nores, W. L., & Mauk, M. D. (2003). Stimulus generalization of conditioned eyelid responses produced without cerebellar cortex: implications for plasticity in the cerebellar nuclei. *Learning & Memory, 10*, 346–354.

Ohyama, T., Nores, W. L., Medina, J. F., Riusech, F. A., & Mauk, M. D. (2006). Learning-induced plasticity in deep cerebellar nucleus. *The Journal of Neuroscience, 26*, 12656–12663.

Palkovits, M., Mezey, E., Hamori, J., & Szentagothai, J. (1977). Quantitative histological analysis of the cerebellar nuclei in the cat. I. Numerical data on cells and on synapses. *Experimental Brain Research, 28*, 189–209.

Parenti, R., Zappala, A., Serapide, M. F., Panto, M. R., & Cicirata, F. (2002). Projections of the basilar pontine nuclei and nucleus reticularis tegmenti pontis to the cerebellar nuclei of the rat. *Journal of Comparative Neurology, 452*, 115–127.

Parker, K. L., Zbarska, S., Carrel, A. J., & Bracha, V. (2009). Blocking GABAA neurotransmission in the interposed nuclei: effects on conditioned and unconditioned eyeblinks. *Brain Research, 1292*, 25–37.

Passey, G. E. (1948). The influence of intensity of unconditioned stimulus upon acquisition of a conditioned response. *Journal of Experimental Psychology, 38*, 420–428.

Pavlov, I. P. (1927). In G. V. Anrep (Ed.), *Conditioned reflexes, an investigation of the physiological activity of the cerebral cortex.*

Pellegrini, J. J., Horn, A. K., & Evinger, C. (1995). The trigeminally evoked blink reflex. I. Neuronal circuits. *Experimental Brain Research, 107*, 166–180.

Perrett, S. P., Ruiz, B. P., & Mauk, M. D. (1993). Cerebellar cortex lesions disrupt learning-dependent timing of conditioned eyelid responses. *The Journal of Neuroscience, 13*, 1708–1718.

Pijpers, A., Voogd, J., & Ruigrok, T. J. (2005). Topography of olivo-cortico-nuclear modules in the intermediate cerebellum of the rat. *Journal of Comparative Neurology, 492*, 193–213.

Piochon, C., Kruskal, P., Maclean, J., & Hansel, C. (2012). Non-Hebbian spike-timing-dependent plasticity in cerebellar circuits. *Frontiers in Neural Circuits, 6*, 124.

Plakke, B., Freeman, J. H., & Poremba, A. (2009). Metabolic mapping of rat forebrain and midbrain during delay and trace eyeblink conditioning. *Neurobiology of Learning and Memory, 92*, 335–344.

Prokasy, W. F., Ebel, H. C., & Thompson, D. D. (1963). Response shaping at long interstimulus intervals in classical eyelid conditioning. *Journal of Experimental Psychology, 66*, 138–141.

Prokasy, W. F., & Papsdorf, J. D. (1965). Effects of increasing the interstimulus interval during classical conditioning of the albino rabbit. *Journal of Comparative and Physiological Psychology, 60*, 249–252.

Pugh, J. R., & Raman, I. M. (2008). Mechanisms of potentiation of mossy fiber EPSCs in the cerebellar nuclei by coincident synaptic excitation and inhibition. *The Journal of Neuroscience, 28*, 10549–10560.

Raman, I. M., & Bean, B. P. (1997). Resurgent sodium current and action potential formation in dissociated cerebellar Purkinje neurons. *The Journal of Neuroscience, 17*, 4517–4526.

Raman, I. M., & Bean, B. P. (1999). Ionic currents underlying spontaneous action potentials in isolated cerebellar Purkinje neurons. *The Journal of Neuroscience, 19,* 1663–1674.

Rasmussen, A., & Hesslow, G. (2014). Feedback control of learning by the cerebello-olivary pathway. *Progress in Brain Research, 210,* 103–119.

Rasmussen, A., Jirenhed, D. A., & Hesslow, G. (2008). Simple and complex spike firing patterns in purkinje cells during classical conditioning. *Cerebellum, 7,* 563–566.

Rasmussen, A., Jirenhed, D. A., Wetmore, D. Z., & Hesslow, G. (2014). Changes in complex spike activity during classical conditioning. *Frontiers in Neural Circuits, 8,* 90.

Rasmussen, A., Jirenhed, D. A., Zucca, R., Johansson, F., Svensson, P., & Hesslow, G. (2013). Number of spikes in climbing fibers determines the direction of cerebellar learning. *The Journal of Neuroscience, 33,* 13436–13440.

Rosenfield, M. E., & Moore, J. W. (1983). Red nucleus lesions disrupt the classically conditioned nictitating membrane response in rabbits. *Behavioural Brain Research, 10,* 393–398.

Rosenfield, M. E., & Moore, J. W. (1985). Red nucleus lesions impair acquisition of the classically conditioned nictitating membrane response but not eye-to-eye savings or unconditioned response amplitude. *Behavioural Brain Research, 17,* 77–81.

Rosenfield, M. E., & Moore, J. W. (1995). Connections to cerebellar cortex (Larsell's HVI) in the rabbit: a WGA-HRP study with implications for classical eyeblink conditioning. *Behavioral Neuroscience, 109,* 1106–1118.

Ruigrok, T. J. (2011). Ins and outs of cerebellar modules. *Cerebellum, 10,* 464–474.

Ruigrok, T. J., Hensbroek, R. A., & Simpson, J. I. (2011). Spontaneous activity signatures of morphologically identified interneurons in the vestibulocerebellum. *The Journal of Neuroscience, 31,* 712–724.

Ruigrok, T. J., & Voogd, J. (1990). Cerebellar nucleo-olivary projections in the rat: an anterograde tracing study with Phaseolus vulgaris-leucoagglutinin (PHA-L). *Journal of Comparative Neurology, 298,* 315–333.

Salafia, W. R., Martino, L. J., Cloutman, K., & Romano, A. G. (1979). Unconditional-stimulus locus and interstimulus-interval shift in rabbit (*Oryctolagus cuniculus*) nictitating membrane conditioning. *The Pavlovian Journal of Biological Science, 14,* 64–71.

Sanchez-Campusano, R., Gruart, A., & Delgado-Garcia, J. M. (2011). Timing and causality in the generation of learned eyelid responses. *Frontiers in Integrative Neuroscience, 5,* 39.

Schmaltz, L. W., & Theios, J. (1972). Acquisition and extinction of a classically conditioned response in hippocampectomized rabbits (*Oryctolagus cuniculus*). *Journal of Comparative and Physiological Psychology, 79,* 328–333.

Schneiderman, N. (1966). Interstimulus interval function of the nictitating membrane response of the rabbit under delay versus trace conditioning. *Journal of Comparative and Physiological Psychology, 57,* 188–195.

Schneiderman, N., & Gormezano, I. (1964). Conditioning of the nictitating membrane of the rabbit as a function of CS-US interval. *Journal of Comparative and Physiological Psychology, 57,* 188–195.

Schonewille, M., Belmeguenai, A., Koekkoek, S. K., Houtman, S. H., Boele, H. J., van Beugen, B. J., et al. (2010). Purkinje cell-specific knockout of the protein phosphatase PP2B impairs potentiation and cerebellar motor learning. *Neuron, 67,* 618–628.

Schonewille, M., Gao, Z., Boele, H. J., Veloz, M. F., Amerika, W. E., Simek, A. A., et al. (2011). Reevaluating the role of LTD in cerebellar motor learning. *Neuron, 70,* 43–50.

Shibuki, K., Gomi, H., Chen, L., Bao, S., Kim, J. J., Wakatsuki, H., et al. (1996). Deficient cerebellar long-term depression, impaired eyeblink conditioning, and normal motor coordination in GFAP mutant mice. *Neuron, 16,* 587–599.

Smith, M. C. (1968). CS-US interval and US intensity in classical conditioning of the rabbit's nictitating membrane response. *Journal of Comparative and Physiological Psychology, 66,* 679–687.

Solomon, P. R., Blanchard, S., Levine, E., Velazquez, E., & Groccia-Ellison, M. (1991). Attenuation of age-related conditioning deficits in humans by extension of the interstimulus interval. *Psychology and Aging, 6*, 36–42.

Song, M., & Messing, R. O. (2005). Protein kinase C regulation of GABAA receptors. *Cellular and Molar Life Sciences, 62*, 119–127.

Sotelo, C., & Llinas, R. (1972). Specialized membrane junctions between neurons in the vertebrate cerebellar cortex. *The Journal of Cell Biology, 53*, 271–289.

Spence, K. W. (1953). Learning and performance in eyelid conditioning as a function of intensity of the UCS. *Journal of Experimental Psychology, 45*.

Steinmetz, A. B., Buss, E. W., & Freeman, J. H. (2013). Inactivation of the ventral lateral geniculate and nucleus of the optic tract impairs retention of visual eyeblink conditioning. *Behavioral Neuroscience, 127*, 690–693.

Steinmetz, A. B., & Freeman, J. H. (2014). Localization of the cerebellar cortical zone mediating acquisition of eyeblink conditioning in rats. *Neurobiology of Learning and Memory, 114C*, 148–154.

Steinmetz, J. E., Lavond, D. G., & Thompson, R. F. (1989). Classical conditioning in rabbits using pontine nucleus stimulation as a conditioned stimulus and inferior olive stimulation as an unconditioned stimulus. *Synapse, 3*, 225–233.

Steinmetz, J. E., Logan, C. G., Rosen, D. J., Thompson, J. K., Lavond, D. G., & Thompson, R. F. (1987). Initial localization of the acoustic conditioned stimulus projection system to the cerebellum essential for classical eyelid conditioning. *Proceedings of the National Academy of Sciences of the United States of America, 84*, 3531–3535.

Steinmetz, J. E., Rosen, D. J., Chapman, P. F., Lavond, D. G., & Thompson, R. F. (1986). Classical conditioning of the rabbit eyelid response with a mossy-fiber stimulation CS: I. Pontine nuclei and middle cerebellar peduncle stimulation. *Behavioral Neuroscience, 100*, 878–887.

Steinmetz, A. B., Skosnik, P. D., Edwards, C. R., Bolbecker, A. R., Steinmetz, J. E., & Hetrick, W. P. (2011). Evaluation of bidirectional interstimulus interval (ISI) shift in auditory delay eye-blink conditioning in healthy humans. *Learning & Behavior, 39*, 358–370.

Sugihara, I., & Shinoda, Y. (2004). Molecular, topographic, and functional organization of the cerebellar cortex: a study with combined aldolase C and olivocerebellar labeling. *The Journal of Neuroscience, 24*, 8771–8785.

Svensson, P., & Ivarsson, M. (1999). Short-lasting conditioned stimulus applied to the middle cerebellar peduncle elicits delayed conditioned eye blink responses in the decerebrate ferret. *The European Journal of Neuroscience, 11*, 4333–4340.

Svensson, P., Ivarsson, M., & Hesslow, G. (1997). Effect of varying the intensity and train frequency of forelimb and cerebellar mossy fiber conditioned stimuli on the latency of conditioned eye-blink responses in decerebrate ferrets. *Learning & Memory, 4*, 105–115.

Svensson, P., Jirenhed, D. A., Bengtsson, F., & Hesslow, G. (2010). Effect of conditioned stimulus parameters on timing of conditioned Purkinje cell responses. *Journal of Neurophysiology, 103*, 1329–1336.

Teune, T. M., van der Burg, J., de Zeeuw, C. I., Voogd, J., & Ruigrok, T. J. (1998). Single Purkinje cell can innervate multiple classes of projection neurons in the cerebellar nuclei of the rat: a light microscopic and ultrastructural triple-tracer study in the rat. *Journal of Comparative Neurology, 392*, 164–178.

Teune, T. M., van der Burg, J., van der Moer, J., Voogd, J., & Ruigrok, T. J. (2000). Topography of cerebellar nuclear projections to the brain stem in the rat. *Progress in brain research, 124*, 141–172.

Titley, H. K., & Hansel, C. (2015). Asymmetries in cerebellar plasticity and motor learning. *Cerebellum*.

Tracy, J. A., & Steinmetz, J. E. (1998). Purkinje cell responses to pontine stimulation CS during rabbit eyeblink conditioning. *Physiology & Behavior, 65*, 381–386.

Trigo, J. A., Gruart, A., & Delgado-Garcia, J. M. (1999). Discharge profiles of abducens, accessory abducens, and orbicularis oculi motoneurons during reflex and conditioned blinks in alert cats. *Journal of Neurophysiology, 81*, 1666–1684.

Uusisaari, M., & Knopfel, T. (2011). Functional classification of neurons in the mouse lateral cerebellar nuclei. *Cerebellum, 10,* 637–646.

Van Der Giessen, R. S., Koekkoek, S. K., van Dorp, S., De Gruijl, J. R., Cupido, A., Khosrovani, S., et al. (2008). Role of olivary electrical coupling in cerebellar motor learning. *Neuron, 58,* 599–612.

Vogel, R. W., Amundson, J. C., Lindquist, D. H., & Steinmetz, J. E. (2009). Eyeblink conditioning during an interstimulus interval switch in rabbits (*Oryctolagus cuniculus*) using picrotoxin to disrupt cerebellar cortical input to the interpositus nucleus. *Behavioral Neuroscience, 123,* 62–74.

Vogel, E. H., Brandon, S. E., & Wagner, A. R. (2003). Stimulus representation in SOP: II. An application to inhibition of delay. *Behavioural Processes, 62,* 27–48.

Voogd, J. (2003). The human cerebellum. *Journal of Chemical Neuroanatomy, 26,* 243–252.

Voogd, J., & Ruigrok, T. J. (2004). The organization of the corticonuclear and olivocerebellar climbing fiber projections to the rat cerebellar vermis: the congruence of projection zones and the zebrin pattern. *Journal of Neurocytology, 33,* 5–21.

Wells, G. R., Hardiman, M. J., & Yeo, C. H. (1989). Visual projections to the pontine nuclei in the rabbit: orthograde and retrograde tracing studies with WGA-HRP. *Journal of Comparative Neurology, 279,* 629–652.

Welsh, J. P. (1992). Changes in the motor pattern of learned and unlearned responses following cerebellar lesions: a kinematic analysis of the nictitating membrane reflex. *Neuroscience, 47,* 1–19.

Welsh, J. P., & Harvey, J. A. (1989). Cerebellar lesions and the nictitating membrane reflex: performance deficits of the conditioned and unconditioned response. *The Journal of Neuroscience, 9,* 299–311.

Welsh, J. P., & Harvey, J. A. (1991). Pavlovian conditioning in the rabbit during inactivation of the interpositus nucleus. *The Journal of Physiology, 444,* 459–480.

Welsh, J. P., & Harvey, J. A. (1998). Acute inactivation of the inferior olive blocks associative learning. *The European Journal of Neuroscience, 10,* 3321–3332.

Welsh, J. P., Yamaguchi, H., Zeng, X. H., Kojo, M., Nakada, Y., Takagi, A., et al. (2005). Normal motor learning during pharmacological prevention of Purkinje cell long-term depression. *Proceedings of the National Academy of Sciences of the United States of America, 102,* 17166–17171.

Wen, Q., Stepanyants, A., Elston, G. N., Grosberg, A. Y., & Chklovskii, D. B. (2009). Maximization of the connectivity repertoire as a statistical principle governing the shapes of dendritic arbors. *Proceedings of the National Academy of Sciences of the United States of America, 106,* 12536–12541.

Wetmore, D. Z., Jirenhed, D. A., Rasmussen, A., Johansson, F., Schnitzer, M. J., & Hesslow, G. (2014). Bidirectional plasticity of Purkinje cells matches temporal features of learning. *The Journal of Neuroscience, 34,* 1731–1737.

Woodruff-Pak, D. S., & Finkbiner, R. G. (1995). Larger nondeclarative than declarative deficits in learning and memory in human aging. *Psychology and Aging, 10,* 416–426.

Wu, G. Y., Yao, J., Hu, B., Zhang, H. M., Li, Y. D., Li, X., et al. (2013). Reevaluating the role of the hippocampus in delay eyeblink conditioning. *PloS One, 8,* e71249.

Wu, G. Y., Yao, J., Zhang, L. Q., Li, X., Fan, Z. L., Yang, Y., et al. (2012). Reevaluating the role of the medial prefrontal cortex in delay eyeblink conditioning. *Neurobiology of Learning and Memory, 97,* 277–288.

Yamazaki, T., & Tanaka, S. (2009). Computational models of timing mechanisms in the cerebellar granular layer. *Cerebellum, 8,* 423–432.

Yeo, C. H. (2004). Memory and the cerebellum. *Current Neurology and Neuroscience Report, 4,* 87–89.

Yeo, C. H., & Hardiman, M. J. (1992). Cerebellar cortex and eyeblink conditioning: a reexamination. *Experimental Brain Research, 88,* 623–638.

Yeo, C. H., Hardiman, M. J., & Glickstein, M. (1985a). Classical conditioning of the nictitating membrane response of the rabbit. I. Lesions of the cerebellar nuclei. *Experimental Brain Research, 60,* 87–98.

Yeo, C. H., Hardiman, M. J., & Glickstein, M. (1985b). Classical conditioning of the nictitating membrane response of the rabbit. II. Lesions of the cerebellar cortex. *Experimental Brain Research, 60,* 99–113.

Yeo, C. H., Hardiman, M. J., & Glickstein, M. (1985c). Classical conditioning of the nictitating membrane response of the rabbit. III. Connections of cerebellar lobule HVI. *Experimental Brain Research, 60,* 114–126.

Yeo, C. H., Hardiman, M. J., & Glickstein, M. (1986). Classical conditioning of the nictitating membrane response of the rabbit. IV. Lesions of the inferior olive. *Experimental Brain Research, 63,* 81–92.

Yeo, C. H., Lobo, D. H., & Baum, A. (1997). Acquisition of a new-latency conditioned nictitating membrane response–major, but not complete, dependence on the ipsilateral cerebellum. *Learning & Memory, 3,* 557–577.

Zbarska, S., Bloedel, J. R., & Bracha, V. (2008). Cerebellar dysfunction explains the extinction-like abolition of conditioned eyeblinks after NBQX injections in the inferior olive. *The Journal of Neuroscience, 28,* 10–20.

Zbarska, S., Holland, E. A., Bloedel, J. R., & Bracha, V. (2007). Inferior olivary inactivation abolishes conditioned eyeblinks: extinction or cerebellar malfunction? *Behavioural Brain Research, 178,* 128–138.

Zhang, W., & Linden, D. J. (2003). The other side of the engram: experience-driven changes in neuronal intrinsic excitability. *Nat Rev Neurosci, 4,* 885–900.

Zhang, W., & Linden, D. J. (2006). Long-term depression at the mossy fiber-deep cerebellar nucleus synapse. *The Journal of Neuroscience, 26,* 6935–6944.

Zhou, H., Lin, Z., Voges, K., Ju, C., Gao, Z., Bosman, L. W., et al. (2014). Cerebellar modules operate at different frequencies. *eLife, 3,* e02536.

CHAPTER

4

How the Vestibulocerebellum Builds an Internal Model of Self-motion

Jean Laurens, Dora E. Angelaki

Department of Neuroscience, Baylor College of Medicine, Houston, TX, USA

INTRODUCTION

The vestibular organs (the ear's "balance organs") send head-motion signals to a network of brain areas, among which the vestibulocerebellum plays a preeminent role. Vestibular signals encode head rotations, head translations, and head orientation relative to gravity (tilt). These signals are important for spatial orientation, locomotion and balance (Agrawal, Carey, Della Santina, Schubert, & Minor, 2009; Crane & Demer, 1998; Maurer, Mergner, & Peterka, 2006), motor activities (Sağlam, Glasauer, & Lehnen, 2014), motion perception (Mayne, 1974), and navigation (Rochefort, Lefort, & Rondi-Reig, 2013). They also drive the vestibulo-ocular reflex that counterrotates the eyes when the head moves, such that the gaze remains stable in space.

Two aspects of vestibular signal processing have attracted considerable attention: the processing of rotation signals and the estimation of head tilt and translation. Processing of rotation signals involves dynamic transformations and multisensory integration, as reviewed in Laurens and Angelaki (2011). Here we focus on the role of the cerebellum in estimating and encoding tilt and translation. This requires solving a sensory ambiguity that originates from the equivalence principle (Einstein, 1907): inertial systems cannot distinguish linear acceleration associated with head translation from gravitational acceleration due to head tilt. Behavioral (Angelaki, McHenry, Dickman, Newlands, & Hess, 1999; Merfeld, Zupan, & Peterka, 1999) and theoretical (Laurens & Angelaki, 2011; Laurens & Droulez, 2007; Merfeld, 1995) research has demonstrated that the brain uses an internal model of motion to solve this ambiguity and build internal estimates of tilt and translation. Physiological studies have probed into the neuronal basis of this internal model, leading to the identification of cell groups in the vestibular nuclei (VN) and vestibulocerebellum that encode translation (Angelaki, Shaikh, Green, & Dickman, 2004; Laurens, Meng, & Angelaki, 2013a; Shaikh, Ghasia, Dickman, & Angelaki, 2005; Shaikh, Green et al., 2005; Yakusheva, Blazquez, & Angelaki 2008, 2010; Yakusheva et al., 2007) and tilt (Laurens, Meng, & Angelaki, 2013b) signals. Cortical neurons in the dorsal medial superior temporal area and the parietoinsular vestibular cortex share many of these properties (Liu & Angelaki, 2009; Liu, Dickman, & Angelaki 2011).

This review describes how cerebellar neurons encode tilt and translation. We start with a brief description of the peripheral vestibular sensors and the signals that they encode and summarize computational models of tilt/translation discrimination. Then we examine how tilt and translation are encoded by individual cerebellar neurons and neuronal populations. Finally we discuss how the underlying neuronal computations can be uncovered experimentally.

BASIC ORGANIZATION OF THE PERIPHERAL VESTIBULAR SYSTEM

The vestibular organs are located in the inner ear (Fig. 1(A)), close to the cochlea (the hearing organ). They are inertial motion sensors and they can be compared, to a certain extent, to the gyroscope systems that are commonly used in model aircrafts. The two main components of the vestibular system are the semicircular canals, which detect rotations, and the otolithic organs that detect linear accelerations (Fig. 1(A)).

The semicircular canals are tubes filled with a freely flowing liquid, the endolymph (Fig. 1(B)). A cavity contains a gelatinous membrane (cupula) within which hair cells are embedded. Whenever the head rotates, the endolymph flows within the canals due to its inertia. This flow deflects the cupula, bending the hair bundles of receptor cells, thus changing the firing rate of canal afferents in the eighth cranial nerve. Note that the semicircular canals are driven by angular accelerations, differing from human-made gyroscopes that detect angular velocity. Each ear contains three mutually orthogonal canals, altogether detecting rotations around all head axes (Fig. 1(C)). The horizontal canals detect yaw rotations, whereas the vertical canals detect combinations of pitch and roll rotations.

The otolithic organs are endolymph-filled cavities. Within each organ, a layer of crystals (the otochonia) rests on a gelatinous membrane that contains hair cells (Fig. 1(D)). The otochonia are heavier than the surrounding endolymph. As a consequence, when the head accelerates or when the head tilts (Fig. 1(D)), the otochonia's weight displaces them, bending

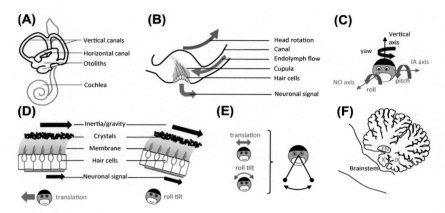

FIGURE 1   **Description of the vestibular system.** (A) Schematic of the labyrinth in the inner ear. (B) Operating principle of the semicircular canals. (C) Definition of the head's translation (NO, naso-occipital; IA, interaural) and rotation (yaw, pitch, roll) axes. (D) Operating principle of the otolithic organs. (E) Analogy between the otolith organs and a pendulum. A head-fixed pendulum would swing relative to the head when the head tilts or translates; therefore a pendulum detects both tilt and translation, similar to the otoliths. (F) Sagittal section of the cerebellum and main vestibular regions (lobules X and IX, nodulus and uvula; FN, rostral fastigial nuclei).

the hair bundles of receptor cells, thus changing the firing rate of otolith afferents in the eighth cranial nerve. The signal carried by otolith afferents is ambiguous, since they detect both tilt and translation. This is analogous to a pendulum attached to the head (Fig. 1(E)) that swings when the head tilts or translates. The otolithic organs can also be compared to human-made accelerometers. Two otolithic organs exist in each ear, together encoding acceleration and gravity in three dimensions.

Vestibular signals are processed centrally in the VN and in the cerebellum. Here we focus on a specific element of the vestibulocerebellum. The nodulus and uvula (referred to as NU) are lobules X and IX of the cerebellar vermis (Fig. 1(F)). These regions receive more than 70% of primary vestibular afferents directly, as well as indirectly through the VN. The Purkinje cell layers of the NU have been extensively studied (Laurens et al., 2013a,b; Yakusheva et al., 2008, 2010, 2007). In vivo recordings in the granular layers of the NU are challenging but have been performed (Meng, Laurens, Blazquez, & Angelaki, in press). The NU projects back to the VN both directly and indirectly through the fastigial nuclei (FN).

FRAMEWORK OF THE INTERNAL MODEL

The key principles of vestibular information processing have been established through decades of behavioral and modeling work (Angelaki et al., 1999, 2004; Borah, Young, & Curry, 1988; Bos & Bles, 2002;

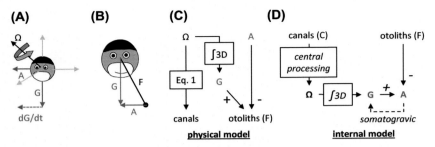

FIGURE 2   **Basics of central vestibular processing.** (A) Motion variables used to describe head motion. (B) Vector representation of Eq. (2). (C) Physical model of motion and sensory variables. (D) Principle of an internal model of tilt/translation discrimination. See the text for the definition of the variables.

Glasauer & Merfeld, 1997; Green & Angelaki, 2007; Holly, 2004; Laurens & Angelaki, 2011; Laurens & Droulez, 2007; Laurens, Strauman, & Hess, 2011; Mayne, 1974; Merfeld, 1995; Merfeld et al., 1999; Zupan, Merfeld, & Darlot, 2002). The head-motion variables can be thoroughly described by three quantities: rotational velocity, Ω; linear acceleration, A; and orientation relative to gravity (i.e., head tilt, which can be described by expressing the orientation of the gravity vector, G, in head-fixed coordinates; Fig. 2(A)).

Extracting these motion variables from vestibular signals requires central processing because head tilt, translation, and rotations are not detected directly by the vestibular organs. Specifically, generating angular velocity signals requires a temporal integration from acceleration to velocity that is performed in part by the canals and in part centrally by the brain using multisensory integration (Laurens & Angelaki, 2011; Raphan, Matsuo, & Cohen, 1977). For simplicity, we can assume that the brain obtains an accurate estimate of Ω during the motion protocols covered in this review (see Laurens & Angelaki, 2011 for a broader approach).

On the other hand, the otolithic organs detect the net gravitoinertial acceleration (GIA), F (which is the vectorial sum of gravity and linear acceleration, Fig. 2(B)), and do not distinguish whether the head is tilting and/or translating (Fig. 1(E)). This reflects the equivalence principle (Einstein, 1907): a linear inertial sensor alone cannot distinguish gravity from linear acceleration. However, tilt movements are rotations that can be detected by the semicircular canals. By tracking head rotations relative to gravity, the brain can estimate the head tilt (G in Fig. 2(B)) and subsequently extract the translational component (A in Fig. 2(B)) from the net otolithic signal (F in Fig. 2(B)).

The associated central processing can be modeled mathematically, as outlined in Fig. 2(C) and (D). This model (Laurens & Angelaki, 2011) produces internal estimates of head-motion variables (**Ω, G,** and **A**); for clarity these estimates are represented using bold characters. The semicircular canals perform a leaky integration of angular acceleration,

$$dC/dt = d\Omega/dt - 1/\tau_c \cdot C \quad (1)$$

where C is the signal from the canals, $d\Omega/dt$ is the angular acceleration, and τ_c is a time constant with a value of ~4s in monkeys and humans. Equation (1) describes how the canal signal C is converted into a central rotation signal Ω. As shown in Fig. 2(B), the gravitoinertial acceleration, F, encoded by otolith afferents is

$$F = G - A \quad (2)$$

Head orientation relative to gravity (i.e., G) changes when the head rotates around an axis that is not aligned with G (Fig. 2(A)), according to

$$dG/dt = G \times \Omega \quad (3)$$

Theoretical work (Laurens & Angelaki, 2011; Merfeld, 1995; Zupan et al., 2002) has proposed that the brain solves these equations (Fig. 2(D)) and constructs internal estimates of tilt and translation, G and A, using the following two equations:

$$G = \int (G \times \Omega + 1/\tau_S (F-G)) \cdot dt \quad (4)$$

$$A = G - F \quad (5)$$

In Eq. (4), the first term tracks the orientation of the gravity vector by integrating head rotation signals Ω (Eq. (3)). The second term, $(1/\tau_S(F - G))$, drives the G estimate toward F continuously. This mechanism, named "somatogravic feedback" in Laurens & Angelaki (2011), optimizes the estimation of G. Indeed, rotation signals (Ω) are noisy and inaccurate at low frequencies. Without correction mechanisms, errors in Ω would create errors in G that would accumulate over time. The somatogravic feedback prevents this by progressively aligning G with F. This mechanism is efficient because natural linear accelerations are typically of short duration: over a few seconds, the average acceleration is generally close to zero and G is close to F. Therefore, the net otolith afferent signal, F, can be used as a reference for G at low frequencies under natural conditions. The downside of this mechanism is that unnatural sustained accelerations, such as those experienced in an aircraft, create erroneous tilt perception. This well-documented phenomenon is called somatogravic or oculogravic illusion (Graybiel, 1952; Paige & Seidman, 1999).

Once G is computed, the estimate A is obtained using Eq. (5), that is, a straightforward inversion of Eq. (2). Note that Eqs (4) and (5) form the basis of the model in Laurens & Angelaki (2011). Although other models (Bos & Bles, 2002; Merfeld, 1995; Zupan et al., 2002) have used alternative mathematical formulations, they share the key concepts represented by Eqs (4) and (5). As summarized next, the neuronal correlates of these computations have been found in the vestibulocerebellum.

TILT- AND TRANSLATION-SELECTIVE NEURONS IN THE CEREBELLUM

A series of studies (Angelaki et al., 2004; Barmack, 2003; Barmack & Shojaku, 1995; Barmack & Yakhnista, 2008; Kitama, Komagata, Ozawa, Suzuki, & Sato, 2014; Laurens et al., 2013a,b; Shaikh, Ghasia et al., 2005; Shaikh, Green et al., 2005; Yakusheva et al., 2008, 2010, 2007; Zhou, Tang, Newlands, & King, 2006) have identified tilt and translation signals in the brain stem and vestibulocerebellum, thus demonstrating that the gravitoinertial ambiguity is resolved by subcortical processing. These studies have used specifically designed motion protocols and analyses that are described here, together with a brief summary of experimental results.

The original experimental protocols, fundamental in identifying the behavioral (Angelaki et al., 1999) and neurophysiological (Angelaki et al., 2004) signature of the postulated computations, are illustrated in Fig. 3. Most importantly, these tilt and translation stimuli are matched, both eliciting an identical GIA and the same activation of the otolith organs. In the tilt–translation protocol, tilt and translation stimuli

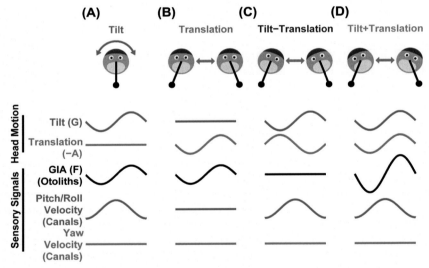

FIGURE 3   **Motion protocols used in the two-dimensional tilt/translation paradigms.** (A) Tilt. (B) Translation. (C) Tilt–translation. (D) Tilt+translation. Tilt stimuli are shown around the roll axis (A) and translation around the interaural axis (B); however, the same protocols were also applied around the pitch/naso-occipital axes, as well as intermediate axes. During Tilt–translation, only semicircular canals are activated. In the Tilt+translation protocol, tilt and translation sum up, such that the activation of the otoliths is doubled compared to tilt or translation alone. These sinusoidal motions are commonly performed at 0.5 Hz, with a peak tilt of 11.5° and a translation amplitude of 20 cm (both corresponding to a peak gravitoinertial acceleration of 0.2 G).

are applied with opposite phases, such that they cancel each other out and the net GIA in the horizontal plane is nearly zero. Hence, tilt–translation stimulates sinusoidally only the canals and not the otolith organs. The ability of central cells in both the VN/FN and the NU to encode translation during tilt–translation is a direct demonstration that the brain uses canal signals to compute the translation of the head (Laurens et al., 2013a,b; Meng et al., in press; Meng et al., 2014; Yakusheva et al., 2007). Inactivation of the semicircular canals largely eliminates this modulation (Shaikh, Ghasia et al., 2005; Yakusheva et al., 2007).

Systematic neuronal recordings in the vestibulocerebellum using these protocols have uncovered populations of neurons that respond preferentially to tilt, translation, or the raw otolithic signal (i.e., the GIA). These neurons, called tilt-, translation-, and GIA-selective, are classified by comparing each neuron's response to three models (Angelaki et al., 2004; Laurens et al., 2013b). One model assumes that the neuron responds to tilt only (i.e., it does not respond to translation). Another model assumes that the neuron responds to translation only. The third model assumes that it responds to the GIA, that is, identically to tilt and translation. A statistical procedure (see below) is used to determine if the neuron's response is significantly closer to one of these models. We begin with an overview of the population responses in the NU (Fig. 4(A), n = 221 cells, including data shown in Laurens et al., 2013b, and additional recordings) and the FN (Fig. 4(B), n = 229 cells, not previously published).

Because the tilt and translation stimuli are matched (Fig. 3), cells that encode the GIA exhibit similar response gains during tilt and translation and cluster along the diagonal (Fig. 4, black symbols). In contrast, tilt-selective cells have higher responses to tilt than to translation and appear above the diagonal (Fig. 4, green symbols). Similarly, translation-selective cells appear below the diagonal (Fig. 4, red symbols). Cells that cannot be classified into one of these categories are called "composite" (Fig. 4, gray symbols). These cells may be encountered along the diagonal (e.g., cells that respond to tilt and translation with similar gains but different phases) or between the diagonal and the tilt- or translation-selective cells (i.e., cells that have intermediate responses, between GIA and tilt or translation).

Tilt-selective cells represent one-third of the NU population, and translation-selective cells represent another third (Fig. 4(A)). Few cells appear along the diagonal, as shown by projecting the population responses onto an axis perpendicular to the diagonal. The resulting histogram (tilt–translation ratio, TTR) shows two peaks separated by a valley in the center that corresponds to the small number of cells along the diagonal (Fig. 4(A)). This distribution suggests that NU Purkinje cells form two discrete functional groups, tilt- and translation-selective cells, and each group forms one cloud of dots on the tilt/translation response gain plot. The GIA and composite cells represent the borders of these clouds, rather than a distinct functional group.

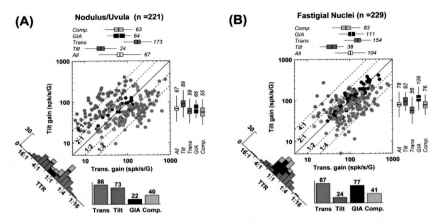

FIGURE 4   **Population responses in (A) nodulus/uvula and (B) fastigial nuclei.** The scatter plots show the response gain of all recorded cells during tilt and translation along the cells' preferred direction. The box plots on the top and right show the average response gains (±confidence interval) of various cell types. The histograms on the lower left show the tilt–translation ratio (TTR), that is, the ratio of tilt gain to translation gain. The bottom histogram shows the repartition of the cells in to four categories.

Cell distribution in the FN is fundamentally different (Fig. 4(B)): one-third are translation-selective and another third are GIA-selective. Tilt-selective cells represent a scarce 10% of the population. The TTR is asymmetrically distributed, with a peak at a value of 1:1 and extended toward translation-selective cells.

The existence of tilt- and translation-selective neurons in the vestibulocerebellum suggests that the brain resolves the gravitoinertial ambiguity. We now provide a more complete description of their response to combined motion stimuli around various axes.

SPATIOTEMPORAL TUNING

Central vestibular neurons in the vestibulocerebellum exhibit a common form of tuning (Green, Shaikh, & Angelaki, 2005; Laurens et al., 2013b). A formal description of this tuning is a powerful tool for studying neuronal responses, decoding the internal tilt and translation signals they encode, and elucidating the underlying neuronal computations. We will describe an example neuron and then present the mathematical framework of spatiotemporal tuning.

Let us consider an example tilt-selective neuron (Fig. 5). Sinusoidal tilt around the roll and pitch axes elicits a modulation of the neuron's firing rate (Fig. 5(B) and (D)), with approximately the same gain (25 spikes per seconds; spk/s) and a slightly different phase (58° vs 27° phase lead). These responses

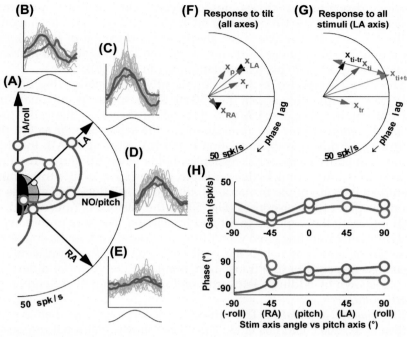

FIGURE 5 **Spatiotemporal tuning of central vestibular cells.** (A–E) Response of a tilt-selective cell during tilt (green) and translation (red) along the head's NO, IA, and the intermediate axes (LA, left–anterior; RA, right–anterior axes). Note that pitch rotations (*around* the IA axis) cause the head to tilt forward/backward and activate the otoliths *along* the NO axis: therefore the response to pitch (x_p) is shown on the NO axis. Similarly, the response to roll (x_r) is shown on the IA axis. (A) Polar-plot representation of the gain of the response to tilt and translation. Circles: response gain measured experimentally along the four axes. Lines: model fit. (B–E) Average response during tilt (green) and translation (red). Gray traces represent the response to individual motion cycles during tilt. (F) Polar plot of the responses to tilt along all four axes. The upward- and downward-pointing black triangles represent the responses predicted along the LA and RA axes by linear combinations of x_p and x_r. (G) Polar plot of the response to tilt/translation stimuli along the LA axis. x_{ti}, response to tilt. x_{tr}, response to translation. x_{ti-tr}, response to tilt–translation. x_{ti+tr}, response to tilt+translation. The rightward- and leftward-pointing red vectors at the end of x_{ti} represent the vectorial sums $x_{ti}+x_{tr}$ and $x_{ti}-x_{tr}$. (H) Gain and phase of the responses to tilt (green) and translation (red) as a function of the stimulation axis. Circles: experimental data. Lines: model fit.

can be represented as vectors on a polar plot (Fig. 5(F)), where the length of the vectors represents the gain and their orientation represents the phase.

The tuning of this neuron is linear: tilt stimuli along the RA and LA axes can be expressed as combinations of pitch and roll. This is illustrated by comparing the actual neuronal responses to RA/LA (combined pitch and roll; vectors x_{LA} and x_{RA} in Fig. 5) with the sum of the responses to pitch and roll (Fig. 5(F), compare green arrows with upward- and downward-pointing triangles, respectively). This neuron's preferred direction to tilt is the LA axis (Fig. 5(C); see also Fig. 5(H)). Orthogonal to the LA axis, the RA axis is the antipreferred direction of the cell, but not a null direction. Indeed, rotation along the RA axis elicits a nonzero response (Fig. 5(E); 10 spk/s modulation; x_{RA} in Fig. 5(F)).

This example cell also responds significantly to translation (Fig. 5(B–E), red curves), with a lower gain (Fig. 5(H)). The response is maximal during translation along the LA axis (Fig. 5(C)); therefore this cell's preferred directions to tilt and translation are the same. Similar to tilt, the antipreferred direction to translation is the RA axis (Fig. 5(A)). In addition, the linearity of neuronal responses holds when tilt and translation are combined. According to this principle, the response to tilt + translation should be the sum of the responses to tilt and translation. This applies to the polar plot of the responses (Fig. 5(G)): the vectors x_{ti} (green) and x_{tr} (red) represent the response to tilt and translation. The sum of these vectors is shown by adding a red vector (pointing rightward) at the end of x_{ti}. This sum is closely equal to the vector x_{ti+tr} (cyan) that represents the measured response to tilt + translation. Similarly, the vectorial difference $x_{ti} - x_{tr}$ (shown by adding a leftward pointing red vector at the end of x_{ti}) nearly matches x_{ti-tr}.

Mathematical formulation. This tuning can be formalized mathematically (Green et al., 2005; Laurens et al., 2013b) as follows. Neuronal responses are represented using complex numbers (to account for both gain and phase as a function of frequency). A sinusoidal motion stimulus with a profile $A_s \times \cos(2 \times \pi \times \omega \cdot t + \varphi_s)$ (where A_s is the peak amplitude in units of G ($= 9.81$ m/s^2), ω is the frequency in Hz, and φ_s is the phase in radians) is represented by the complex number $s = A_s \cdot \exp(i \cdot \varphi_s)$. Similarly, the neuron's response is fitted with a sine function $A_x \times \cos(2 \times \pi \times \omega \cdot t + \varphi_x) + B$. The term B represents the average firing rate of the neuron and the modulation is expressed as a complex number $x = A_x \cdot \exp(i \cdot \varphi_x)$. Figure 5(F) and (G) presents polar plot representations of these complex numbers.

The neuron's response during tilt can be expressed as $x_{tilt} = h_r \cdot s_r + h_p \cdot s_p$, where h_p and h_r are the transfer functions to pitch and roll tilt, and s_p and s_r are the pitch and roll components of the tilt stimulus. Tilt around an axis that forms an angle α with the pitch/NO axis can be decomposed into $s_p = 0.2 \cdot \sin(\alpha)$ and $s_r = 0.2 \cdot \cos(\alpha)$, and the corresponding response is $x = 0.2 \cdot (h_p \cdot \sin(\alpha) + h_r \cdot \cos(\alpha))$. This formula is used to compute the gain and phase of the neuron's response to tilt at multiple values of α (Fig. 5(A), green line), as well as the predicted response to tilt around LA and RA in Fig. 5(F) (with $\alpha = 45°$ and $\alpha = -45°$, respectively).

Similar to the responses to tilt, the cell's tuning function to translation can be expressed as $x_{trans} = h_{NO} \cdot s_{NO} + h_{IA} \cdot s_{IA}$, where s_{NO} and s_{IA} describe the translation stimulus along the NO and IA axes, and h_{NO} and h_{IA} are the transfer functions of the cell's response to NO and IA translation.

Combining both the equations, one obtains a full characterization of the cell's response that can be used to describe its response to combined tilt and translation stimuli (corresponding to the composite model):

$$x = h_r \cdot s_r + h_p \cdot s_p + h_{NO} \cdot s_{NO} + h_{IA} \cdot s_{IA} \qquad (6)$$

Fitting the composite model. The models can be fit to data recorded during a series of tilt/translation trials (Table 1). Each motion stimulus can be written as a function of s_p, s_r, s_{NO}, and s_{IA}, and each trial yields one measured response x. By repeating Eq. (6), one creates a set of equations in which the four unknowns are h_p, h_r, h_{NO}, and h_{IA} and each motion trial provides one equation. Finding the least-square solution of this system allows computation of the best estimate of h_p, h_r, h_{NO}, and h_{IA}.

Cell classification. The classification of the cells in Fig. 4 has been based on fitting their responses with models that assume that it responds to tilt

TABLE 1   Composite Model Fit for the Tilt-Selective Cell in Fig. 5. The Neuronal Responses and the Stimuli Used in 12 Motion Trials are Indicated in the Form of Complex Numbers and Collectively Represented by Two Matrices, X and S. Neuronal Responses are also Expressed in the Form of Gain and Phase. The Equations Used for Fitting the Composite Model are Indicated, as well as the Best-Fit Values

Trial n°	Response			Stimulus (G)				Stimulus type	Stimulation axis
	x (spk/s)	gain (spk/s)	phase (°)	s_r	s_p	s_{NO}	s_{IA}		
1	22+11.i	25	27	0.2	0	0	0	tilt	roll/NO
2	13+21.i	25	58	0.14	-0.14	0	0	tilt	pitch/IA
3	29+27.i	40	43	0	0.2	0	0	tilt	LA
4	7-7.i	10	-45	0.14	0.14	0	0	tilt	RA
5	19+0.i	19	0	0	0	0	0.2	translation	roll/NO
6	11-8.i	14	-36	0	0	0.14	-0.14	translation	pitch/IA
7	14-2.i	14	-8	0	0	0.14	0.14	translation	LA
8	2+4.i	4	63	0	0	0.2	0	translation	RA
9	13+13.i	18	45	0.2	0	-0.2	0	tilt-translation	roll/NO
10	15+29.i	33	63	0.14	0.14	-0.14	-0.14	tilt-translation	LA
11	36+9.i	37	14	0.14	0.14	0.14	0.14	tilt+translation	roll/NO
12	51+22.i	56	23	0.2	0	0.2	0	tilt+translation	LA

X	S
12 equations with form:	$x = h_r \cdot s_r + h_p \cdot s_p + h_{NO} \cdot s_{NO} + h_{IA} \cdot s_{IA}$
Matrix notation:	$H = (h_r, h_p, h_{NO}, h_{IA})$ X=H*S
Solution:	$H = (S'*S)^{-1}*S'*X$
Matlab command:	$H = inv(S'*S)*S'*X$
Alternative:	$H = regress(X,S)$
Best-fit values:	$h_r = 127+60i$ $h_p = 84+116i$
(in spk/s/G)	$h_{NO} = 69-2i$ $h_{IA} = 53-28i$

only (i.e., $h_{NO} = h_{IA} = 0$), translation only ($h_p = h_r = 0$), or the GIA ($h_p = h_{IA}$ and $h_r = h_{NO}$). A statistical test is used to determine which model (if any) fits each cell significantly better than the others. In Angelaki et al. (2004), the goodness of fit was evaluated using a partial correlation measure, and the statistical test was based on a Z-score. In Laurens et al. (2013b), we used a simple VAF (variance accounted for) measure and the statistical test was based on a bootstrapping method.

This analysis has been used successfully to describe the sinusoidal tuning of NU Purkinje cells (Laurens et al., 2013a,b; Yakusheva et al., 2008, 2010, 2007), interneurons and putative mossy fibers in the granular layer of the cerebellar cortex (Meng et al., 2014), FN cells (Angelaki et al., 2004; Shaikh, Ghasia et al., 2005; Shaikh, Green et al., 2005), VN cells (Angelaki et al., 2004; Shaikh, Ghasia et al., 2005), and canal and otolith afferents in the eighth cranial nerve (Yu et al., 2012).

Note also that, while the cells encode sinusoidal tilt and translation in a linear manner, the underlying computations are not linear, as shown next.

REVEALING THE INTERNAL MODEL COMPUTATIONS

The tilt/translation protocols (Fig. 3) have demonstrated that the brain segregates tilt from translation (Fig. 4) and provided detailed information about how these variables are encoded (Figs 5 and 6). However, they provide only a limited insight into the underlying computations and thus limited support for the neural implementation of the internal model. We show next how additional experiments and analyses reveal that vestibulocerebellar neurons encode internal estimates of tilt and translation computed using an internal model of head motion (Fig. 2(D)). Specifically, we examine three crucial components of the internal model's computational predictions: (1) the somatogravic effect, (2) the three-dimensional integration of rotation signals, and (3) that these neurons encode motion illusions predicted by the internal model.

Somatogravic effect. The somatogravic loop is part of the internal model (Fig. 2(D)) and generates an illusory estimate of tilt during middle- or low-frequency translation. Based on the model in Fig. 2(D) (with $\tau_s = 0.9\,s$), the tilt illusion during translation at 0.5 Hz should have a gain of 0.33 and a phase lag of $-70°$ (Fig. 6(A), bottom traces, green versus red curve), represented by a complex number, h_{soma}. Next, we show how the internal tilt signal follows the dynamics of the somatogravic effect.

The internal tilt signal is decoded as follows (Fig. 6(B)): consider for instance a tilt-selective neuron whose preferred direction is the IA/roll axis. We assume that its firing rate (x) encodes the internal tilt signal (t) through its transfer function h_r, such that $x = h_r \cdot t$. During any stimulation along the IA/roll axis, the internal tilt estimate can be decoded by

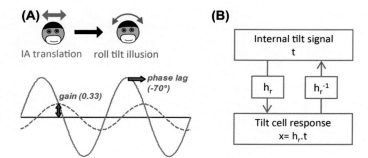

FIGURE 6   **Somatogravic effect.** (A) Illustration of the illusion. (B) Neural encoding and decoding of the internal tilt signal.

a simple inversion of the transfer function: $t = h_r^{-1} \cdot x$. For better accuracy, one can use several roll-selective neurons to decode t. Knowing their transfer function, h_r, and their response, x, a linear regression $x = t \cdot h_r$ gives the regression coefficient, t, as the least-square error estimate of the internal tilt signal.

The internal model predicts that the somatogravic effect generates a tilt signal during translation stimuli, with gain and phase that follows $t = h_{soma} \cdot s_{trans}$. In Laurens et al. (2013b), we pooled all tilt-selective neurons and decoded the neuronal tilt signal during translation. We found that h_{soma} had a gain of 0.19 and a lag of $-71°$, a close match with the predicted values. Thus, cerebellar neurons carry the correlates of one of the internal model equations. However, the full extent of the computations performed by central vestibular networks is revealed through additional three-dimensional motion protocols, as described next.

Using three-dimensional stimuli to reveal the underlying computations. The two-dimensional tilt/translation protocols (Fig. 3; reillustrated in Fig. 7(A–D)) are not sufficient to demonstrate that the brain implements the nonlinear computations shown in Fig. 2(D) and, in particular, the three-dimensional integrator. As an alternative to the internal model hypothesis, one may instead propose that each cerebellar neuron sums linearly inputs from the vertical semicircular canals and the otoliths (Fig. 7(G), transformed through transfer functions h_{canals} and h_{oto}). When using the stimuli shown in Fig. 3 (reillustrated in Fig. 7(A–D)), tilt-like, translation-like, and GIA-like responses can still be observed, even for random choices of h_{canals} and h_{oto}. For example, neurons that receive predominantly canal inputs (i.e., $|h_{canals}| \gg |h_{oto}|$) would respond predominantly to tilt and appear tilt-selective (Fig. 7(A–D)). Similarly, neurons that receive predominantly otolith inputs (i.e., $|h_{canals}| \ll |h_{oto}|$) would appear GIA-selective. Neurons with opposite canal and otolith inputs (i.e., $h_{canals} \approx -h_{oto}$) would have reduced responses during tilt compared to translation (Fig. 7(A–D)) and be classified as translation-selective. In short, responses like those in Figs 3, 4, and 7(A–D)

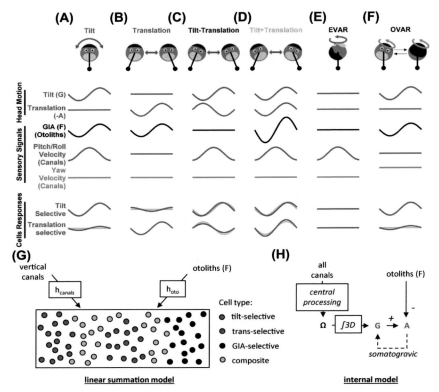

FIGURE 7   **Generalization of three-dimensional (3D) motion protocols necessary to quantitatively support the internal model hypothesis.** (A–F) Illustration of (A–D) 2D and (E–F) 3D motion protocols, summarizing the corresponding sensory signals and responses of stereotyped tilt- and translation-selective cells. (G) Linear summation model (alternative to internal model) having the same predictions as the internal model when testing using the 2D motion protocols (A–D; see also Fig. 3). (H) Computations underlying tilt- and translation-selective cells, revealed by 3D motion protocols.

can still be observed in cells that have little to do with predictions of the internal model. Furthermore, this reasoning highlights a limitation of the two-dimensional tilt/translation protocols (Fig. 3): they do not allow one to distinguish neurons that encode tilt from neurons that encode rotations. Many neurons in the central vestibular system respond to rotations irrespective of head orientation relative to gravity. Such neurons would always be classified as tilt-selective based on the classification scheme of Fig. 3 (reillustrated in Fig. 7(A–D)). Three-dimensional experimental protocols, such as those illustrated in Fig. 7(E) and (F), have been purposely designed to address these limitations and demonstrate that cerebellar cells implement an internal model of motion (Fig. 7(H)) rather than a random otolith/canal convergence scheme (Fig. 7(G)).

Yakusheva et al. (2007) used an earth-vertical axis rotation protocol (EVAR, Fig. 7(E); Green & Angelaki, 2007), in which the subject is tilted (e.g., nose-up) and rotated around an earth-vertical axis. Figure 7(E) shows EVAR performed with a tilt angle of 90°—a smaller angle (10°–45°) is used in practice. EVAR activates the canals in a similar manner compared to tilt and does not activate sinusoidally the otoliths; thus it mimics the tilt–translation protocol. However, translation-selective cells, which respond during tilt–translation, do not respond to EVAR. This is because the brain detects that the rotation axis is parallel to gravity and thus distinguishes there is no translation during EVAR. Purkinje cell responses during the EVAR protocol presented the first indication that the brain performs three-dimensional computations, as suggested by the model (Green & Angelaki, 2007; Yakusheva et al., 2007).

More recently, we used the off-vertical axis rotation protocol (OVAR, Fig. 7(F); Laurens et al., 2013b) to test responses of tilt- and translation-selective cells. OVAR is performed by rotating the animal at a constant speed around a tilted yaw axis. As a result, the animal tilts periodically from side to side. Therefore, OVAR produces the same tilt as in the two-dimensional protocols, but through constant velocity rotation around the yaw head axis instead of sinusoidal rotation around the pitch or roll axis. This rotation is detected by the horizontal semicircular canals. If tilt-selective cells relayed semicircular afferent-like rotation signals, they would respond in a radically different fashion during sinusoidal tilt and OVAR since (1) sinusoidal tilt and OVAR are performed using rotations around different axes and (2) OVAR, being a constant velocity rotation, would not produce a sinusoidal response. Instead, we found that responses of tilt-selective cells are the same, irrespective of whether tilt is archieved through the two-dimensional protocols or OVAR (Fig. 7(F); Laurens et al., 2013b). Because the only common stimulus is tilt orientation relative to gravity, this demonstrates that tilt-selective cells encode a central estimate of tilt rather than rotation velocity.

Thus, in summary, both EVAR and OVAR three-dimensional motion paradigms have demonstrated that the brain implements the three-dimensional integration (Eqs (3) and (4)) by integrating rotations around all head axes to track head orientation relative to gravity (Laurens et al., 2013b).

Motion illusions. Beyond encoding real motion, tilt- and translation-encoding neurons respond during illusory motion, as predicted by the internal model hypothesis (Laurens & Angelaki, 2011; Laurens et al., 2013a,b). Three observations are of relevance here. First, we have already shown that tilt-selective cell responses reflect the somatogravic effect (Fig. 6). As mentioned earlier, low-frequency translation induces an illusion of tilt; and tilt-selective cells respond accordingly (Laurens et al., 2013b).

A second motion illusion was created in Laurens et al., (2013a), in which the vertical canals were artificially activated although the animal was in fact upright. The semicircular canal activation causes an illusory tilt and, through Eq. (5), an illusory translation. We found that translation-selective cells responded to this illusion. We controlled the magnitude and duration of canal activation, allowing us to simulate the illusion through the model shown in Fig. 2(D); the simulation matched the translation signals decoded from the population of translation-selective cells (Laurens et al., 2013a).

A third motion illusion was induced during the steady-state OVAR protocol in Laurens et al. (2013b). We measured neuronal responses to 1 min of continuous OVAR. During constant-velocity OVAR, rotation signals decrease with a time constant of about 20 s (Laurens et al., 2013b). When the yaw velocity signal (Fig. 7(F)) vanishes, human subjects or animals progressively develop an illusion of translation (Vingerhoets et al., 2005). We found that translation-selective cells in the NU and FN responded after the first seconds of OVAR. This response built up with a time constant that could be simulated using the model in Fig. 2(D). The responses of tilt-selective cells decreased in parallel. We found that the decrease and buildup of tilt- and translation-selective cell modulation matched each other, in agreement with Eqs (2) and (5).

Together, these findings have demonstrated that neuronal computations in the vestibulocerebellum follow the theoretical principles of the internal model (Fig. 7(H)).

DISCUSSION

In this brief review, we have summarized the three building blocks of the gravity internal model hypothesis: (1) the ability to integrate semicircular canals signals in three dimensions (Eq. (3)), (2) the creation of tilt and translation signals whose sum equals the GIA (Eq. (2)), and (3) the somatogravic effect (Eq. (4)). Specifically designed experimental protocols show that all the three principles underlie the properties of tilt- and translation-selective cells in the NU and FN.

Furthermore, these studies bring solutions to the fundamental problem of interpreting neuronal responses. The three motion variables that are manipulated during the tilt/translation protocol (tilt, translation, and GIA) are interdependent, since each variable is a combination of the other two. For instance, a neuron that responds (preferentially) to tilt could arguably be responding to a mixture of translation and GIA. Thus, drawing meaningful interpretations is a fundamental problem that was addressed by the classification method explained above. Its rationale, based on fitting the neuron's response with tilt, translation, or GIA models, may appear oversimplified. For instance, the assumption that a translation-selective neuron responds to translation only is incorrect: all translation-selective cells did respond to tilt to a limited but significant extent. Yet, this simplistic scheme yielded an efficient classification technique, whose validity was confirmed by subsequent studies (Laurens et al., 2013a,b).

Many fundamental aspects of tilt/translation discrimination remain to be investigated. For example, the neural circuit that performs the computations that discriminate tilt from translations remains to be dissected. Translation-selective cells have been found in the responses of granular layer interneurons (Meng et al, 2014) and in the vestibular/fastigial nuclei (Angelaki et al., 2004; Shaikh, Ghasia et al., 2005; Shaikh, Green et al., 2005), indicating that these computations may be distributed across brain regions.

LIST OF ABBREVIATIONS

EVAR Earth-vertical axis rotation (motion protocol)
FN Fastigial nuclei
GIA Gravitoinertial acceleration
IA Interaural (head axis)
LA Left anterior (head axis)
NO Naso-occipital (head axis)
NU Nodulus–uvula complex
OVAR Off-vertical axis rotation (motion protocol)
RA Right anterior (head axis)
SPK Spikes
TTR Tilt–translation ratio
VN Vestibular nuclei

MATHEMATICAL VARIABLES

A Linear acceleration vector
C Semicircular canals signal
F Gravitoinertial acceleration
G Gravity vector
H Complex number representation of a transfer function
s Complex number representation of a stimulus
x Complex number representation of a neuronal response
τ_c Time constant of the semicircular canals
τ_s Time constant of the somatogravic effect
Ω Angular velocity vector

References

Agrawal, Y., Carey, J., Della Santina, C., Schubert, M., & Minor, L. (2009). Disorders of balance and vestibular function in us adults. *Archives of Internal Medicine, 169*, 938–944.
Angelaki, D. E., McHenry, M. Q., Dickman, J. D., Newlands, S. D., & Hess, B. J. (1999). Computation of inertial motion: neural strategies to resolve ambiguous otolith information. *The Journal of Neuroscience, 19*, 316–327.
Angelaki, D. E., Shaikh, A. G., Green, A. M., & Dickman, J. D. (2004). Neurons compute internal models of the physical laws of motion. *Nature, 430*, 560–564.

Barmack, N. H. (2003). Central vestibular system: vestibular nuclei and posterior cerebellum. *Brain Research Bulletin, 60,* 511–541.

Barmack, N. H., & Shojaku, H. (1995). Vestibular and visual climbing fiber signals evoked in the uvula-nodulus of the rabbit cerebellum by natural stimulation. *Journal of Neurophysiology, 74,* 2573–2589.

Barmack, N. H., & Yakhnista, V. (2008). Functions of interneurons in mouse cerebellum. *The Journal of Neuroscience, 28,* 1140–1152.

Borah, J., Young, L. R., & Curry, R. E. (1988). Optimal estimator model for human spatial orientation. *Annals of the New York Academy of Sciences, 545,* 51–73.

Bos, J. E., & Bles, W. (2002). Theoretical considerations on canal-otolith interaction and an observer model. *Biological Cybernetics, 86,* 191–207.

Crane, B. T., & Demer, J. L. (1998). Gaze stabilization during dynamic posturography in normal and vestibulopathic humans. *Experimental Brain Research, 122,* 235–246.

Einstein, A. (1907). Über das Relativitätsprinzip und die aus demselben gezogenen Folgerungen. *Jahrbuch der Radioaktivität und Elektronik, 4,* 411–462.

Glasauer, S., & Merfeld, D. M. (1997). Modelling three-dimensional vestibular responses during complex motion stimulation. In M. Fetter, T. Haslwanter, & H. Misslisch (Eds.), *Three-dimensional kinematics of eye, head and limb movements* (pp. 387–398). Amsterdam: Harwood Academic.

Graybiel, A. (1952). Oculogravic illusion. *Archives of Ophthalmology, 48,* 605–615.

Green, A. M., & Angelaki, D. E. (2007). Coordinate transformations and sensory integration in the detection of spatial orientation and self-motion: from models to experiments. *Progress in Brain Research, 165,* 155–180.

Green, A. M., Shaikh, A. G., & Angelaki, D. E. (2005). Sensory vestibular contributions to constructing internal models of self-motion. *Journal of Neural Engineering, 2,* S164–S179.

Holly, J. E. (2004). Vestibular coriolis effect differences modeled with three-dimensional linear-angular interactions. *Journal of Vestibular Research, 14,* 443–460.

Kitama, T., Komagata, J., Ozawa, K., Suzuki, Y., & Sato, Y. (2014). Plane-specific Purkinje cell responses to vertical head rotations in the cat cerebellar nodulus and uvula. *Journal of Neurophysiology, 112,* 644–659.

Laurens, J., & Angelaki, D. E. (2011). The functional significance of velocity storage and its dependence on gravity. *Experimental Brain Research, 210,* 407–422.

Laurens, J., & Droulez, J. (2007). Bayesian processing of vestibular information. *Biological Cybernetics, 96,* 389–404.

Laurens, J., Meng, H., & Angelaki, D. E. (2013a). Computation of linear acceleration through an internal model in the macaque cerebellum. *Nature Neuroscience, 16,* 1701–1708.

Laurens, J., Meng, H., & Angelaki, D. E. (2013b). Neural representation of gravity in the macaque vestibulocerebellum. *Neuron, 80,* 1508–1518.

Laurens, J., Strauman, D., & Hess, B. J. (2011). Spinning versus wobbling: how the brain solves a geometry problem. *The Journal of Neuroscience, 31,* 8093–8101.

Liu, S., & Angelaki, D. E. (2009). Vestibular signals in macaque extrastriate visual cortex are functionally appropriate for heading perception. *The Journal of Neuroscience, 29,* 8936–8945.

Liu, S., Dickman, J. D., & Angelaki, D. E. (2011). Response dynamics and tilt versus translation discrimination in parietoinsular vestibular cortex. *Cerebral Cortex, 21,* 563–573.

Maurer, C., Mergner, T., & Peterka, R. J. (2006). Multisensory control of human upright stance. *Experimental Brain Research, 171,* 231–250.

Mayne, R. (1974). A systems concept of the vestibular organs. In H. H. Kornhuber (Ed.), *Handbook of sensory physiology IV/2: The vestibular system* (pp. 493–580). Berlin: Springer.

Meng, H., Laurens, J., Blazquez, P. M., & Angelaki, D. E. In-vivo properties of cerebellar interneurons in the macaque caudal vestibular vermis. *The Journal of Physiology,* in press.

Meng, H., Laurens, J., Blazquez, P. M., Dickman, J. D., & Angelaki, D. E. (2014). Diversity of vestibular nuclei neurons targeted by cerebellar nodulus inhibition. *The Journal of Physiology, 592,* 171–188.

Merfeld, D. M. (1995). Modeling the vestibulo-ocular reflex of the squirrel monkey during eccentric rotation and roll tilt. *Experimental Brain Research, 106*, 123–134.

Merfeld, D. M., Zupan, L. H., & Peterka, R. J. (1999). Humans use internal models to estimate gravity and linear acceleration. *Nature, 398*, 615–618.

Paige, G., & Seidman, S. (1999). Characteristics of the VOR in response to linear acceleration. *Annals of the New York Academy of Sciences, 871*, 123–135.

Raphan, T., Matsuo, V., & Cohen, B. (1977). A velocity storage mechanism responsible for optokinetic nystagmus (OKN), optokinetic after-nystagmus (OKAN) and vestibular nystagmus. In R. Baker, & A. Berthoz (Eds.), *Control of gaze by brain stem neurons* (pp. 37–47). Amsterdam: Elsevier.

Rochefort, C., Lefort, J. M., & Rondi-Reig, L. (2013). The cerebellum: a new key structure in the navigation system. *Frontiers in Neural Circuits, 13*, 7–35.

Sağlam, M., Glasauer, S., & Lehnen, N. (2014). Vestibular and cerebellar contribution to gaze optimality. *Brain, 137*, 1080–1094.

Shaikh, A. G., Ghasia, F. F., Dickman, J. D., & Angelaki, D. E. (2005). Properties of cerebellar fastigial neurons during translation, rotation, and eye movements. *Journal of Neurophysiology, 93*, 853–863.

Shaikh, A. G., Green, A. M., Ghasia, F. F., Newlands, S. D., Dickman, J. D., & Angelaki, D. E. (2005). Sensory convergence solves a motion ambiguity problem. *Current Biology, 15*, 1657–1662.

Vingerhoets, R. A., Medendorp, W. P., & Van Gisbergen, J. A. (2005). Time course and magnitude of illusory translation perception during off-vertical axis rotation. *Journal of Neurophysiology, 95*, 1571–1587.

Yakusheva, T., Blazquez, P. M., & Angelaki, D. E. (2008). Frequency-selective coding of translation and tilt in macaque cerebellar nodulus and uvula. *The Journal of Neuroscience, 28*, 9997–10009.

Yakusheva, T., Blazquez, P. M., & Angelaki, D. E. (2010). Relationship between complex and simple spike activity in macaque caudal vermis during three-dimensional vestibular stimulation. *The Journal of Neuroscience, 30*, 8111–8126.

Yakusheva, T., Shaikh, A. G., Green, A. M., Blazquez, P. M., Dickman, J. D., & Angelaki, D. E. (2007). Purkinje cells in posterior cerebellar vermis encode motion in an inertial reference frame. *Neuron, 54*, 973–985.

Yu, X. J., Dickman, J. D., & Angelaki, D. E. (2012). Detection thresholds of macaque otolith afferents. *The Journal of Neuroscience, 32*, 8306–8316.

Zhou, W., Tang, B. F., Newlands, S. D., & King, W. M. (2006). Responses of monkey vestibular-only neurons to translation and angular rotation. *Journal of Neurophysiology, 96*, 2915–2930.

Zupan, L. H., Merfeld, D. M., & Darlot, C. (2002). Using sensory weighting to model the influence of canal, otolith and visual cues on spatial orientation and eye movements. *Biological Cybernetics, 86*, 209–230.

Modeling the Generation of Cerebellar Nuclear Spike Output

Volker Steuber

Science and Technology Research Institute, University of Hertfordshire, Hatfield, UK

INTRODUCTION

The cerebellum is involved in a large number of complex tasks, ranging from the coordination of movements to language processing, spatial cognition, and other higher cognitive and affective functions (Baudouin et al., 2012; Schmahmann, 2010; Tsai et al., 2012). Lesions of or other damage to the cerebellum typically lead to motor deficits, but they can also result in cognitive impairments such as loss of working memory and verbal fluency, and they are associated with conditions such as autism and dyslexia. The cerebellum is often seen as a powerful computational machine (Raymond, Lisberger, & Mauk, 1996), and a large number of experimental and modeling studies have investigated information processing in the cerebellar cortex. However, with the sole exception of a projection to the vestibular nuclei, all output from the cerebellar cortex has to be processed by the cerebellar nuclei (CN) before it can affect neuronal activity in other brain structures, and our understanding of information processing at the cerebellar output stage is still very limited. The number of modeling studies that specifically address the computational role of the CN is relatively small, and there is no general consensus about the nature of integration of cerebellar cortical output by neurons in the CN.

CN neurons receive input from the cerebellar cortex in the form of an inhibitory projection from cerebellar cortical Purkinje cells through GABAergic synapses. All neurons in the CN that have been recorded fire spontaneous action potentials. For example, in cerebellar slices at near-physiological temperatures, excitatory CN projection neurons exhibit intrinsic firing rates close to 90 Hz (Person & Raman, 2012a), and

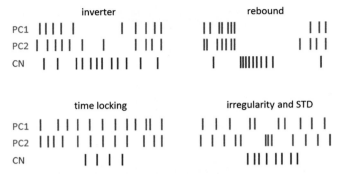

FIGURE 1   Possible forms of cerebellar corticonuclear communication. Top left: CN neurons as inverters of Purkinje cell spike rates. Top right: Rebound responses after the synchronized cessation of strong inhibitory Purkinje cell input. Bottom left: Time-locking of CN neuron spikes to synchronized Purkinje cell spikes. Bottom right: Short-term depression (STD) at Purkinje cell–CN neuron synapses enables the translation of Purkinje cell irregularity into the CN neuron spike rate (see also Person & Raman, 2012b).

inhibitory nucleo-olivary projection neurons are spontaneously active at rates of approximately 30 Hz (Najac & Raman, 2015). The presence of spontaneous activity, together with the inhibitory input from Purkinje cells, has inspired the obvious prediction that CN neurons are simple inverters of Purkinje cell activity, by increasing their spike rate in response to decreased Purkinje cell firing, and vice versa. However, the idea that CN neurons simply invert their Purkinje cell input rate is in apparent conflict with some experimental data that show both correlated and anticorrelated changes in CN neuron and Purkinje cell spike rates during motor behaviors (Armstrong & Edgley, 1984a,b; Thach, 1970a,b). Thus, alternative mechanisms for Purkinje cell input to shape CN neuron spike patterns have been suggested.

Figure 1 compares the commonly assumed inversion of Purkinje cell spike output by their target neurons in the CN with three other possible scenarios for CN spike output modulation by Purkinje cell inhibition. CN neurons exhibit characteristic rebound spike responses at the offset of hyperpolarizing current injections or inhibitory synaptic bursts (Aizenman & Linden, 1999; Llinas & Muhlethaler, 1988; Molineux et al., 2006, 2008; Sangrey & Jaeger, 2010; Tadayonnejad et al., 2010) (Fig. 2), and it has long been assumed that the firing of rebound spikes in response to a synchronized cessation of Purkinje cell input is an important component of the cerebellar output (Fig. 1, top right). Moreover, more recent experimental and modeling studies have suggested other forms of CN spike modulation by Purkinje cell input that are based on time-locking of the CN output spikes to the Purkinje cell input spikes (Fig. 1, bottom left) and on the decoding of irregular Purkinje cell spike trains by short-term depression at Purkinje cell–CN neuron synapses (Fig. 1, bottom right). This chapter provides an overview of existing computer simulations with spiking neuron models

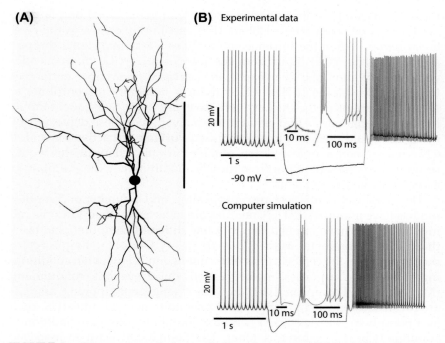

FIGURE 2   CN neuron morphology and rebound response. (A) Morphology of a recon-structed CN neuron used for the model in Steuber et al. (2011). The scale bar indicates 100 μm. (B) Top: Whole-cell recording of a CN neuron in a brain slice during a 1.5-s current injection of −150 pA. Two distinct components of the rebound response can be discriminated: a fast spike burst and a prolonged period of spike rate acceleration. Bottom: The computer model described in Steuber et al. (2011) can replicate these rebound response components based on the activation of CaT current for the fast rebound burst and NaP current for the slow rebound period. *Adapted from Steuber et al. (2011).*

that have explored these four different forms of communication between Purkinje cells and CN neurons and links this to the suggested involvement of the CN in various computational functions and pathological conditions. A subset of these computer simulations has previously been reviewed by Steuber and Jaeger (2013), looking at them from a slightly different angle and categorizing them as forms of rate coding, temporal coding, or both.

CEREBELLAR NUCLEUS NEURONS AS SIMPLE INVERTERS

The assumption that the output firing rate of the CN is an inverted version of their inhibitory Purkinje cell input firing rate has been fueled by the classic Marr–Albus–Ito theory of cerebellar learning (Albus, 1971; Ito, Sakurai, & Tongroach, 1982; Marr, 1969). According to the Marr–Albus–Ito theory in its simplest instantiation, motor learning is based on plasticity at synapses between parallel fibers (PF) and Purkinje cells in the cerebellar cortex. When the Purkinje cell receives a teaching signal through a climbing fiber (CF) input from the inferior olive (IO) that coincides with the activation of a PF synapse, the activated PF synapse undergoes long-term depression (LTD), which reduces its ability to contribute to future activations of the Purkinje cell (Ito et al., 1982). Subsequent inputs to the cerebellar cortex that result in the activation of these depressed PF synapses would then lead to a diminished Purkinje cell activation and, if CN neurons were simple inverters of their Purkinje cell input, this would result in an increased output from the CN and ultimately the execution of a newly learned movement.

The simplicity of this scenario is appealing, and a number of computer models have assumed that CN neurons are inverters of their Purkinje cell input rate and have applied this to a few different computational tasks that are extensions of the Marr–Albus–Ito theory. One of the simplest computational tasks the cerebellum is often implied in is Pavlovian conditioning of eyeblink responses, more precisely, delay eyeblink conditioning (McCormick & Thompson, 1984). In delay eyeblink conditioning, animals are presented repeatedly with a short unconditioned stimulus (US; such as a periorbital electrical shock) and a coterminating longer conditioned stimulus (CS; for example, a tone). The animal can learn to associate the CS with the US, and it can also learn the interstimulus interval (ISI) between the CS and the US onset: after training with paired CS and US, the CS alone triggers conditioned eyeblink responses (CRs) that are timed adaptively so that the peak of the CR coincides with the time of the US during training.

If we assume that the CS and US result in PF and CF input to Purkinje cells, respectively (McCormick & Thompson, 1984), the Marr–Albus–Ito theory can explain how CS and US pairing-induced PF LTD can underlie the formation of the association between the CS and the US: PF LTD will result in a decreased Purkinje cell response to CS presentations and, based on the Purkinje spike rate inverter model, this will lead to an increased output from the CN and trigger an eyeblink CR. The only additional ingredient that is required to explain the adaptive timing of the CR is for the CS to leave activity traces in the cerebellar cortical network that last long enough so that a subset of the PF synapses is active when the US-induced CF signal arrives at the Purkinje cell.

A number of computational studies of cerebellum-dependent eyeblink conditioning have modeled how the cerebellar connectivity and plasticity could result in the generation of adaptively timed CN spike responses. The model by Medina and collaborators (Medina, Garcia, Nores, Taylor, & Mauk, 2000) is an extension of the cerebellar cortical network model by Buonomano and Mauk (1994), with the addition of six CN neuron models.

In the Medina model, LTD and long-term potentiation (LTP) at PF–Purkinje cell synapses, together with LTP at mossy fiber (MF)–CN neuron synapses, enables the CN neurons to learn spike responses with temporal profiles that match experimentally recorded eyeblink responses. The adaptive timing of the CN spike responses in the Medina model is based on the existence of different subpopulations of granule cells that are active at different times during the CS. The representation of time by granule cells was investigated further in the network model by Yamazaki and Tanaka (2007), who found that random recurrent connections between granule and Golgi cells could result in the generation of nonrecurring temporal sequences of active granule cell groups. In a follow-up study, the model was then adapted by Yamazaki and Nagao (2012) to show that in addition to learning adaptively timed eyeblink responses, the model could also explain gain adaptations during optokinetic response eye movements. In both the original and the adapted Yamazaki models, the output from the cerebellum is generated by a single model of a CN neuron.

Another application domain that is based on the Marr–Albus–Ito theory of cerebellar learning, and that typically assumes a simple inversion of Purkinje cell spike rates by the CN, is cerebellar robotics. A series of computational studies have used cerebellar network models to control simulated and real robot arms (Carrillo, Ros, Boucheny, & Coenen, 2008; Casellato et al., 2014; Hofstötter, Mintz, & Verschure, 2002; Luque, Garrido, Carrillo, Tolu, & Ros, 2011; Schweighofer, Spoelstra, Arbib, & Kawato, 1998; Spoelstra, Schweighofer, & Arbib, 2000). In these studies, the cerebellar network learns the inverse dynamics of a robot arm, with MF input providing information about the target position and desired positions and speed of the joints, CF input providing an error signal, and the CN neuron output carrying information about torque corrections that are applied to the joints. For example, in the cerebellar network model by Carrillo et al. (2008), 16 CN neuron models represent positive and negative torque corrections for a shoulder and an elbow joint of a two-joint robotic arm. However, although these models have usually been designed for the control of robot arms, they are deeply rooted in the general Marr–Albus–Ito theory and, as a consequence, in principle applicable to a multitude of learning tasks. An example of such a widely applicable model is the cerebellar network model by Casellato et al. (2014), which was successfully applied to arm reaching, eyeblink conditioning, and vestibulo-ocular reflex (VOR) adaptation in simulations and real robots.

Although these network models have been applied to a variety of computational tasks, they are all based on the common assumption that CN neurons simply invert the spike rate of their Purkinje cell output, which has direct consequences on the choice of CN neuron models that are used in these networks. All of these models use simple leaky-integrate-and-fire (LIF) models to represent CN neurons, and they assume that any specific biophysical properties of the CN neurons are irrelevant. The next section describes a different approach to modeling CN neurons that takes into account how their response properties are determined by their characteristic ensemble of ion channels.

MODELING REBOUND RESPONSES

CN neurons are characterized by their ability to generate rebound spike responses at the offset of hyperpolarizing current injections and after bursts of inhibitory synaptic inputs (Fig. 2). These rebound responses are composed of fast rebound spike bursts and often also longer lasting periods of accelerated spiking (Aizenman & Linden, 1999; Engbers et al., 2011; Llinas & Muhlethaler, 1988; Molineux et al., 2006, 2008; Sangrey & Jaeger, 2010; Steuber, Schultheiss, Silver, De Schutter, & Jaeger, 2011; Tadayonnejad et al., 2010), and they are based on the hyperpolarization-induced de-inactivation of low-voltage-activated (LVA) T-type calcium channels and probably also persistent sodium (NaP) channels and the activation of hyperpolarization-activated cyclic nucleotide (HCN) gated channels (Engbers et al., 2011; Sangrey & Jaeger, 2010; Steuber et al., 2011). Although the ability of negative current injections to elicit rebound responses in CN neurons is well established, the conditions that lead to the firing of robust rebound responses in vivo are still a matter of debate (Alvina, Walter, Kohn, Ellis-Davies, & Khodakhah, 2008; Bengtsson, Ekerot, & Jorntell, 2011; Engbers et al., 2011; Tadayonnejad et al., 2010). In cerebellar slices, bursts of Purkinje cell inputs are more effective at triggering rebound responses than hyperpolarizing current injections (Aizenman & Linden, 1999). However, many neurons in vivo operate under high-conductance conditions that are caused by a constant bombardment from the background synaptic input (Destexhe, Rudolph, & Pare, 2003; Stern, Jaeger, & Wilson, 1998), and the intrinsic activity of Purkinje cells in vivo, together with the large number of Purkinje cell synapses onto CN neurons (Person & Raman, 2012a,b), suggests that this might also be the case for CN neurons. An elevated membrane conductance could lead to shunting and prevent the generation of rebound responses in vivo. Moreover, while negative current injections in vitro can hyperpolarize CN neurons down to voltages below −100 mV, the level of hyperpolarization that can be achieved by GABAergic input from Purkinje cells is constrained by the chloride reversal potential E_{Cl} of the $GABA_A$ receptors, which could limit the de-inactivation of T-type calcium and NaP channels and activation of HCN channels and further prohibit the expression of rebound responses in vivo.

The conditions that could lead to the generation of rebound spike responses in vivo, and how different ion channels in CN neurons interact to shape rebound responses, have been subjects of two modeling studies by Steuber et al. (2011) and Engbers et al. (2011). The work by Steuber and collaborators has used a morphologically realistic model of a CN neuron with 517 compartments. The model has a large soma with a diameter of 22 μm and a total capacitance of 203 pF, similar to measurements for excitatory CN projection neurons (Uusisaari, Obata, & Knopfel, 2007). The model includes eight Hodgkin–Huxley-type ion channels that are distributed differentially across the axon, soma, and proximal and distal dendrites: a fast sodium (NaF) current, a mixture of fast Kv3 (fKdr) and slow Kv2 (sKdr) delayed rectifiers, an small conductance (Sk) type calcium-gated potassium current, an HCN current, a high-voltage-activated (HVA) calcium current, a Cav3.1-type LVA calcium (CaT) current, an NaP current, and a tonic nonspecific cation (TNC) current. The model was tuned to replicate whole-cell recordings from 129 CN neurons (including data from Gauck & Jaeger, 2000), aiming to reproduce characteristic behaviors of excitatory projection neurons such as a narrow spike waveform and a postspike sequence of fast after-hyperpolarization (AHP), after-depolarization (ADP), and slow AHP (Uusisaari et al., 2007). The TNC current in the model drives the membrane repolarization during spikes, which results in rhythmic pacemaking in the absence of synaptic input (Raman, Gustafson, & Padgett, 2000). At a simulated temperature of 37 °C, this causes spontaneous activity at a rate of 26 Hz (Luthman et al., 2011); however, based on more recent data from Person and Raman (2012a), this underestimates spike rates of excitatory CN projection neurons under physiological conditions. The early tuning of the model resulted in the requirement for selective coupling of the SK channel to the HVA calcium channel; this prediction was confirmed by an independent experimental study (Alvina & Khodakhah, 2008).

The model by Steuber and collaborators (2011) makes several predictions about the mechanisms that shape the spontaneous activity and its modulation by synaptic input. For example, the ADP in the model is caused by current flowing back from the dendrites into the soma, which suggests that a reduction in the size of the dendrites would reduce the ADP. Moreover, the intrinsic currents are much smaller than the synaptic currents, resulting in a spike pattern and rate that are very sensitive to modulation by synaptic input. The model predicts that CN neurons can implement a rate code, where small changes in excitatory MF input rate or inhibitory Purkinje cell input rate result in smooth changes in the CN output rate. Inhibitory input from Purkinje cells has a purely additive effect on the relationship between the MF input rate and the CN neuron output rate, resulting in shifts of the MF input–CN output curves along the MF input axis. Such an additive operation has been implicated in computational functions such as VOR reflex adaptation (Medina & Lisberger, 2009).

The main aim of the modeling study by Steuber and collaborators (2011) was to investigate factors contributing to the generation of rebound responses under in vitro and in vivo conditions. The whole-cell slice recordings from the 129 CN neurons that served as a target for the model tuning showed very heterogeneous rebound responses at the offset of negative current injections. In these recordings, rebounds contained varying amounts of fast bursts that were often followed by short pauses and longer increases in firing rate (Fig. 2). Similar patterns of rebound responses have been described before, but the fast bursts seem to occur more commonly than the prolonged periods of accelerated spiking (Aizenman & Linden, 1999; Engbers et al., 2011; Llinas & Muhlethaler, 1988; Molineux et al., 2006, 2008; Sangrey & Jaeger, 2010; Steuber et al., 2011; Tadayonnejad et al., 2010). In the CN neuron model, the fast bursts, short pauses, and prolonged accelerated spiking were shaped differentially by the CaT, NaP, and HCN currents. Unsurprisingly, increasing the conductance of the faster CaT channels increased the extent of the fast rebound bursts, while increasing the slower NaP conductance resulted in more pronounced long-lasting increases in firing rate. Increasing the HCN conductance could eliminate pauses between the fast bursts and the following period of accelerated spiking, but it could also lead to reduced rebound responses by decreasing the extent of pre-rebound hyperpolarization and therefore diminishing the de-inactivation of the CaT and NaP channels. For longer (≥250 ms) current injections, the HCN conductance also affected the latency of rebound responses, with larger hyperpolarizations that resulted in more HCN channel activation leading to smaller delays between the offset of the current injections and the rebound response. Furthermore, a series of simulations explored the generation of rebound responses in vivo for various rates of synaptic background and various E_{Cl} values. These in vivo simulations predict that rebound responses are robust against shunting by synaptic background input, but that they require sufficiently negative E_{Cl} values of −75 mV or below.

The extent of hyperpolarization, however, and therefore the value of E_{Cl} that is required to elicit rebound response in vivo depend on the half-inactivation voltages of the CaT and NaP currents and the half-activation voltage of the HCN current. In the model by Steuber and colleagues, these voltages were set to −80 mV, which might overestimate the extent of required hyperpolarization. A combined experimental and modeling study by Engbers et al. (2011) found that it is sufficient to hyperpolarize CN neurons in slices to −72 mV to de-inactivate and activate a small fraction of CaT and HCN channels, respectively. The same study also performed simulations of a two-compartmental model of a CN neuron with NaF, Kdr, and HCN conductances in a soma compartment and CaT and slow potassium conductances in a dendrite compartment. To replicate their experimental data, the CaT half-inactivation voltage and the HCN half-activation voltage in the Engbers model were set to −64 and −92 mV, respectively. Like the model by Steuber et al. (2011), the Engbers model predicts that the HCN current contributes to a reduction in the rebound latency. Another prediction of the model is that the HCN current decreases the variability of the rebound latency and that it acts synergistically with the CaT current to increase the spike rate in the rebound burst.

In addition to the computational studies that have investigated cellular mechanisms that underlie the generation of rebound responses, there are also a number of models that study the computational function of rebound spiking in CN neurons. A series of articles by Kistler and collaborators have suggested that postinhibitory rebounds in CN neurons could form the basis of reverberatory cerebellar loops through the IO and the nucleus reticularis tegmenti pontis (Kistler & De Zeeuw, 2003; Kistler & van Hemmen, 1999; Kistler, van Hemmen, & De Zeeuw, 2000). The CN neuron model that has been used in these simulations has been derived from a single-compartmental model of a thalamocortical relay neuron (McCormick & Huguenard, 1992), which has been adapted by decreasing the size of the model and changing the kinetics of the CaT and HCN conductances. Kistler and colleagues show that rebound responses in CN neurons could provide the cerebellar network with the ability to store and recall spatiotemporal activity patterns. However, the storage and recall of the spatiotemporal pattern seem to depend on the ability of the CN neuron model to generate precisely timed rebound responses that occur 100 ms after the inhibitory Purkinje cell input, independently of the number or synchronicity of the Purkinje cell spikes. The required lack of dependence of the rebound latency on the strength of the inhibitory input is in contrast to the results of the study by Steuber et al. (2011), which suggest that the strength of inhibitory input affects the delay between the offset of inhibition and rebound response.

Two other modeling studies have implicated rebound responses in CN neurons in Pavlovian delay eyeblink conditioning. According to the "lock-and-key" hypothesis by Wetmore, Mukamel, and Schnitzer (2008), the generation of rebound responses is necessary for the expression of correctly timed eyeblink CRs after training. Wetmore and colleagues suggest that the training with paired CS–US presentations results in LTP and LTD at subsets of PF synapses onto Purkinje cells that are activated early and late during the CS, respectively. As a consequence, CS presentations after training will result in an increase in the Purkinje cell spike rate that is followed by a decrease. Such a temporal Purkinje spike pattern (a "key") can elicit a rebound response in the CN neurons and trigger an appropriately timed eyeblink CR, while training with the opposite order of stimuli (US before CS) will be ineffective. The lock-and-key hypothesis is investigated with three CN neuron models with different degrees of complexity: their Model 1 is a single compartment with a CaT conductance, Model 2 also includes an HVA calcium conductance, and Model 3 consists of two compartments with NaF and Kdr conductances in the soma and an SK conductance in both compartments. All three models can learn adaptively timed rebound responses; these are low-threshold calcium spikes in Model 1, high-threshold calcium spikes in Model 2, and sodium spike bursts in Model 3. Moreover, Models 2 and 3 exhibit a probability of rebound responses as a function of the CS–US ISI that resembles the relationship between the ISI and the reliability of eyeblink CRs in experiments.

The assumption that rebound responses in CN neurons are the basis of appropriately timed CRs is also at the center of a study by Hofstötter et al. (2002). Hofstötter and colleagues use a modified version of an integrate-and-fire model to simulate the generation of rebound responses in CN neurons. They apply their model to two different Pavlovian conditioning tasks, a simulated one and one in which a mobile robot learns obstacle avoidance with detection of collision as US and visual identification of the obstacle as CS.

TIME-LOCKING, SYNCHRONY CODING, AND THE EFFECT OF IRREGULARITY

Although rebound responses in the CN provide an attractive mechanism for the cerebellum to provide well-timed output signals, they introduce a time lag between stimuli that result in an increase in the Purkinje cell spike rate and the generation of output signals from the cerebellum (Person & Raman, 2012b). Moreover, a cerebellar code that relies on CN rebound responses does not convey information about Purkinje cell firing rates as easily as a scenario in which CN neurons are simple inverters of their Purkinje cell input spike rates (Person & Raman, 2012b). However, a previous modeling study has suggested that information about PF inputs to Purkinje cells can be carried by pauses in the Purkinje cell spike trains (Steuber et al., 2007), and the firing of a rebound response would provide a fast way to signal the onset of synchronized pauses in the Purkinje cell activity. Interestingly, it has been shown that pauses in Purkinje cell spiking synchronize more readily than spikes that are not associated with pauses (Shin et al., 2007). Moreover, the rate of Purkinje cell spikes before a pause will determine the depth of the hyperpolarization in the CN neuron and therefore also the strength of the rebound response (De Schutter & Steuber, 2009; Steuber et al., 2011). Thus, rebound responses provide a mechanism to combine temporal coding based on the timing of Purkinje cell pauses with rate coding based on Purkinje cell spike rates (De Schutter & Steuber, 2009). However, evidence for signaling based on rebound responses in vivo is still lacking, and other forms of CN neuron spike modulation by Purkinje cell input have been suggested and investigated in experiments and computer simulations. One possibility is that the precise timing of CN neuron spikes is determined by synchronous inhibition from the presynaptic Purkinje cells (Fig. 1, bottom left). When the population of inhibitory Purkinje cells that converge onto a CN neuron synchronizes their activity, the synchronized gaps between the Purkinje cell input spikes will allow precisely timed CN output spikes. This possibility was explored in dynamic clamp studies (Gauck & Jaeger, 2000, 2003), which showed that increases in the Purkinje cell synchrony led to increases in the CN neuron spike rate. A limitation of these dynamic clamp studies is that all the input is applied at the soma, but an accompanying computer simulation of a morphologically realistic CN neuron model (Steuber et al., 2011) has indicated that the spike response of CN neurons is very similar for both somatic and dendritically distributed synaptic input (Lin & Jaeger, 2011). A similar time-locking of CN neuron spikes to synchronized Purkinje cell input spikes has been found in another experimental study (Person & Raman, 2012a). This time-locking is facilitated by the fast kinetics of the Purkinje cell synapses at near-physiological temperatures, and it can even be observed when only a small fraction (5%) of afferent Purkinje cells synchronize. The study also indicates that the number of Purkinje cells converging onto a single CN neuron is around 50, which is considerably smaller than previous estimates (Palkovits, Mezey, Hamori, & Szentagothai, 1977).

Time-locking of CN neuron activity to synchronized Purkinje cell inputs has also been investigated in a modeling study that tried to explain the effect of 4-aminopyridine (4-AP) in treating downbeat nystagmus (DBN) and cerebellar ataxia (Glasauer, Rossert, & Strupp, 2011). Glasauer and colleagues used a model of a medial vestibular nucleus neuron (Av-Ron & Vidal, 1999; Weaver & Wearne, 2008) with Fitzhugh–Nagumo-type models of NaF and Kdr channels and Hodgkin–Huxley type-models of NaP, HVA calcium, A-type potassium, and calcium-dependent potassium channels, and they presented this model with regular versus irregular and synchronized versus desynchronized Purkinje cell inputs. The study showed that regular Purkinje cell firing resulted in increased CN activity, but only when the Purkinje cell input was synchronized. However, these results are in apparent conflict with experimental data, indicating that the therapeutic effect of 4-AP is based on a regularization of Purkinje cell activity that decreases the spike rate in the CN (Alvina & Khodakhah, 2010). The discrepancy between the modeling results by Glasauer et al. (2011) and the experimental results can be explained by the absence of short-term depression (STD) at the Purkinje cell synapses in the model, as will be explained below.

Several other experimental studies indicate that maintaining a sufficient degree of regularity of Purkinje cell spiking is important for intact cerebellar functioning and motor control. Tottering mice, which suffer from a natural mutation in the *Cacna1a* gene that encodes the α1A subunit of P/Q calcium channels, show an increased degree of irregularity in their Purkinje cell activity (Hoebeek et al., 2005; Walter, Alvina, Womack, Chevez,

& Khodakhah, 2006). These mice exhibit impaired motor behavior and abnormal optokinetic reflexes, and they show increased CN neuron firing rates (Hoebeek, Khosrovani, Witter, & De Zeeuw, 2008), although this has as of this writing been shown only for anesthetized mice and should also be confirmed by recordings from awake behaving mice. Moreover, regular electrical stimulation of the cerebellum can alleviate these motor deficits, which suggests a functional link between irregular Purkinje cell activity, increased CN spiking, and impaired motor control. Prompted by these experimental results, a modeling study by Luthman et al. (2011) used a modification of the morphologically realistic CN neuron model (Steuber et al., 2011) to investigate the effect of irregular Purkinje cell input on CN neurons, by applying both artificially generated Purkinje cell spike trains and spike trains from tottering and wild-type mice. Luthman and collaborators found that an increased degree of irregularity in the Purkinje cell input did indeed lead to an increased output firing in the CN neuron model. The increase in the CN neuron spike rate occurred for both synchronized and desynchronized Purkinje cell input, but the degree of synchronization affected the underlying mechanism. When the Purkinje cell input was desynchronized, even by only a small extent, the irregularity-driven spike rate increase was based on STD at the synapses between Purkinje cells and CN neurons (Pedroarena & Schwarz, 2003; Telgkamp & Raman, 2002), which resulted in a decrease in inhibitory synaptic conductance in response to irregular inputs. Only when the Purkinje cell input to the CN neuron was fully synchronized did the CN neuron spike rate acceleration occur independently of STD. These results suggest that the causal link between irregular Purkinje cell firing and impaired motor control is mediated by STD at Purkinje cell–CN neuron synapses, and they also provide a potential explanation for the beneficial effect of 4-AP in treating DBN and ataxia.

CONCLUSIONS

This chapter has described a number of computational models of CN neurons that have addressed, directly or indirectly, one of the most important questions in cerebellar neuroscience: how is the output from the cerebellar cortex processed by the CN? Neurons in the CN receive inhibitory GABAergic input from Purkinje cells in the cerebellar cortex, but there is as yet no consensus on how exactly the Purkinje cell spike output shapes the spike patterns in CN neurons that are transmitted to the rest of the brain and that are ultimately responsible for cerebellum-dependent behaviors. As illustrated in Fig. 1, four different scenarios for the modulation of CN neuron spiking by Purkinje cell input have been proposed. In the simplest case, the inhibitory input from Purkinje cells could simply result in an inversion of Purkinje cell spike rate by spike rates in the CN, with an deceleration of Purkinje cell spiking resulting in an acceleration of CN neuron spiking, and vice versa. Alternatively, the relevant output from CN neurons might be formed by rebound responses that follow the synchronized cessation of strong inhibitory input from Purkinje cells. More recently, it has been suggested that spikes in CN neurons time-lock to Purkinje cell input spikes; this requires partial synchronization of the Purkinje cell inputs and at the same time provides a mechanism to read out the extent of this synchronization (Gauck & Jaeger, 2000, 2003; Person & Raman, 2012a,b). Finally, a computational study has indicated that CN neurons can translate increases in the irregularity of their Purkinje cell input into increases in their firing rate, a phenomenon that is based on STD at the Purkinje cell–CN neuron synapse (Luthman et al., 2011).

The type and level of complexity of the computational models of CN neurons that have been used to simulate these four scenarios depend both on the scenario that is being simulated and on the particular computational function and the research question that is being addressed. A simulation study that investigates the generation of rebound responses requires the use of a conductance-based neuronal model that includes Hodgkin–Huxley-type or Markov models of ion channels. Thus, all computational models that have been used to study rebound responses have been of this type, with the sole exception of the work by Hofstötter et al. (2002), in which the focus of the work was robot control, and rebound responses were effectively pasted into an integrate-and-fire model. In contrast, all studies that have assumed a simple inversion of Purkinje cell spike rates by CN neurons have used LIF models, given that there is no need to include ion channel models if all that is required is synaptic inhibition and integration. In fact, using a LIF, Izhikevich (Izhikevich, 2003), or adaptive exponential integrate-and-fire model (Brette & Gerstner, 2005) is often the best strategy if the data on ion channel kinetics are very sparse (Herz, Gollisch, Machens, & Jaeger, 2006). However, although we do not yet have a complete set of kinetic data for all ion channels in CN neurons, the large amount of available data justifies the use of conductance-based models of CN neurons, especially since it is not possible to exclude that rebound responses play a role in information processing in the CN.

Although computational models can be used to explore the possibility of any of the four scenarios of spike modulation operating in the CN, they cannot be used to prove which of the modulation scenarios is in fact in operation in the real cerebellum. Simulations of the morphologically realistic CN neuron model (Steuber et al., 2011) indicate that the available connectivity and physiology can implement all four possible types of modulation: inversion, rebound, time-locking, and irregularity decoding. It is not unlikely that depending on the particular conditions and the computational task, all of these forms of modulation are utilized. Moreover, it is likely that the form of CN spike modulation by Purkinje cell input depends on the particular type of CN neurons and the origin of its Purkinje cell input. For example, inhibitory projection neurons that project to the IO exhibit slower synaptic kinetics and lower firing rates and are more likely to be inverters of Purkinje cell spike rates (Najac & Raman, 2015), while excitatory projection neurons are more suited to synchrony-dependent time-locking (Person & Raman, 2012a). Similarly, CN neurons that receive input from very fast (100 Hz) spiking Purkinje cells located in zebrin-negative modules may be better equipped to generate rebound responses, while those that receive input from moderately (50–80 Hz) spiking zebrin-positive Purkinje cells might be more prone to time-locking (Zhou et al., 2014). To fully understand the modulation of CN spike output by their Purkinje cell input, and importantly also how it is affected by excitatory input from MFs and CFs, we will need more data on the types and physiology of CN neurons, their afferents from outside the CN, and the intrinsic circuitry within the CN (Uusisaari & De Schutter, 2011; Uusisaari & Knopfel, 2012).

References

Aizenman, C. D., & Linden, D. J. (1999). Regulation of the rebound depolarization and spontaneous firing patterns of deep nuclear neurons in slices of rat cerebellum. *Journal of Neurophysiology, 82,* 1697–1709.

Albus, J. S. (1971). A theory of cerebellar function. *Mathematical Biosciences, 10*(1–2), 25–61.

Alvina, K., & Khodakhah, K. (2008). Selective regulation of spontaneous activity of neurons of the deep cerebellar nuclei by N-type calcium channels in juvenile rats. *Journal of Physiology, 586*(10), 2523–2538. http://dx.doi.org/10.1113/jphysiol.2007.148197.

Alvina, K., & Khodakhah, K. (2010). The therapeutic mode of action of 4-aminopyridine in cerebellar ataxia. *Journal of Neuroscience, 30*(21), 7258–7268. http://dx.doi.org/10.1523/JNEUROSCI.3582-09.2010.

Alvina, K., Walter, J. T., Kohn, A., Ellis-Davies, G., & Khodakhah, K. (2008). Questioning the role of rebound firing in the cerebellum. *Nature Neuroscience, 11*(11), 1256–1258. http://dx.doi.org/10.1038/nn.2195.

Armstrong, D. M., & Edgley, S. A. (1984a). Discharges of nucleus interpositus neurones during locomotion in the cat. *Journal of Physiology, 351,* 411–432.

Armstrong, D. M., & Edgley, S. A. (1984b). Discharges of Purkinje cells in the paravermal part of the cerebellar anterior lobe during locomotion in the cat. *Journal of Physiology, 352,* 403–424.

Av-Ron, E., & Vidal, P. P. (1999). Intrinsic membrane properties and dynamics of medial vestibular neurons: a simulation. *Biological Cybernetics, 80*(6), 383–392.

Baudouin, S. J., Gaudias, J., Gerharz, S., Hatstatt, L., Zhou, K., Punnakkal, P., et al. (2012). Shared synaptic pathophysiology in syndromic and nonsyndromic rodent models of autism. *Science, 338*(6103), 128–132. http://dx.doi.org/10.1126/science.1224159.

Bengtsson, F., Ekerot, C. F., & Jorntell, H. (2011). In vivo analysis of inhibitory synaptic inputs and rebounds in deep cerebellar nuclear neurons. *PLoS One, 6*(4), e18822. http://dx.doi.org/10.1371/journal.pone.0018822.

Brette, R., & Gerstner, W. (2005). Adaptive exponential integrate-and-fire model as an effective description of neuronal activity. *Journal of Neurophysiology, 94*(5), 3637–3642. http://dx.doi.org/10.1152/jn.00686.2005.

Buonomano, D. V., & Mauk, M. D. (1994). Neural network model of the cerebellum: temporal discrimination and the timing of motor responses. *Neural Computation*, 6, 38–55.

Carrillo, R. R., Ros, E., Boucheny, C., & Coenen, O. J. (2008). A real-time spiking cerebellum model for learning robot control. *Biosystems*, 94(1–2), 18–27. http://dx.doi.org/10.1016/j.biosystems.2008.05.008.

Casellato, C., Antonietti, A., Garrido, J. A., Carrillo, R. R., Luque, N. R., Ros, E., et al. (2014). Adaptive robotic control driven by a versatile spiking cerebellar network. *PLoS One*, 9(11), e112265. http://dx.doi.org/10.1371/journal.pone.0112265.

De Schutter, E., & Steuber, V. (2009). Patterns and pauses in Purkinje cell simple spike trains: experiments, modeling and theory. *Neuroscience*, 162(3), 816–826. http://dx.doi.org/10.1016/j.neuroscience.2009.02.040.

Destexhe, A., Rudolph, M., & Pare, D. (2003). The high-conductance state of neocortical neurons in vivo. *Nature Reviews Neuroscience*, 4(9), 739–751.

Engbers, J. D. T., Anderson, D., Tadayonnejad, R., Mehaffey, W. H., Molineux, M. L., & Turner, R. W. (2011). Distinct roles for IT and IH in controlling the frequency and timing of rebound spike responses. *Journal of Physiology*, 589(22), 5391–5413. http://dx.doi.org/10.1113/jphysiol.2011.215632.

Gauck, V., & Jaeger, D. (2000). The role of intrinsic currents in determining the spike pattern of deep cerebellar nucleus neurons with synaptic input. *Society for Neuroscience Abstract*, 26, 93.

Gauck, V., & Jaeger, D. (2003). The contribution of NMDA and AMPA conductances to the control of spiking in neurons of the deep cerebellar nuclei. *Journal of Neuroscience*, 23(22), 8109–8118.

Glasauer, S., Rossert, C., & Strupp, M. (2011). The role of regularity and synchrony of cerebellar Purkinje cells for pathological nystagmus. *Annals of New York Academy of Sciences*, 1233, 162–167. http://dx.doi.org/10.1111/j.1749-6632.2011.06149.x.

Herz, A. V., Gollisch, T., Machens, C. K., & Jaeger, D. (2006). Modeling single-neuron dynamics and computations: a balance of detail and abstraction. *Science*, 314(5796), 80–85. http://dx.doi.org/10.1126/science.1127240.

Hoebeek, F. E., Khosrovani, S., Witter, L., & De Zeeuw, C. I. (2008). Purkinje cell input to cerebellar nuclei in tottering: ultrastructure and physiology. *Cerebellum*, 7(4), 547–558. http://dx.doi.org/10.1007/s12311-008-0086-0.

Hoebeek, F. E., Stahl, J. S., van Alphen, A. M., Schonewille, M., Luo, C., Rutteman, M., et al. (2005). Increased noise level of purkinje cell activities minimizes impact of their modulation during sensorimotor control. *Neuron*, 45(6), 953–965. http://dx.doi.org/10.1016/j.neuron.2005.02.012 pii: S0896-6273(05)00129-7.

Hofstötter, C., Mintz, M., & Verschure, P. F. (2002). The cerebellum in action: a simulation and robotics study. *European Journal of Neuroscience*, 16(7), 1361–1376.

Ito, M., Sakurai, M., & Tongroach, P. (1982). Climbing fibre induced depression of both mossy fibre responsiveness and glutamate sensitivity of cerebellar Purkinje cells. *Journal of Physiology*, 324, 113–134.

Izhikevich, E. M. (2003). Simple model of spiking neurons. *IEEE Transactions on Neural Networks*, 14(6), 1569–1572. http://dx.doi.org/10.1109/TNN.2003.820440.

Kistler, W. M., & De Zeeuw, C. I. (2003). Time windows and reverberating loops: a reverse-engineering approach to cerebellar function. *Cerebellum*, 2(1), 44–54.

Kistler, W. M., & van Hemmen, J. L. (1999). Delayed reverberation through time windows as a key to cerebellar function. *Biological Cybernetics*, 81, 373–380.

Kistler, W. M., van Hemmen, J. L., & De Zeeuw, C. I. (2000). Time window control: a model for cerebellar function based on synchronization, reverberation, and time slicing. *Progress in Brain Research*, 124, 275–297.

Lin, R. J., & Jaeger, D. (2011). Using computer simulations to determine the limitations of dynamic clamp stimuli applied at the soma in mimicking distributed conductance sources. *Journal of Neurophysiology*, 105(5), 2610–2624. http://dx.doi.org/10.1152/jn.00968.2010.

Llinas, R., & Muhlethaler, M. (1988). Electrophysiology of Guinea-pig cerebellar nuclear cells in the in vitro brain stem-cerebellar preparation. *Journal of Physiology, 404,* 241–258.

Luque, N. R., Garrido, J. A., Carrillo, R. R., Tolu, S., & Ros, E. (2011). Adaptive cerebellar spiking model embedded in the control loop: context switching and robustness against noise. *International Journal of Neural Systems, 21*(5), 385–401. http://dx.doi.org/10.1142/S0129065711002900.

Luthman, J., Hoebeek, F. E., Maex, R., Davey, N., Adams, R., De Zeeuw, C. I., et al. (2011). STD-dependent and independent encoding of input irregularity as spike rate in a computational model of a cerebellar nucleus neuron. *Cerebellum, 10*(4), 667–682. http://dx.doi.org/10.1007/s12311-011-0295-9.

Marr, D. (1969). A theory of cerebellar cortex. *Journal of Physiology, 202*(2), 437–470.

McCormick, D. A., & Huguenard, J. R. (1992). A model of the electrophysiological properties of thalamocortical relay neurons. *Journal of Neurophysiology, 68*(4), 1384–1400.

McCormick, D. A., & Thompson, R. F. (1984). Cerebellum: essential involvement in the classically conditioned eyelid response. *Science, 223*(4633), 296–299.

Medina, J. F., Garcia, K. S., Nores, W. L., Taylor, N. M., & Mauk, M. D. (2000). Timing mechanisms in the cerebellum: testing predictions of a large-scale computer simulation. *Journal of Neuroscience, 20*(14), 5516–5525.

Medina, J. F., & Lisberger, S. G. (2009). Encoding and decoding of learned smooth-pursuit eye movements in the floccular complex of the monkey cerebellum. *Journal of Neurophysiology, 102*(4), 2039–2054. http://dx.doi.org/10.1152/jn.00075.2009.

Molineux, M. L., McRory, J. E., McKay, B. E., Hamid, J., Mehaffey, W. H., Rehak, R., et al. (2006). Specific T-type calcium channel isoforms are associated with distinct burst phenotypes in deep cerebellar nuclear neurons. *Proceedings of the National Academy of Sciences of the United States of America, 103*(14), 5555–5560.

Molineux, M. L., Mehaffey, W. H., Tadayonnejad, R., Anderson, D., Tennent, A. F., & Turner, R. W. (2008). Ionic factors governing rebound burst phenotype in rat deep cerebellar neurons. *Journal of Neurophysiology, 100*(5), 2684–2701. http://dx.doi.org/10.1152/jn.90427.2008.

Najac, M., & Raman, I. M. (2015). Integration of Purkinje cell inhibition by cerebellar nucleo-olivary neurons. *Journal of Neuroscience, 35*(2), 544–549. http://dx.doi.org/10.1523/JNEUROSCI.3583-14.2015.

Palkovits, M., Mezey, E., Hamori, J., & Szentagothai, J. (1977). Quantitative histological analysis of the cerebellar nuclei in the cat. I. Numerical data on cells and on synapses. *Experimental Brain Research, 28*(1–2), 189–209.

Pedroarena, C. M., & Schwarz, C. (2003). Efficacy and short-term plasticity at GABAergic synapses between Purkinje and cerebellar nuclei neurons. *Journal of Neurophysiology, 89*(2), 704–715.

Person, A. L., & Raman, I. M. (2012a). Purkinje neuron synchrony elicits time-locked spiking in the cerebellar nuclei. *Nature, 481*(7382), 502–505. http://dx.doi.org/10.1038/nature10732.

Person, A. L., & Raman, I. M. (2012b). Synchrony and neural coding in cerebellar circuits. *Frontiers in Neural Circuits, 6,* 97. http://dx.doi.org/10.3389/fncir.2012.00097.

Raman, I. M., Gustafson, A. E., & Padgett, D. (2000). Ionic currents and spontaneous firing in neurons isolated from the cerebellar nuclei. *Journal of Neuroscience, 20*(24), 9004–9016.

Raymond, J. L., Lisberger, S. G., & Mauk, M. D. (1996). The cerebellum: a neuronal learning machine? *Science, 272*(5265), 1126–1131.

Sangrey, T., & Jaeger, D. (2010). Multiple components of rebound spiking in deep cerebellar nucleus neurons. *European Journal of Neuroscience, 32,* 1646–1657.

Schmahmann, J. D. (2010). The role of the cerebellum in cognition and emotion: personal reflections since 1982 on the dysmetria of thought hypothesis, and its historical evolution from theory to therapy. *Neuropsychology review, 20*(3), 236–260.

Schweighofer, N., Spoelstra, J., Arbib, M. A., & Kawato, M. (1998). Role of the cerebellum in reaching movements in humans. II. A neural model of the intermediate cerebellum. *European Journal of Neuroscience, 10*(1), 95–105.

Shin, S. L., Hoebeek, F. E., Schonewille, M., De Zeeuw, C. I., Aertsen, A., & De Schutter, E. (2007). Regular patterns in cerebellar Purkinje cell simple spike trains. *PLoS One, 2*(5), e485. http://dx.doi.org/10.1371/journal.pone.0000485.

Spoelstra, J., Schweighofer, N., & Arbib, M. A. (2000). Cerebellar learning of accurate predictive control for fast-reaching movements. *Biological Cybernetics, 82*(4), 321–333.

Stern, E. A., Jaeger, D., & Wilson, C. J. (1998). Membrane potential synchrony of simultaneously recorded striatal spiny neurons in vivo. *Nature, 394*(6692), 475–478.

Steuber, V., & Jaeger, D. (2013). Modeling the generation of output by the cerebellar nuclei. *Neural Networks, 47*, 112–119. http://dx.doi.org/10.1016/j.neunet.2012.11.006.

Steuber, V., Mittmann, W., Hoebeek, F. E., Silver, R. A., De Zeeuw, C. I., Hausser, M., et al. (2007). Cerebellar LTD and pattern recognition by Purkinje cells. *Neuron, 54*(1), 121–136. http://dx.doi.org/10.1016/j.neuron.2007.03.015.

Steuber, V., Schultheiss, N. W., Silver, R. A., De Schutter, E., & Jaeger, D. (2011). Determinants of synaptic integration and heterogeneity in rebound firing explored with data-driven models of deep cerebellar nucleus cells. *Journal of Computational Neuroscience, 30*(3), 633–658. http://dx.doi.org/10.1007/s10827-010-0282-z.

Tadayonnejad, R., Anderson, D., Molineux, M. L., Mehaffey, W. H., Jayasuriya, K., & Turner, R. W. (2010). Rebound discharge in deep cerebellar nuclear neurons in vitro. *Cerebellum, 9*(3), 352–374. http://dx.doi.org/10.1007/s12311-010-0168-7.

Telgkamp, P., & Raman, I. M. (2002). Depression of inhibitory synaptic transmission between Purkinje cells and neurons of the cerebellar nuclei. *Journal of Neuroscience, 22*(19), 8447–8457.

Thach, W. T. (1970a). Discharge of cerebellar neurons related to two maintained postures and two prompt movements. I. Nuclear cell output. *Journal of Neurophysiology, 33*(4), 527–536.

Thach, W. T. (1970b). Discharge of cerebellar neurons related to two maintained postures and two prompt movements. II. Purkinje cell output and input. *Journal of Neurophysiology, 33*(4), 537–547.

Tsai, P. T., Hull, C., Chu, Y., Greene-Colozzi, E., Sadowski, A. R., Leech, J. M., et al. (2012). Autistic-like behaviour and cerebellar dysfunction in Purkinje cell Tsc1 mutant mice. *Nature, 488*(7413), 647–651. http://dx.doi.org/10.1038/nature11310.

Uusisaari, M., & De Schutter, E. (2011). The mysterious microcircuitry of the cerebellar nuclei. *JournalofPhysiology,589*(Pt14),3441–3457.http://dx.doi.org/10.1113/jphysiol.2010.201582 pii: jphysiol.2010.201582.

Uusisaari, M. Y., & Knopfel, T. (2012). Diversity of neuronal Elements and circuitry in the cerebellar nuclei. *Cerebellum*. http://dx.doi.org/10.1007/s12311-011-0350-6.

Uusisaari, M., Obata, K., & Knopfel, T. (2007). Morphological and electrophysiological properties of GABAergic and non-GABAergic cells in the deep cerebellar nuclei. *Journal of Neurophysiology, 97*(1), 901–911. http://dx.doi.org/10.1152/jn.00974.2006 pii: 00974.2006.

Walter, J. T., Alvina, K., Womack, M. D., Chevez, C., & Khodakhah, K. (2006). Decreases in the precision of Purkinje cell pacemaking cause cerebellar dysfunction and ataxia. *Nature Neuroscience, 9*(3), 389–397. http://dx.doi.org/10.1038/nn1648.

Weaver, C. M., & Wearne, S. L. (2008). Neuronal firing sensitivity to morphologic and active membrane parameters. *PLoS Computational Biology, 4*(1), e11. http://dx.doi.org/10.1371/journal.pcbi.0040011.

Wetmore, D. Z., Mukamel, E. A., & Schnitzer, M. J. (2008). Lock-and-key mechanisms of cerebellar memory recall based on rebound currents. *Journal of Neurophysiology, 100*(4), 2328–2347. http://dx.doi.org/10.1152/jn.00344.2007.

Yamazaki, T., & Nagao, S. (2012). A computational mechanism for unified gain and timing control in the cerebellum. *PLoS One, 7*(3), e33319. http://dx.doi.org/10.1371/journal.pone.0033319.

Yamazaki, T., & Tanaka, S. (2007). A spiking network model for passage-of-time representation in the cerebellum. *European Journal of Neuroscience, 26*(8), 2279–2292. http://dx.doi.org/10.1111/j.1460-9568.2007.05837.x.

Zhou, H., Lin, Z., Voges, K., Ju, C., Gao, Z., Bosman, L. W., et al. (2014). Cerebellar modules operate at different frequencies. *Elife, 3*, e02536. http://dx.doi.org/10.7554/eLife.02536.

6

Cerebrocerebellar Loops in the Rodent Brain

Clément Léna, Daniela Popa

Institut de Biologie de l'ENS (IBENS), Inserm U1024, CNRS 8197,
École Normale Supérieure, Paris, France

INTRODUCTION

If one compares the rodent and the human brains, their structure scales up quite differently: while the total number of neurons is multiplied by a factor of 400 between adult rats and humans, the number of hippocampal neurons is increased by a modest factor of 20 (West & Gundersen, 1990; West, Slomianka, & Gundersen, 1991). In contrast, the number of neurons in the cerebellum and in the cerebral cortex (which might represent up to respectively 80 and 19% of human brain neurons) scales up by keeping their ratio constant (Herculano-Houzel, 2010). A complex, polysynaptic circuit reciprocally connects the cerebellum and the cerebral cortex: several mesencephalic and pontine nuclei relay inputs from the cerebral cortex to the cerebellum, and the cerebellum returns projections to portions of the cerebral cortex via multiple diencephalic nuclei. Many behavioral and theoretical studies have led to the general notion that the corticocerebellar circuit subserves the formation of "internal models," which provide representations of the expected outcome of actions or of actions required to obtain a desired outcome (Ito, 2008; Wolpert, Miall, & Kawato, 1998). However, the neurophysiological analysis of the processes that underlie these models has made limited progress since the early recognition of functional cerebrocerebellar and cerebellocerebral connections (reviewed in Allen & Tsukahara, 1974), and the degree of specific reciprocity in these connections has long been unclear. Still, major progress has been achieved in the analysis of the anatomical organization of this circuit and in deciphering the modular structure of the cerebellum; this knowledge, coupled to the

The Neuronal Codes of the Cerebellum
http://dx.doi.org/10.1016/B978-0-12-801386-1.00006-X

advent of massively parallel recordings and optogenetic approaches, shall revolutionize our understanding of the operations taking place between and within the cerebellum and the cerebral cortex. This chapter provides an overview of current knowledge and general principles that seem to govern the organization of these circuits, with a strong emphasis on data obtained from rats and mice.

THE CORTICOCEREBELLAR PATHWAY

The cerebral cortex contributes to the two main types of inputs to the cerebellum, the mossy fibers and the climbing fibers. However, these projections are generally indirect and relayed by structures in the midbrain, pons, and medulla.

Cerebellar mossy fibers relaying cortical inputs emanate primarily from the pontine nuclei and to a lesser extent from a set of nuclei associated with the reticular formation (notably the basal pontine reticulotegmental and the lateral reticular nuclei). Retrograde and anterograde studies indicate that most cortical regions contribute to this descending pathway, although the frontal and parietal areas provide major contributions while the temporal regions provide more modest inputs (Leergaard & Bjaalie, 2007; Legg, Mercier, & Glickstein, 1989; Wiesendanger & Wiesendanger, 1982a, 1982b). The cortical projections to the pontine nuclei emanate from a specific set of glutamatergic pyramidal neurons in layer V. Early retrograde tracing experiments suggested a limited overlap between the pyramidal cell populations contributing to the four major corticopontine, corticorubral, corticostriatal, and corticospinal (pre)motor pathways (Akintunde & Buxton, 1992). Retrograde labeling experiments have revealed that corticopontine cells are found solely in layer Vb, while corticostriatal cells are mostly located in cortical layer Va (with some labeling in layer Vb). These downward projections may be quite divergent since a quarter of the rodent's barrel field corticopontine neurons was estimated to send collaterals to the superior colliculus (Mercier, Legg, & Glickstein, 1990). Single-axon reconstruction studies demonstrated that most pyramidal tract- (Mercier et al., 1990) and cerebral- (Donoghue & Kitai, 1981; Levesque, Charara, Gagnon, Parent, & Deschenes, 1996) projecting neurons in the rat emit collaterals to the striatum. Still, two separated downward-projection channels emanate from layer V of the cortex, projecting respectively either to the brain stem/spinal cord and ipsilateral striatum or bilaterally to the striatum. The cortical neurons projecting bilaterally to the striatum entrain, via excitatory collaterals, the pontine-projecting cortical neurons, suggesting a hierarchical order between these subcircuits, the corticostriatal circuit being situated upstream from the corticopontine circuit (Kiritani, Wickersham, Seung, & Shepherd, 2012;

Morishima & Kawaguchi, 2006; Morishima, Morita, Kubota, & Kawaguchi, 2011). It shall be noted that the brain-stem/spinal cord-projecting pathways in rodents are probably less differentiated in rodents than in primates (see the comment in Smith, Wichmann, & DeLong, 2014).

The corticopontine projections exhibit a high level of topographical organization (Leergaard & Bjaalie, 2007; Legg et al., 1989; Panto, Cicirata, Angaut, Parenti, & Serapide, 1995; Wiesendanger & Wiesendanger, 1982b). Pontine territories receiving from the motor and sensory cortices are generally distinct, even when they are related to the same body area: barrel field cortex terminals and vibrissae motor cortex terminate in separate fields (Leergaard et al., 2004; Mihailoff, Lee, Watt, & Yates, 1985; Proville et al., 2014; Schwarz & Mock, 2001); interestingly, the strength of corticopontine projections, measured as an estimated number of terminal varicosities, is higher for the vibrissae sensory cortex input than for the vibrissae motor cortex input. Cortical projections to the basal pontine nuclei are typically organized as predominantly ipsilateral lamellar structures organized by a combination of mediolateral and inside-out arrangement rules (Leergaard & Bjaalie, 2007). Whereas different cortical regions generally end up in different lamellae, evidence points toward some occasional convergence: projections from cortical barrels corresponding to a single row of vibrissae—but not to different rows (Hoffer, Arantes, Roth, & Alloway, 2005; Leergaard, Alloway, Mutic, & Bjaalie, 2000; Schwarz & Mock, 2001)—or from several anteroposterior regions in the medial prefrontal cortex (Moya et al., 2014) exhibit some degree of overlap in the same lamellae. Moreover, the primary and secondary sensory vibrissae cortices exhibit a strikingly high degree of convergence in the pontine nuclei (Leergaard et al., 2004).

The basal pontine nuclei also receive inputs from a number of subcortical brain structures (Mihailoff, Kosinski, Azizi, & Border, 1989), allowing the convergence of direct and indirect corticopontine pathways; evidence for such convergence has been observed in tracing studies for medial–prefrontal cortex and hypothalamic inputs to the pontine nuclei (Allen & Hopkins, 1998). Similarly, cuneo- and gracilopontine fibers partially overlap with corticopontine projections from forelimb sensory and hind-limb sensorimotor cortical regions, respectively (Kosinski, Azizi, & Mihailoff, 1988; Kosinski, Neafsey, & Castro, 1986). In contrast, while the superior colliculus receives inputs from the somatosensory and visual cortices, the colliculopontine projections reach different pontine compartments than the somatosensory and visual cortices (Schwarz, Horowski, Mock, & Thier, 2005). In monkeys, transsynaptic retrograde tracings have provided evidence for a corticosubthalamic–pontine pathway (Bostan, Dum, & Strick, 2010), but there has been so far little evidence for such a circuit in the rat brain, although projections from the subthalamic area to the pontine and reticulotegmental nuclei have been found to emanate from the zona incerta and fields of Forel (Mihailoff et al., 1989; Ricardo, 1981; Torigoe, Blanks, & Precht, 1986b).

The nature of the integration taking place in the pontine nuclei is still unresolved. The functional integration of inputs from different cortical regions has been suggested by single-unit electrophysiological studies in the rat (Potter, Ruegg, & Wiesendanger, 1978). However, the dendritic trees of single pontine neurons rarely cross the borders of cortical afferent fields, suggesting that they remain within the terminal fields of a single cortical area (Schwarz et al., 2005; Schwarz & Thier, 1995), leaving the early electrophysiological data unexplained. Little coupling between pontine neurons seems to take place via pontopontic connections, but reciprocal connections between pontine and cerebellar nuclei neurons could permit the integration of information across pontine areas (Lee & Mihailoff, 1990; Mock, Butovas, & Schwarz, 2006; Watt & Mihailoff, 1983).

The reticulotegmental nucleus of the pons is another relay of cortical inputs to the cerebellum, mostly from ipsilateral prefrontal, sensorimotor, and cingular cortices (Torigoe, Blanks, & Precht, 1986a). The rostromedial part of the lateral reticular nucleus also provides a (modest) relay of inputs mostly from the contralateral sensorimotor cortex (Rajakumar, Hrycyshyn, & Flumerfelt, 1992; Shokunbi, Hrycyshyn, & Flumerfelt, 1986). The vestibulocerebellum may receive cortical inputs via the pontine nuclei and potentially via reticular areas (Eisenman & Noback, 1980; Ruigrok, 2003), and via the vestibular nuclei, which receive direct projections from a parietotemporal region and a few more sensorimotor areas (Nishiike, Guldin, & Baurle, 2000) their.

Overall, the available evidence suggests that these descending pathways from the cortex are organized into numerous parallel channels, with occasional convergence for specific inputs allowing a limited degree of integration.

MOSSY FIBERS

Mossy fibers carrying cerebral cortex information emanate primarily from the pontine, reticulotegmental, and lateral reticular nuclei. The topography of these projections is complex and its connection with the modular organization of the cerebellum (e.g., Apps & Hawkes, 2009) is not yet fully understood.

In the pontine nuclei, retrograde tracing from the cerebellar cortex often results in patchy patterns reminiscent of the lamellar organization of corticopontine terminal fields, each cerebellar area receiving inputs from distinct pontine sources, which relay separate cortical inputs (e.g., Eisenman, 1981; Leergaard, Lillehaug, De Schutter, Bower, & Bjaalie, 2006; Odeh, Ackerley, Bjaalie, & Apps, 2005; Pijpers & Ruigrok, 2006). In the rat, the pontine nuclei project predominantly to the posterior cerebellar cortex (Serapide, Panto, Parenti, Zappala, & Cicirata, 2001). Projections from the pontine, reticulotegmental, and lateral reticular nuclei produce bilateral patterns of terminals with various degrees of preference: mostly contralateral for the pontine and reticulotegmental nuclei and ipsilateral for the lateral reticular nucleus. Ipsi- and contralateral projections emanate from largely distinct pools of pontine neurons (Herrero, Pardoe, & Apps, 2002; Mihailoff, 1983; Serapide, Zappala, Parenti, Panto, & Cicirata, 2002; Wu, Sugihara, & Shinoda, 1999). Small retrograde tracer injections in the cerebellum-labeled cells spread over relatively extended territories, which are more densely populated by larger tracer injections at the same site, suggesting that pontocerebellar projections are specified between territories rather than in a point-to-point manner (Mihailoff, Burne, Azizi, Norell, & Woodward, 1981).

The mapping of the cerebral cortex on the cerebellar cortex is not fully resolved. Transsynaptic retrograde labeling from various target areas in the posterior cerebellum of the rat revealed that each area receives inputs from widespread albeit different sets of cortical regions. Paravermal and hemispheric portions of lobules VIII (copula), VII (paramedian lobule), and crus II receive convergent inputs from motor and sensory areas of the cortical regions involved respectively in hind-limb, forelimb, and face sensorimotor processing, corresponding broadly to the distribution of peripheral inputs to these lobules; a mediolateral gradient of sensory versus motor cortex inputs was also noted in these lobules (Suzuki, Coulon, Sabel-Goedknegt, & Ruigrok, 2012). The posterior cerebellum also receives peripheral inputs via the mossy fiber system, and electrophysiological mapping demonstrated that they are distributed in patches with substantial redundancy, but little somatotopy (Shambes, Gibson, & Welker, 1978). This segmentation is conditioned by the modular, mediolateral, zonal organization of the cerebellum characterized by zebrin immunoreactivity, but also by a supplementary anteroposterior segmentation (Hallem et al., 1999): the same zebrin band may thus receive peripheral inputs from different body parts in different lobules. Electrophysiological recordings have documented the convergence of peripheral and cerebral inputs: recordings from the granular layer of crus II following various facial sensory stimuli revealed topographically organized, spatially confined, biphasic responses with an early component due to direct trigeminal inputs and a late component relayed by the corresponding facial part of the sensory cortex (Morissette & Bower, 1996). Superior colliculus inputs may also converge with these sensory inputs with a high degree of specificity (Kassel, 1980). Convergence at the level of single Golgi cells (i.e., interneurons of the granular layer) of inputs from the trigeminal nucleus and sensory and motor cortices of the mystacial vibrissae have been observed in the lateral hemisphere of crus I; a similar sensorimotor convergence for the perioral cortical regions was also found in crus II (Proville et al., 2014). Anatomical reconstruction also revealed that single granule cells may integrate peripheral and pontine inputs (Huang et al., 2013). All these elements argue for a strong convergence of peripheral and cerebral sensorimotor inputs in the cerebellar hemispheres.

Injections of anterograde tracers in the pons occasionally reveal an organization of mossy fiber terminals from the pontine nuclei arrayed in sagittal stripes extending across more than one lobule (Mihailoff, 1993). These stripes are often bilateral and symmetric, with a preference for the side contralateral to the tracer injection site; pairs of small injections may reveal complementary terminal stripes, while wider injection sites produce diffuse labeling as expected if multiple sets of stripes were targeted (Serapide et al., 2001). Stripes are also observed for reticulotegmental projections (Serapide, Parenti, Panto, Zappala, & Cicirata, 2002) and for lateral reticular projections (Wu et al., 1999). Autoradiographic mapping of glucose uptake following stimulation of the vibrissae or the forelimb motor cortices revealed an increased metabolism in a large network encompassing distinct subterritories of the pontine nuclei, different patterns in the cerebellar nuclei, and distinct stripes in the granule layer of the lobules crus I and II and (for the forelimb motor cortex) copula (Sharp & Evans, 1982; Sharp & Ryan, 1984).

One of the best markers of the modular zonation of the cerebellar cortex is provided by the climbing fiber receptive fields and by their anatomical origin (Apps & Hawkes, 2009). Injections of retrograde tracers in defined zones of the copula, paramedian lobule, and crus II showed that the topography of the pontocerebellar projections is not only constrained by the zonal target, but is also distributed according to the lobules, with pontine areas relaying hind-limb, forelimb, and face sensory cortices projecting respectively to the copula, lateral paramedian lobule, and crus II/medial paramedial lobule (Odeh et al., 2005; Pijpers & Ruigrok, 2006). Interestingly, the redundancy of climbing fiber receptive fields is not reflected in the pontocerebellar projections: injections of retrograde tracers in the forelimb C1 zone of distant lobules (simplex and paramedian) reveals overlapping climbing fiber origin in the inferior olive but very limited shared pontine inputs (Herrero et al., 2002). Small injections of retrograde tracers, targeting individual zebrin zones of the copula, provided a finer description of the topography of pontocerebellar projections and demonstrated that pontine afferents to different zebrin zones (either positive or negative) emanate from largely distinct territories and cell populations (Cerminara, Aoki, Loft, Sugihara, & Apps, 2013). Similarly, retrograde injections from the C and D2 zone of the vibrissae-related area of crus I emanate from largely distinct (but intermingled) pontine populations (Proville et al., 2014).

In humans, the topography of cerebrocerebellar functional connectivity has been examined in studies of resting state brain activity; these studies have revealed a multiplicity of cerebrocerebellar patterns of covariance in the blood oxygen-level-dependent (BOLD) signal (Bernard et al., 2012; Buckner, Krienen, Castellanos, Diaz, & Yeo, 2011; Habas et al., 2009; Kipping et al., 2013; Krienen & Buckner, 2009; O'Reilly, Beckmann, Tomassini, Ramnani, & Johansen-Berg, 2010; Sang et al., 2012). The meaning of these patterns is not fully known, but since the BOLD signal is probably dominated by the granular layer signal (Howarth, Peppiatt-Wildman, & Attwell, 2010; discussion in Diedrichsen, Verstynen, Schlerf, & Wiestler, 2010), these patterns probably reveal the topography of the mossy fiber inputs to the cerebellar cortex. They show both segregation and redundancy of cerebrocerebellar connections; moreover the cerebellar areas are coupled to whole cortical circuits, which could result from the convergence of cortical inputs from regions belonging to these defined circuits (sensorimotor, visual, default mode, etc.). Patterns of activations in the cerebellum during behavior also vary as a function of the task (e.g., see Stoodley & Schmahmann, 2009 for a meta-analysis); the comparison between the resting-state and the task-related cerebrocerebellar activation patterns supports that they both reflect preferential cerebrocerebellar connectivity patterns (Balsters, Laird, Fox, & Eickhoff, 2014; Buckner et al., 2011).

Overall, these studies point to a complex and refined topography of the pontocerebellar projections, which exhibit some degree of convergence but are constrained according to the zonal segmentation and the functional segmentation of the granular layer. It shall be noted that the cerebellar nuclei also receive direct projections: anterograde tracing from the pontine nuclei revealed a predominantly (~90%) contralateral projection to the lateral (or dentate) nucleus and to portions of the intermediate nucleus, while the reticulotegmental projections target areas distributed across all cerebellar nuclei with a more bilateral pattern (Mihailoff, 1993; Parenti, Zappala, Serapide, Panto, & Cicirata, 2002). Reconstruction of single pontocerebellar axons in the cat revealed that they systematically gave rise to mossy fibers in the granular layer but only half of them exhibited pontonuclear collaterals (Shinoda, Sugiuchi, Futami, & Izawa, 1992). Such a study has not been replicated in the rat. How these pontonuclear projections converge with Purkinje cell inputs in the cerebellar nuclei remains to be investigated.

CLIMBING FIBERS

The cerebral cortex also exerts some control over the climbing fiber afferents to the cerebellum. However, the organization of the cerebro-olivary pathways in the rat is far less characterized compared to the corticopontocerebellar mossy fiber pathway. Experiments conducted in the rat paramedian lobule and crus II demonstrated that the activation of corticofugal fibers by stimulation in the pyramidal tract triggers, with diverse latencies, climbing fiber discharge throughout the explored hemispheric and paravermal portions of these lobules (Ackerley, Pardoe, & Apps, 2006; Baker, Javid, & Edgley, 2001). Anterograde tracing experiments suggested the existence of broad direct olivary projections from the sensorimotor cortices, with a labeling pattern in the inferior olive subnuclei depending heavily on the cortical region injected (Swenson, Sievert, Terreberry, Neafsey, & Castro, 1989). However, more recent tracing experiments failed to evidence direct afferents from the forelimb and hind-limb motor cortices and forelimb sensory cortex to the inferior olive (Ackerley et al., 2006; Lee & Kim, 2012), but revealed discrete direct projections from the dysgranular zone of the cortex, a region involved in processing deep somatic inputs, to the dorsal inferior olive (Lee & Kim, 2012). An area situated ventral to the dorsal column nuclei was found to relay motor cortex inputs to the inferior olive (Ackerley et al., 2006). This area could indeed correspond to the dorsal column nucleus relay to the C1 and C3 zones formerly identified in the cat (Andersson, 1984). The inferior olive also receives afferents from a number of brain structures, such as the red nucleus, situated around the mesodiencephalic junction (Ruigrok, 2004; Swenson & Castro, 1983), which receives input from the cerebral cortex. The convergence of mesodiencephalic inputs with cerebellar (GABAergic) inputs to single glomeruli has been reported in the rostral medial accessory and posterior olive (respectively innervating the C2 and D zones) of the rat (de Zeeuw, Holstege, Ruigrok, & Voogd, 1990). How ascending sensory inputs and cerebral (direct or indirect) inputs are combined in the inferior olive is unknown. Studies in cats and monkeys support a refined functional organization of the cerebro-olivary pathway (see the review in Voogd, 2014) but the detailed functional organization of the cerebro-olivary pathway in the rat remains still largely unexplored.

PARALLEL FIBERS

The excitation provided by the mossy fibers to the granule cells is propagated to the Purkinje cells via the parallel fibers and entrains the simple spike firing of these cells. The parallel fibers may extend over the whole transverse axis of the hemispheres and therefore propagate the variety of granule cell inputs to all the Purkinje cells they encounter in the mediolateral axis. The Purkinje cells could be potentially entrained—via the parallel fibers—by all the mossy fiber inputs found in the mediolateral axis of the lobule and, therefore, the topography of the mossy fiber inputs to the granule cells could be totally absent in the overlying Purkinje cell layer.

The examination of sensory simple spike receptive fields of Purkinje cells in the rat hemisphere reveals instead a strong resemblance to the granule cell layer receptive field underneath (Bower & Woolston, 1983). This has led to the proposal that simple spike responses are entrained by the ascending axon of granule cells (Gundappa-Sulur, De Schutter, & Bower, 1999). Ex vivo inspection of connections between single granule cells and Purkinje cells (in the vermis and paravermal areas) confirmed that most parallel fibers do not trigger measurable synaptic currents in the Purkinje cells they contact, but these data do not support the hypothesis of distinct inputs from the ascending axon (Isope & Barbour, 2002). The global mapping of granule cell layer inputs (stimulated by glutamate uncaging in the vermis) to neighboring Purkinje cells also supports a substantial entrainment by the local granule layer via the parallel fiber system but little bias in favor of the ascending axon (Walter, Dizon, & Khodakhah, 2009). In the C3 zone of the decerebrated cat cerebellum, there is a good correspondence only between the receptive fields of mossy fibers and climbing fibers impinging on the overlying Purkinje cells, but these are anticorrelated with—or spatially distant from—the simple spike receptive field (Ekerot & Jorntell, 2001), indicating a dominant contribution of distant granule cells located in a neighboring microzone in the modulation of Purkinje cell firing. The correspondence between mossy fiber and climbing sensory receptive fields is also observed in the rat cerebellum (Brown & Bower, 2001). The mapping of the single vibrissae sensory response in the mouse crus lobules demonstrated that the climbing fiber receptive fields exhibited no systematic relation with the simple spike receptive fields (Bosman et al., 2010), suggesting that the correspondence between mossy and climbing fiber receptive fields is valid only at the regional level. A regional confinement of incoming mossy fiber excitation following white matter stimulation was observed with voltage-sensitive dyes (Cohen & Yarom, 1998; Rokni, Llinas, & Yarom, 2007). Although the studies cited above do not single out the pontine inputs, the available evidence is consistent with the notion that Purkinje cells are primarily driven (as far as the receptive fields approach can reveal) by mossy fibers emanating from a neighboring territory. For pontine inputs, evidence indeed showed that in crus I of mice, the predominance of responses to the stimulation of the vibrissae sensory and motor cortices was observed in the granule and Purkinje cell layers in the lateral but not in the medial part of the lobule (Proville et al., 2014), consistent with the limited spread of pontine mossy fiber excitation to distant Purkinje cells via parallel fibers.

CEREBELLOCEREBRAL CONNECTIONS

Purkinje cell inhibitory projections from the cerebellar cortex to the nuclei are highly organized following the zonal organization of the cerebellum as reviewed elsewhere (e.g., Ruigrok, 2011); injections of small amounts of a retrograde tracer in to the cerebellar nuclei indeed label ipsilateral narrow bands of Purkinje cells, consistent with a precise mapping of cerebellar cortical microzones in the nuclei (Ruigrok, 2011; Sugihara et al., 2009). The cerebellum then projects to the cerebral cortex via nucleodiencephalic, primarily contralateral, excitatory projections. All the cerebellar nuclei contribute differentially to these projections, and a small subset of diencephalic structures concentrate most of the cerebellar inputs: ventrolateral and posterior medial thalamic nuclei, intralaminar nuclei (centrolateral, centromedial, parafascicular), zona incerta, ventromedial nuclei (Angaut, Cicirata, & Serapide, 1985; Aumann, Rawson, Finkelstein, & Horne, 1994; Teune, van der Burg, van der Moer, Voogd, & Ruigrok, 2000). The cerebellar inputs are never very abundant: even in the ventrolateral thalamus, which receives strong cerebellar projections, cerebellar synapses are estimated to represent less than 10% of the synapses, the others coming principally from the cerebral cortex and the reticular thalamus (Aumann & Horne, 1999; Sawyer, Tepper, & Groves, 1994). However, these inputs are rather powerful: cerebellar stimulations produce, in the ventrolateral thalamocortical neurons, relatively large excitatory synaptic potentials (several millivolts) with little gradation of the responses, suggesting that they emanate from few axons (Sawyer, Young, Groves, & Tepper, 1994). Cerebellar terminals exhibit a similar ultrastructural appearance (large boutons, packed with synaptic vesicles and mitochondria, with perforated synaptic densities) in all diencephalic structures examined so far (Aumann & Horne, 1996; Aumann et al., 1994), suggesting that they share the same functional properties.

Overall, the main diencephalic structures recipient of cerebellar inputs project primarily to the frontal cortex, dorsal striatum, and sensory cortex. Interestingly, while the cerebellum is, as the basal ganglia, a major afferent of the frontal cortex, the cerebellar and basal ganglia channels remain remarkably segregated in the ventrolateral thalamus (Deniau, Kita, & Kitai, 1992; Kuramoto et al., 2011). The ventrolateral thalamus projects to multiple layers in the cortex (II–V), with a dense innervation to layer VB where it excites pyramidal tract neurons (Kuramoto et al., 2009), therefore allowing the cerebro-ponto-cerebello-thalamo-cerebral loops to close.

The hierarchical structure of the cerebrostriatal and cerebrocerebellar circuit (see above) is not entirely respected: the cerebellum provides excitatory inputs to the striatum via the centrolateral (Chen, Fremont, Arteaga-Bracho, & Khodakhah, 2014) and possibly the parafascicular nuclei, which receive a cerebellar innervation from the lateral and medial nuclei. Moreover the ventromedial thalamus, which provides extensive projections to cortical layer I, might exhibit convergent inputs from the basal ganglia and cerebellum, although in contrast to the cat (Steriade, 1995), these afferents seem to be weak in the rat (Aumann et al., 1994; Deniau et al., 1992; Kuramoto et al., 2011). The zona incerta could also be an area of convergence with the basal ganglia inputs, and a relay toward layer I of the cortex (Lin, Nicolelis, & Chapin, 1997), but very few data are available on these connections.

Single-axon tracing from the ventrolateral thalamus revealed wider projection patterns than found in sensory thalamocortical projections: each axon targets multiple motor and sensory cortical regions (Aumann, Ivanusic, & Horne, 1998; Kuramoto et al., 2009), suggestive of a broad divergence of this pathway. Similarly, single posterior thalamic neurons target multiple cortical regions (Ohno et al., 2012), consistent with a role of the cerebellum in the coordination of neuronal activity between distant cortical sites (Popa et al., 2013).

FUNCTIONAL MAPPING OF THE CEREBELLOCEREBRAL CONNECTIONS

So far, there has been still little functional mapping of the cerebellar cortex onto the cerebral cortex. In the cat, microstimulations in the cerebellar nuclei at sites receiving from a distinct cerebellar microzone revealed wide but distinct patterns of activation in the motor cortex (Jorntell & Ekerot, 1999). In the monkey, transsynaptic retrograde tracing from cortical regions tend to label broad cerebellar territories (Kelly & Strick, 2003; Lu, Miyachi, Ito, Nambu, & Takada, 2007; Prevosto, Graf, & Ugolini, 2010), and functionally distinct cortical regions receive inputs from overlapping cerebellar territories (Lu et al., 2007). Testing the specificity of the connections requires functional approaches. The functional mapping of cerebellar projections to the cerebral cortex is complicated by the inhibitory nature of the projections from the cerebellar cortex. In mice, the functional input from crus I to the motor cortex has been investigated using the rebound activity taking place in the cerebellocerebral network following Purkinje cell optogenetic stimulation (Proville et al., 2014); stimulation of the Purkinje cells in the area receiving dense inputs from the vibrissae motor cortex, the lateral crus I, but not of the adjacent cerebellar areas triggered an activation of the vibrissae motor cortex; this demonstrates the existence of specific corticocerebrocortical loops, as suggested by transsynaptic viral tracing (Kelly & Strick, 2003).

Functional synchronization of population activity between the cerebral cortex and the cerebellar cortex and nuclei has indeed been reported in unanesthetized animals (O'Connor, Berg, & Kleinfeld, 2002; Ros, Sachdev, Yu, Sestan, & McCormick, 2009), but they exhibit a rather loose temporal relationship (100 ms time scale). Coherent activities are also found in anesthetized animals and directed transfer function analysis points rather toward an entrainment of the cerebellar circuit by the cerebral cortex than the reverse (Rowland, Goldberg, & Jaeger, 2010), but this might be due to the disruption of the mossy fiber excitation by anesthesia (Bengtsson & Jorntell,

2007), which would thus prevent cerebellar computations from being generated before being fed back to the cortex. Indeed, in the unanesthetized condition, the optogenetic interruption of the cerebrocerebellar loop resulted in a change in the whisking behavior, an effect that required an intact motor thalamus (Proville et al., 2014). Moreover, the selective disruption of a single parameter of whisking in this study suggests that, despite the apparent divergence of the cerebellocerebral pathways (see above), there is a rather sharp functional selectivity in the target of these pathways.

CONCLUSION

One of the striking features of the cerebellocerebral connections is their asymmetry: most of the cortex projects to the cerebellum, but fewer cortical regions concentrate most of the inputs from the cerebellum. The studies of the sensorimotor system indicate that some of this reduction takes place in the cerebellar cortex where sensory and motor cortical inputs, together with peripheral and tectal inputs, may converge. However, the cerebellar cortex seems to primarily combine inputs of various origins but linked to the same body part. The ascending cerebellocerebral pathway is certainly less characterized and might seem to be more divergent. Indeed, the wide divergence of single thalamic cells relaying cerebellar inputs to the sensorimotor cortex contrasts with the functional evidence of selective cerebrocerebellar loops and with the discrete, specific, behavioral effects observed by the targeted disruption of these loops. Therefore the topographic divergence of the cerebellocerebral connections might rather reflect the topographically-distributed nature of sensorimotor representations in the cortex than a lack of specificity of cerebrocerebellar loops. In rodents, most of the principles of the functional organization of the cerebrocerebellar circuitry have been (and probably will continue to be) derived in the sensorimotor system. A major task now is to understand the computations performed in this circuit. Finally, a significant portion of the cerebrocerebellar loops in humans might be involved in higher-order, associative or cognitive functions (Buckner, 2013); finding and studying such loops in the rodent brain is certainly also an important challenge for the coming years.

References

Ackerley, R., Pardoe, J., & Apps, R. (2006). A novel site of synaptic relay for climbing fibre pathways relaying signals from the motor cortex to the cerebellar cortical C1 zone. *The Journal of Physiology, 576*(Pt 2), 503–518.
Akintunde, A., & Buxton, D. F. (1992). Origins and collateralization of corticospinal, corticopontine, corticorubral and corticostriatal tracts: a multiple retrograde fluorescent tracing study. *Brain Research, 586*(2), 208–218.

Allen, G. V., & Hopkins, D. A. (1998). Convergent prefrontal cortex and mamillary body projections to the medial pontine nuclei: a light and electron microscopic study in the rat. *Journal of Comparative Neurology, 398*(3), 347–358.

Allen, G. I., & Tsukahara, N. (1974). Cerebrocerebellar communication systems. *Physiological Reviews, 54*(4), 957–1006.

Andersson, G. (1984). Demonstration of a cuneate relay in a cortico-olivo-cerebellar pathway in the cat. *Neuroscience Letters, 46*(1), 47–52.

Angaut, P., Cicirata, F., & Serapide, F. (1985). Topographic organization of the cerebellothalamic projections in the rat. An autoradiographic study. *Neuroscience, 15*(2), 389–401.

Apps, R., & Hawkes, R. (2009). Cerebellar cortical organization: a one-map hypothesis. *Nature Reviews Neuroscience, 10*(9), 670–681.

Aumann, T. D., & Horne, M. K. (1996). A comparison of the ultrastructure of synapses in the cerebello-rubral and cerebello-thalamic pathways in the rat. *Neuroscience Letters, 211*(3), 175–178.

Aumann, T. D., & Horne, M. K. (1999). Ultrastructural change at rat cerebellothalamic synapses associated with volitional motor adaptation. *Journal of Comparative Neurology, 409*(1), 71–84.

Aumann, T. D., Ivanusic, J., & Horne, M. K. (1998). Arborisation and termination of single motor thalamocortical axons in the rat. *Journal of Comparative Neurology, 396*(1), 121–130.

Aumann, T. D., Rawson, J. A., Finkelstein, D. I., & Horne, M. K. (1994). Projections from the lateral and interposed cerebellar nuclei to the thalamus of the rat: a light and electron microscopic study using single and double anterograde labelling. *Journal of Comparative Neurology, 349*(2), 165–181.

Baker, M. R., Javid, M., & Edgley, S. A. (2001). Activation of cerebellar climbing fibres to rat cerebellar posterior lobe from motor cortical output pathways. *The Journal of Physiology, 536*(Pt 3), 825–839.

Balsters, J. H., Laird, A. R., Fox, P. T., & Eickhoff, S. B. (2014). Bridging the gap between functional and anatomical features of cortico-cerebellar circuits using meta-analytic connectivity modeling. *Human Brain Mapping, 35*(7), 3152–3169.

Bengtsson, F., & Jorntell, H. (2007). Ketamine and xylazine depress sensory-evoked parallel fiber and climbing fiber responses. *Journal of Neurophysiology, 98*(3), 1697–1705.

Bernard, J. A., Seidler, R. D., Hassevoort, K. M., Benson, B. L., Welsh, R. C., Wiggins, J. L., et al. (2012). Resting state cortico-cerebellar functional connectivity networks: a comparison of anatomical and self-organizing map approaches. *Frontiers in Neuroanatomy, 6*, 31.

Bosman, L. W., Koekkoek, S. K., Shapiro, J., Rijken, B. F., Zandstra, F., van der Ende, B., et al. (2010). Encoding of whisker input by cerebellar Purkinje cells. *The Journal of Physiology, 588*(Pt 19), 3757–3783.

Bostan, A. C., Dum, R. P., & Strick, P. L. (2010). The basal ganglia communicate with the cerebellum. *Proceedings of the National Academy of Sciences of the United States of America, 107*(18), 8452–8456.

Bower, J. M., & Woolston, D. C. (1983). Congruence of spatial organization of tactile projections to granule cell and Purkinje cell layers of cerebellar hemispheres of the albino rat: vertical organization of cerebellar cortex. *Journal of Neurophysiology, 49*(3), 745–766.

Brown, I. E., & Bower, J. M. (2001). Congruence of mossy fiber and climbing fiber tactile projections in the lateral hemispheres of the rat cerebellum. *Journal of Comparative Neurology, 429*(1), 59–70.

Buckner, R. L. (2013). The cerebellum and cognitive function: 25 years of insight from anatomy and neuroimaging. *Neuron, 80*(3), 807–815.

Buckner, R. L., Krienen, F. M., Castellanos, A., Diaz, J. C., & Yeo, B. T. (2011). The organization of the human cerebellum estimated by intrinsic functional connectivity. *Journal of Neurophysiology, 106*(5), 2322–2345.

Cerminara, N. L., Aoki, H., Loft, M., Sugihara, I., & Apps, R. (2013). Structural basis of cerebellar microcircuits in the rat. *Journal of Neuroscience, 33*(42), 16427–16442.

Chen, C. H., Fremont, R., Arteaga-Bracho, E. E., & Khodakhah, K. (2014). Short latency cerebellar modulation of the basal ganglia. *Nature Neuroscience, 17*(12), 1767–1775.

Cohen, D., & Yarom, Y. (1998). Patches of synchronized activity in the cerebellar cortex evoked by mossy-fiber stimulation: questioning the role of parallel fibers. *Proceedings of the National Academy of Sciences of the United States of America, 95*(25), 15032–15036.

Deniau, J. M., Kita, H., & Kitai, S. T. (1992). Patterns of termination of cerebellar and basal ganglia efferents in the rat thalamus. Strictly segregated and partly overlapping projections. *Neuroscience Letters, 144*(1–2), 202–206.

Diedrichsen, J., Verstynen, T., Schlerf, J., & Wiestler, T. (2010). Advances in functional imaging of the human cerebellum. *Current Opinion Neurology, 23*(4), 382–387.

Donoghue, J. P., & Kitai, S. T. (1981). A collateral pathway to the neostriatum from corticofugal neurons of the rat sensory-motor cortex: an intracellular HRP study. *Journal of Comparative Neurology, 201*(1), 1–13.

Eisenman, L. M. (1981). Pontocerebellar projections to the pyramis and copula pyramidis in the rat: evidence for a mediolateral topography. *Journal of Comparative Neurology, 199*(1), 77–86.

Eisenman, L. M., & Noback, C. R. (1980). The ponto-cerebellar projection in the rat: differential projections to sublobules of the uvula. *Experimental Brain Research, 38*(1), 11–17.

Ekerot, C. F., & Jorntell, H. (2001). Parallel fibre receptive fields of Purkinje cells and interneurons are climbing fibre-specific. *European Journal of Neuroscience, 13*(7), 1303–1310.

Gundappa-Sulur, G., De Schutter, E., & Bower, J. M. (1999). Ascending granule cell axon: an important component of cerebellar cortical circuitry. *Journal of Comparative Neurology, 408*(4), 580–596.

Habas, C., Kamdar, N., Nguyen, D., Prater, K., Beckmann, C. F., Menon, V., et al. (2009). Distinct cerebellar contributions to intrinsic connectivity networks. *Journal of Neuroscience, 29*(26), 8586–8594.

Hallem, J. S., Thompson, J. H., Gundappa-Sulur, G., Hawkes, R., Bjaalie, J. G., & Bower, J. M. (1999). Spatial correspondence between tactile projection patterns and the distribution of the antigenic Purkinje cell markers anti-zebrin I and anti-zebrin II in the cerebellar folium crus IIA of the rat. *Neuroscience, 93*(3), 1083–1094.

Herculano-Houzel, S. (2010). Coordinated scaling of cortical and cerebellar numbers of neurons. *Frontiers in Neuroanatomy, 4*, 12.

Herrero, L., Pardoe, J., & Apps, R. (2002). Pontine and lateral reticular projections to the c1 zone in lobulus simplex and paramedian lobule of the rat cerebellar cortex. *Cerebellum, 1*(3), 185–199.

Hoffer, Z. S., Arantes, H. B., Roth, R. L., & Alloway, K. D. (2005). Functional circuits mediating sensorimotor integration: quantitative comparisons of projections from rodent barrel cortex to primary motor cortex, neostriatum, superior colliculus, and the pons. *Journal of Comparative Neurology, 488*(1), 82–100.

Howarth, C., Peppiatt-Wildman, C. M., Attwell, D. (2010). The energy use associated with neural computation in the cerebellum. *Journal of Cerebral Blood Flow Metabolism, 30*(2), 403–414.

Huang, C. C., Sugino, K., Shima, Y., Guo, C., Bai, S., Mensh, B. D., et al. (2013). Convergence of pontine and proprioceptive streams onto multimodal cerebellar granule cells. *Elife, 2*, e00400.

Isope, P., & Barbour, B. (2002). Properties of unitary granule cell-->Purkinje cell synapses in adult rat cerebellar slices. *Journal of Neuroscience, 22*(22), 9668–9678.

Ito, M. (2008). Control of mental activities by internal models in the cerebellum. *Nature Reviews Neuroscience, 9*(4), 304–313.

Jorntell, H., & Ekerot, C. F. (1999). Topographical organization of projections to cat motor cortex from nucleus interpositus anterior and forelimb skin. *The Journal of Physiology, 514*(Pt 2), 551–566.

Kassel, J. (1980). Superior colliculus projections to tactile areas of rat cerebellar hemispheres. *Brain Research, 202*(2), 291–305.

Kelly, R. M., & Strick, P. L. (2003). Cerebellar loops with motor cortex and prefrontal cortex of a nonhuman primate. *Journal of Neuroscience, 23*(23), 8432–8444.

Kipping, J. A., Grodd, W., Kumar, V., Taubert, M., Villringer, A., & Margulies, D. S. (2013). Overlapping and parallel cerebello-cerebral networks contributing to sensorimotor control: an intrinsic functional connectivity study. *Neuroimage, 83*, 837–848.

Kiritani, T., Wickersham, I. R., Seung, H. S., & Shepherd, G. M. (2012). Hierarchical connectivity and connection-specific dynamics in the corticospinal-corticostriatal microcircuit in mouse motor cortex. *Journal of Neuroscience, 32*(14), 4992–5001.

Kosinski, R. J., Azizi, S. A., & Mihailoff, G. A. (1988). Convergence of cortico- and cuneopontine projections onto components of the pontocerebellar system in the rat: an anatomical and electrophysiological study. *Experimental Brain Res, 71*(3), 541–556.

Kosinski, R. J., Neafsey, E. J., & Castro, A. J. (1986). A comparative topographical analysis of dorsal column nuclear and cerebral cortical projections to the basilar pontine gray in rats. *Journal of Comparative Neurology, 244*(2), 163–173.

Krienen, F. M., & Buckner, R. L. (2009). Segregated fronto-cerebellar circuits revealed by intrinsic functional connectivity. *Cerebral Cortex, 19*(10), 2485–2497.

Kuramoto, E., Fujiyama, F., Nakamura, K. C., Tanaka, Y., Hioki, H., & Kaneko, T. (2011). Complementary distribution of glutamatergic cerebellar and GABAergic basal ganglia afferents to the rat motor thalamic nuclei. *European Journal of Neuroscience, 33*(1), 95–109.

Kuramoto, E., Furuta, T., Nakamura, K. C., Unzai, T., Hioki, H., & Kaneko, T. (2009). Two types of thalamocortical projections from the motor thalamic nuclei of the rat: a single neuron-tracing study using viral vectors. *Cerebral Cortex, 19*(9), 2065–2077.

Lee, H. S., & Mihailoff, G. A. (1990). Convergence of cortical and cerebellar projections on single basilar pontine neurons: a light and electron microscopic study in the rat. *Neuroscience, 39*(3), 561–577.

Lee, T., & Kim, U. (2012). Descending projections from the dysgranular zone of rat primary somatosensory cortex processing deep somatic input. *Journal of Comparative Neurology, 520*(5), 1021–1046.

Leergaard, T. B., Alloway, K. D., Mutic, J. J., & Bjaalie, J. G. (2000). Three-dimensional topography of corticopontine projections from rat barrel cortex: correlations with corticostriatal organization. *Journal of Neuroscience, 20*(22), 8474–8484.

Leergaard, T. B., Alloway, K. D., Pham, T. A., Bolstad, I., Hoffer, Z. S., Pettersen, C., et al. (2004). Three-dimensional topography of corticopontine projections from rat sensorimotor cortex: comparisons with corticostriatal projections reveal diverse integrative organization. *Journal of Comparative Neurology, 478*(3), 306–322.

Leergaard, T. B., & Bjaalie, J. G. (2007). Topography of the complete corticopontine projection: from experiments to principal Maps. *Frontiers in Neuroscience, 1*(1), 211–223.

Leergaard, T. B., Lillehaug, S., De Schutter, E., Bower, J. M., & Bjaalie, J. G. (2006). Topographical organization of pathways from somatosensory cortex through the pontine nuclei to tactile regions of the rat cerebellar hemispheres. *European Journal of Neuroscience, 24*(10), 2801–2812.

Legg, C. R., Mercier, B., & Glickstein, M. (1989). Corticopontine projection in the rat: the distribution of labelled cortical cells after large injections of horseradish peroxidase in the pontine nuclei. *Journal of Comparative Neurology, 286*(4), 427–441.

Levesque, M., Charara, A., Gagnon, S., Parent, A., & Deschenes, M. (1996). Corticostriatal projections from layer V cells in rat are collaterals of long-range corticofugal axons. *Brain Research, 709*(2), 311–315.

Lin, R. C., Nicolelis, M. A., & Chapin, J. K. (1997). Topographic and laminar organizations of the incertocortical pathway in rats. *Neuroscience, 81*(3), 641–651.

Lu, X., Miyachi, S., Ito, Y., Nambu, A., & Takada, M. (2007). Topographic distribution of output neurons in cerebellar nuclei and cortex to somatotopic map of primary motor cortex. *European Journal of Neuroscience, 25*(8), 2374–2382.

Mercier, B. E., Legg, C. R., & Glickstein, M. (1990). Basal ganglia and cerebellum receive different somatosensory information in rats. *Proceedings of the National Academy of Sciences of the United States of America, 87*(11), 4388–4392.

Mihailoff, G. A. (1983). Intra- and interhemispheric collateral branching in the rat pontocerebellar system, a fluorescence double-label study. *Neuroscience, 10*(1), 141–160.

Mihailoff, G. A. (1993). Cerebellar nuclear projections from the basilar pontine nuclei and nucleus reticularis tegmenti pontis as demonstrated with PHA-L tracing in the rat. *Journal of Comparative Neurology, 330*(1), 130–146.

Mihailoff, G. A., Burne, R. A., Azizi, S. A., Norell, G., & Woodward, D. J. (1981). The pontocerebellar system in the rat: an HRP study. II. Hemispheral components. *Journal of Comparative Neurology, 197*(4), 559–577.

Mihailoff, G. A., Kosinski, R. J., Azizi, S. A., & Border, B. G. (1989). Survey of noncortical afferent projections to the basilar pontine nuclei: a retrograde tracing study in the rat. *Journal of Comparative Neurology, 282*(4), 617–643.

Mihailoff, G. A., Lee, H., Watt, C. B., & Yates, R. (1985). Projections to the basilar pontine nuclei from face sensory and motor regions of the cerebral cortex in the rat. *Journal of Comparative Neurology, 237*(2), 251–263.

Mock, M., Butovas, S., & Schwarz, C. (2006). Functional unity of the ponto-cerebellum: evidence that intrapontine communication is mediated by a reciprocal loop with the cerebellar nuclei. *Journal of Neurophysiology, 95*(6), 3414–3425.

Morishima, M., & Kawaguchi, Y. (2006). Recurrent connection patterns of corticostriatal pyramidal cells in frontal cortex. *Journal of Neuroscience, 26*(16), 4394–4405.

Morishima, M., Morita, K., Kubota, Y., & Kawaguchi, Y. (2011). Highly differentiated projection-specific cortical subnetworks. *Journal of Neuroscience, 31*(28), 10380–10391.

Morissette, J., & Bower, J. M. (1996). Contribution of somatosensory cortex to responses in the rat cerebellar granule cell layer following peripheral tactile stimulation. *Experimental Brain Research, 109*(2), 240–250.

Moya, M. V., Siegel, J. J., McCord, E. D., Kalmbach, B. E., Dembrow, N., Johnston, D., et al. (2014). Species-specific differences in the medial prefrontal projections to the pons between rat and rabbit. *Journal of Comparative Neurology, 522*(13), 3052–3074.

Nishiike, S., Guldin, W. O., & Baurle, J. (2000). Corticofugal connections between the cerebral cortex and the vestibular nuclei in the rat. *Journal of Comparative Neurology, 420*(3), 363–372.

O'Connor, S. M., Berg, R. W., & Kleinfeld, D. (2002). Coherent electrical activity between vibrissa sensory areas of cerebellum and neocortex is enhanced during free whisking. *Journal of Neurophysiology, 87*(4), 2137–2148.

Odeh, F., Ackerley, R., Bjaalie, J. G., & Apps, R. (2005). Pontine maps linking somatosensory and cerebellar cortices are in register with climbing fiber somatotopy. *Journal of Neuroscience, 25*(24), 5680–5690.

Ohno, S., Kuramoto, E., Furuta, T., Hioki, H., Tanaka, Y. R., Fujiyama, F., et al. (2012). A morphological analysis of thalamocortical axon fibers of rat posterior thalamic nuclei: a single neuron tracing study with viral vectors. *Cerebral Cortex, 22*(12), 2840–2857.

O'Reilly, J. X., Beckmann, C. F., Tomassini, V., Ramnani, N., & Johansen-Berg, H. (2010). Distinct and overlapping functional zones in the cerebellum defined by resting state functional connectivity. *Cerebral Cortex, 20*(4), 953–965.

Panto, M. R., Cicirata, F., Angaut, P., Parenti, R., & Serapide, F. (1995). The projection from the primary motor and somatic sensory cortex to the basilar pontine nuclei. A detailed electrophysiological and anatomical study in the rat. *Journal für Hirnforschung, 36*(1), 7–19.

Parenti, R., Zappala, A., Serapide, M. F., Panto, M. R., & Cicirata, F. (2002). Projections of the basilar pontine nuclei and nucleus reticularis tegmenti pontis to the cerebellar nuclei of the rat. *Journal of Comparative Neurology, 452*(2), 115–127.

Pijpers, A., & Ruigrok, T. J. (2006). Organization of pontocerebellar projections to identified climbing fiber zones in the rat. *Journal of Comparative Neurology, 496*(4), 513–528.

Popa, D., Spolidoro, M., Proville, R. D., Guyon, N., Belliveau, L., & Lena, C. (2013). Functional role of the cerebellum in gamma-band synchronization of the sensory and motor cortices. *Journal of Neuroscience, 33*(15), 6552–6556.

Potter, R. F., Ruegg, D. G., & Wiesendanger, M. (1978). Responses of neurones of the pontine nuclei to stimulation of the sensorimotor, visual and auditory cortex of rats. *Brain Research Bulletin, 3*(1), 15–19.

Prevosto, V., Graf, W., & Ugolini, G. (2010). Cerebellar inputs to intraparietal cortex areas LIP and MIP: functional frameworks for adaptive control of eye movements, reaching, and arm/eye/head movement coordination. *Cerebral Cortex, 20*(1), 214–228.

Proville, R. D., Spolidoro, M., Guyon, N., Dugue, G. P., Selimi, F., Isope, P., et al. (2014). Cerebellum involvement in cortical sensorimotor circuits for the control of voluntary movements. *Nature Neuroscience, 17*(9), 1233–1239.

Rajakumar, N., Hrycyshyn, A. W., & Flumerfelt, B. A. (1992). Afferent organization of the lateral reticular nucleus in the rat: an anterograde tracing study. *Anatomy and Embryology (Berlin), 185*(1), 25–37.

Ricardo, J. A. (1981). Efferent connections of the subthalamic region in the rat. II. The zona incerta. *Brain Research, 214*(1), 43–60.

Rokni, D., Llinas, R., & Yarom, Y. (2007). Stars and stripes in the cerebellar cortex: a voltage sensitive dye study. *Frontiers in Systems Neuroscience, 1*, 1.

Ros, H., Sachdev, R. N., Yu, Y., Sestan, N., & McCormick, D. A. (2009). Neocortical networks entrain neuronal circuits in cerebellar cortex. *Journal of Neuroscience, 29*(33), 10309–10320.

Rowland, N. C., Goldberg, J. A., & Jaeger, D. (2010). Cortico-cerebellar coherence and causal connectivity during slow-wave activity. *Neuroscience, 166*(2), 698–711.

Ruigrok, T. J. (2003). Collateralization of climbing and mossy fibers projecting to the nodulus and flocculus of the rat cerebellum. *Journal of Comparative Neurology, 466*(2), 278–298.

Ruigrok, T. J. (2004). Precerebellar nuclei and red nucleus. In G. Paxinos (Ed.), *The rat nervous system* (3rd ed.) (pp. 167–204). San Diego: Elsevier/Academic Press.

Ruigrok, T. J. (2011). Ins and outs of cerebellar modules. *Cerebellum, 10*(3), 464–474.

Sang, L., Qin, W., Liu, Y., Han, W., Zhang, Y., Jiang, T., et al. (2012). Resting-state functional connectivity of the vermal and hemispheric subregions of the cerebellum with both the cerebral cortical networks and subcortical structures. *Neuroimage, 61*(4), 1213–1225.

Sawyer, S. F., Tepper, J. M., & Groves, P. M. (1994). Cerebellar-responsive neurons in the thalamic ventroanterior-ventrolateral complex of rats: light and electron microscopy. *Neuroscience, 63*(3), 725–745.

Sawyer, S. F., Young, S. J., Groves, P. M., & Tepper, J. M. (1994). Cerebellar-responsive neurons in the thalamic ventroanterior-ventrolateral complex of rats: in vivo electrophysiology. *Neuroscience, 63*(3), 711–724.

Schwarz, C., Horowski, A., Mock, M., & Thier, P. (2005). Organization of tectopontine terminals within the pontine nuclei of the rat and their spatial relationship to terminals from the visual and somatosensory cortex. *Journal of Comparative Neurology, 484*(3), 283–298.

Schwarz, C., & Mock, M. (2001). Spatial arrangement of cerebro-pontine terminals. *Journal of Comparative Neurology, 435*(4), 418–432.

Schwarz, C., & Thier, P. (1995). Modular organization of the pontine nuclei: dendritic fields of identified pontine projection neurons in the rat respect the borders of cortical afferent fields. *Journal of Neuroscience, 15*(5 Pt 1), 3475–3489.

Serapide, M. F., Panto, M. R., Parenti, R., Zappala, A., & Cicirata, F. (2001). Multiple zonal projections of the basilar pontine nuclei to the cerebellar cortex of the rat. *Journal of Comparative Neurology, 430*(4), 471–484.

Serapide, M. F., Parenti, R., Panto, M. R., Zappala, A., & Cicirata, F. (2002). Multiple zonal projections of the nucleus reticularis tegmenti pontis to the cerebellar cortex of the rat. *European Journal of Neuroscience, 15*(11), 1854–1858.

Serapide, M. F., Zappala, A., Parenti, R., Panto, M. R., & Cicirata, F. (2002). Laterality of the pontocerebellar projections in the rat. *European Journal of Neuroscience, 15*(9), 1551–1556.

Shambes, G. M., Gibson, J. M., & Welker, W. (1978). Fractured somatotopy in granule cell tactile areas of rat cerebellar hemispheres revealed by micromapping. *Brain, Behavior,and Evolution, 15*(2), 94–140.

Sharp, F. R., & Evans, K. (1982). Regional (^{14}C) 2-deoxyglucose uptake during vibrissae movements evoked by rat motor cortex stimulation. *Journal of Comparative Neurology, 208*(3), 255–287.

Sharp, F. R., & Ryan, A. F. (1984). Regional (^{14}C) 2-deoxyglucose uptake during forelimb movements evoked by rat motor cortex stimulation: pons, cerebellum, medulla, spinal cord, muscle. *Journal of Comparative Neurology, 224*(2), 286–306.

Shinoda, Y., Sugiuchi, Y., Futami, T., & Izawa, R. (1992). Axon collaterals of mossy fibers from the pontine nucleus in the cerebellar dentate nucleus. *Journal of Neurophysiology, 67*(3), 547–560.

Shokunbi, M. T., Hrycyshyn, A. W., & Flumerfelt, B. A. (1986). A horseradish peroxidase study of the rubral and cortical afferents to the lateral reticular nucleus in the rat. *Journal of Comparative Neurology, 248*(3), 441–454.

Smith, Y., Wichmann, T., & DeLong, M. R. (2014). Corticostriatal and mesocortical dopamine systems: do species differences matter? *Nature Reviews Neuroscience, 15*(1), 63.

Steriade, M. (1995). Two channels in the cerebellothalamocortical system. *Journal of Comparative Neurology, 354*(1), 57–70.

Stoodley, C. J., & Schmahmann, J. D. (2009). Functional topography in the human cerebellum: a meta-analysis of neuroimaging studies. *Neuroimage, 44*(2), 489–501.

Sugihara, I., Fujita, H., Na, J., Quy, P. N., Li, B. Y., & Ikeda, D. (2009). Projection of reconstructed single Purkinje cell axons in relation to the cortical and nuclear aldolase C compartments of the rat cerebellum. *Journal of Comparative Neurology, 512*(2), 282–304.

Suzuki, L., Coulon, P., Sabel-Goedknegt, E. H., & Ruigrok, T. J. (2012). Organization of cerebral projections to identified cerebellar zones in the posterior cerebellum of the rat. *Journal of Neuroscience, 32*(32), 10854–10869.

Swenson, R. S., & Castro, A. J. (1983). The afferent connections of the inferior olivary complex in rats. An anterograde study using autoradiographic and axonal degeneration techniques. *Neuroscience, 8*(2), 259–275.

Swenson, R. S., Sievert, C. F., Terreberry, R. R., Neafsey, E. J., & Castro, A. J. (1989). Organization of cerebral cortico-olivary projections in the rat. *Neuroscience Research, 7*(1), 43–54.

Teune, T. M., van der Burg, J., van der Moer, J., Voogd, J., & Ruigrok, T. J. (2000). Topography of cerebellar nuclear projections to the brain stem in the rat. *Progress in Brain Research, 124*, 141–172.

Torigoe, Y., Blanks, R. H., & Precht, W. (1986a). Anatomical studies on the nucleus reticularis tegmenti pontis in the pigmented rat. I. Cytoarchitecture, topography, and cerebral cortical afferents. *Journal of Comparative Neurology, 243*(1), 71–87.

Torigoe, Y., Blanks, R. H., & Precht, W. (1986b). Anatomical studies on the nucleus reticularis tegmenti pontis in the pigmented rat. II. Subcortical afferents demonstrated by the retrograde transport of horseradish peroxidase. *Journal of Comparative Neurology, 243*(1), 88–105.

Voogd, J. (2014). What we do not know about cerebellar systems neuroscience. *Frontiers in Systems Neuroscience, 8*, 227.

Walter, J. T., Dizon, M. J., & Khodakhah, K. (2009). The functional equivalence of ascending and parallel fiber inputs in cerebellar computation. *Journal of Neuroscience, 29*(26), 8462–8473.

Watt, C. B., & Mihailoff, G. A. (1983). The cerebellopontine system in the rat. I. Autoradiographic studies. *Journal of Comparative Neurology, 215*(3), 312–330.

West, M. J., & Gundersen, H. J. (1990). Unbiased stereological estimation of the number of neurons in the human hippocampus. *Journal of Comparative Neurology, 296*(1), 1–22.

West, M. J., Slomianka, L., & Gundersen, H. J. (1991). Unbiased stereological estimation of the total number of neurons in the subdivisions of the rat hippocampus using the optical fractionator. *Anatomical Record, 231*(4), 482–497.

Wiesendanger, R., & Wiesendanger, M. (1982a). The corticopontine system in the rat. I. Mapping of corticopontine neurons. *Journal of Comparative Neurology, 208*(3), 215–226.

Wiesendanger, R., & Wiesendanger, M. (1982b). The corticopontine system in the rat. II. The projection pattern. *Journal of Comparative Neurology, 208*(3), 227–238.

Wolpert, D. M., Miall, R. C., & Kawato, M. (1998). Internal models in the cerebellum. *Trends in Cognitive Science, 2*(9), 338–347.

Wu, H. S., Sugihara, I., & Shinoda, Y. (1999). Projection patterns of single mossy fibers originating from the lateral reticular nucleus in the rat cerebellar cortex and nuclei. *Journal of Comparative Neurology, 411*(1), 97–118.

de Zeeuw, C. I., Holstege, J. C., Ruigrok, T. J., & Voogd, J. (1990). Mesodiencephalic and cerebellar terminals terminate upon the same dendritic spines in the glomeruli of the cat and rat inferior olive: an ultrastructural study using a combination of [^{3}H]leucine and wheat germ agglutinin coupled horseradish peroxidase anterograde tracing. *Neuroscience, 34*(3), 645–655.

Cerebellar Neuronal Codes—Perspectives from Intracellular Analysis In Vivo

Henrik Jörntell

Neural Basis of Sensorimotor Control, Department of Experimental Medical Science, Lund University, Lund, Sweden

INTRODUCTION

By the concept of the cerebellar neuronal code, I here refer to the relationship between the spike firing of an individual neuron and the cerebellar contribution to a function exerted by the brain. The spike firing of an individual neuron can hypothetically take many different shapes, but to provide an explanation for its contribution one will need to consider its spike firing pattern in relation to the spike firing patterns of other neurons and how the relationship could be explained in terms of the known synaptic connections and their respective weights. Hence, the code of a single neuron can be properly understood only if one also understands the codes of the other neurons that participate in the same function. It can safely be assumed that each part of the cerebellum participates in a multitude of brain functions—an understanding of the neuronal code hence implies that it is possible to predict the changes in firing of a given neuron between contexts.

Such an understanding of the participation of a single neuron in brain function requires an understanding of the structure of the local neuronal network, of the position of the neuron in the local network, of the input that drives the local network structure, and of the particular function contributed by the cerebellum (to understand the relationship between the input and the output of the cerebellar network).

With this view, the aim of "cracking" the neuronal code of the cerebellum became realistic already in the 1960s, with the seminal anatomical and physiological characterization of the cerebellar microcircuit summarized in the book of Eccles, Ito, and Szentágothai (1967). The well-known regular, crystalline structure of the cerebellar neuronal circuit seemed ideal to resolve the fundamental cerebellar operation, expressible as an algorithm or a computational unit with specific properties repeated across the entire cerebellar cortex. Even though the path toward this goal has been tortuous, sometimes unexpected, and time-consuming, I personally believe that the field has finally reached the goal of understanding cerebellar processing per se, even though there are details in some experimental findings left to explain. This chapter is an account of the major factors that would influence the flow of information through the network and the format of that information. Through the final step of spike encoding in the individual neurons, this information should be sufficient to understand, in principle, how the spike codes are generated. As will be discussed below, the main problem in deciphering the cerebellar neuronal codes lies in knowing the types and formats of information in the multitude of mossy fiber pathways that reaches the cerebellum. Today, this remains the only major obstacle that prevents us from a full understanding of the cerebellar neuronal code.

This chapter aims at covering the main factors that would influence the cerebellar neuronal encoding of information. It is subdivided into the following subject areas:

1. The configuration of the cerebellar cortical network
2. The flow of information through the cerebellar neuronal network
3. Spike encoding in the cerebellar neurons
4. Distributed neuronal representations
5. Conclusions

THE CONFIGURATION OF THE CEREBELLAR CORTICAL NETWORK

A major factor that would influence the neuronal encoding of the information is naturally the pathway through the neuronal network by which the information reaches the neuron. To know this pathway, one needs to know the structure of the network. In the case of the cerebellum, the anatomy of this structure is known in great detail. In addition, one also needs to be aware of possible gates for the information flow through the anatomically described circuitry structure. Such gates could be generated by plasticity that reduces synaptic weights to zero and by inhibition that shuts off transmission of information.

Anatomical Structure of the Cerebellar Neuronal Network

Numerous excellent accounts of the basic structure of the cerebellar network are already published in the literature (Dean, Porrill, Ekerot, & Jorntell, 2010; Eccles et al., 1967; Ito, 1984, 2006), and another full account is not the aim of this chapter. However, there may be slight differences in the interpretation of the structure and it is hence appropriate to describe the interpretation applied here.

First of all, in this chapter I will assume that climbing fibers do not contribute to the regular information processing of the cerebellar neuronal network. Instead, it is assumed that they contribute to the generation and the maintenance of the network structure by regulating synaptic plasticity and to the maintenance of the overall spike firing level in the cerebellar neurons (Jorntell, 2014). It follows that all fast modulation of spike firing, what most people think of when they hear the term spike encoding, is brought about by the mossy fiber inputs and the direct effects they have on the activity in the network under the performance of a typical behavior or motor program, that is, under the time window of a few hundred milliseconds and certainly not more than 1 s.

In this view, all input information will first of all reach the granule cells via the mossy fibers. The granule cells provide direct excitatory inputs to the output neuron of the cerebellar cortex, the Purkinje cell. But the granule cells also provide excitatory input to the molecular layer interneurons, which in turn provide inhibitory synapses on the Purkinje cells, and this connection makes it hence possible to provide the Purkinje cells also with a sign-inverted version of the mossy fiber information. The only remaining enigma in this part of the circuitry is the basket formation that is contributed to by both basket cells and stellate cells (Jorntell, Bengtsson, Schonewille, & De Zeeuw, 2010), but which has an unclear role as it does not form a regular synaptic formation and the main electrical signal seems to be a weak transmission of the electrical field generated by the axon spike of the interneuron (Blot & Barbour, 2014). Here it is assumed that it is not part of the main transmission of information in the circuitry, but may have long-term effects on the Purkinje cell firing level by regulating the expression of potassium conductances, for example.

The granule cell activity is regulated by inhibition from Golgi cells, which are driven by excitatory input from mossy fibers and granule cells. But Golgi cells appear to primarily provide a slow inhibitory modulation of the granule cells (Brickley, Cull-Candy, & Farrant, 1996; Jorntell & Ekerot, 2006; Wall & Usowicz, 1997), and Golgi cells themselves are under a similar slow modulatory control from Lugaro cells (Dieudonne & Dumoulin, 2000). The cerebellar neuronal network can hence be viewed as a quite simple network structure, with some neuronal elements contributing mainly to slow modulatory effects and a contribution to fast neuronal processing from only three basic elements, the granule cells, the molecular layer interneurons, and the Purkinje cells.

Apart from the anatomical identification of the cerebellar microcircuit, which was relatively advanced already by the mid-1960s, another important early step toward the characterization of the properties of the microcircuit was the anatomical and physiological subdivisioning of the cerebellar cortex into a number of sagittally oriented functional areas or zones (Groenewegen, Voogd, & Freedman, 1979; Oscarsson, 1979). In this chapter I will not spend a lot of energy reviewing this organization. However, the sagittal organization is ontogenetically early defined (Reeber, Loeschel, Franklin, & Sillitoe, 2013), presumably by an interplay of climbing fiber input and molecular markers, which defines a strict parasagittal connectivity in both the olivocortical and the corticonuclear projections (Apps & Garwicz, 2005; Trott & Armstrong, 1987) and corresponds to a functional organization in terms of both nucleofugal projections (Ito, 1984) and afferent pathways to the inferior olive (Armstrong, Harvey, & Schild, 1973; Oscarsson & Sjolund, 1974; Oscarsson & Uddenberg, 1966) and in terms of cortical terminations of the mossy fiber system. Within the overall organization of sagittal zones, there is a more intricate system of microzones, with each microzone being characterized by a set of Purkinje cells whose climbing fibers are driven by the same peripheral input and in some cases are branches of the same climbing fiber axon (Andersson & Oscarsson, 1978; Ekerot, Garwicz, & Schouenborg, 1991). Microzones describe a more detailed pattern in the cerebellar cortex than is currently provided by molecular markers such as zebrin (Apps & Hawkes, 2009; Sugihara & Shinoda, 2004)—however, it is quite possible that the near future will find additional molecular markers that altogether will match the more detailed description. Microzones, which may contain 100–400 Purkinje cells, are likely to be the minimal functional unit of the cerebellar cortex (Dean et al., 2010; Ekerot et al., 1991). As they are defined by the climbing fibers, which in turn regulate plasticity (Jorntell & Ekerot, 2002), the wiring of input from the granule cells to the Purkinje cells and interneurons is relatively stereotyped within the microzone. Since the Purkinje cells of a microzone have a convergent projection to the deep cerebellar nuclei (Apps & Garwicz, 2005), where the Purkinje cells of a microzone innervate the same group of cells, separate from those cells innervated from other microzones, the stereotyped wiring of granule cell input seems to make sense. The Purkinje cells of the microzone can hence be viewed as a super-Purkinje cell, which samples granule cell inputs that are functionally similar and controls a private set of cells in the deep cerebellar nuclei.

Synaptic Plasticity

At least at the parallel fiber synapses on Purkinje cells, and probably also at the parallel fiber synapses on the interneurons, synaptic plasticity appears to have the capacity of reducing synaptic strength to zero (Dean et al., 2010; Ekerot & Jorntell, 2001; Isope & Barbour, 2002; Valera, Doussau, Poulain, Barbour, & Isope, 2012). Such degrees of synaptic plasticity will affect what will here be referred to as the "physiological network structure," in which some synapses in the anatomically defined network structure have been rendered silent or ineffective and hence do not participate in the transmission of information. The physiological network structure can hence be different from the network structure defined by circuitry anatomy alone. But when such network structure effects have been investigated in a systematic fashion against the microzonal organization, it has been found that they occur according to the predictable patterns that are consequences of the input–output relationship of the microzone. It is hence possible to view at least parts of the microcircuitry structure (i.e., the physiological network structure) of the adult cerebellar cortex as a fingerprint of the learning history of the individual—as long as the microzonal location (or the climbing fiber input) of the neuron is the same, the consistent global intraspecies organization of the cerebellar cortex gives us the prediction that the neuron will display similar firing properties.

Physiological Gating Effects

Another potential physiological effect on the effective network structure could, in principle, be imposed by synaptic inhibition. Hypothetically, a powerful inhibition that would completely shut down the transmission of excitatory synaptic input through a particular type of neuron would alter the physiological network structure. If such powerful inhibition was triggered by a particular context or type of event, it would work as a gating element and the network structure would be context-dependent. However, at least for the Golgi cell inhibition of granule cells and interneuron inhibition of Purkinje cells, the inhibition does not appear to be of sufficient magnitude to cause such effects (Jorntell & Ekerot, 2006).

A related mechanism would be supralinear excitation. Supralinear excitation could be claimed if a given synaptic input has a linear input–output relationship over a certain range but at a given point of threshold excitation becomes supralinear (Wang, Denk, & Hausser, 2000). This could, for example, happen if the dendrites of a neuron contain excitable ion channels that are normally not activated by the synaptic input but become so beyond a certain level of excitation. Dendritic spike activation would in that case result in a much more intense (supralinear) spike output at the level of the soma. However, even though supralinearity can be observed in vitro, it has so far not been demonstrated in vivo. In fact, as long as the neurons are driven to frequencies that have been observed under behavior they have been shown to be linear encoders of input (Spanne, Geborek, Bengtsson, & Jorntell, 2014b). Here it is assumed that all transferred information is encoded linearly by the neurons and that the observation of supralinearity in vitro is due to the membrane of the neurons not being in their normal operative state in vitro, due to the absence of normal background synaptic noise (Bengtsson, Ekerot, & Jorntell, 2011) or other factors.

THE FLOW OF INFORMATION THROUGH THE CEREBELLAR NEURONAL NETWORK

When the pathways of information flow are known based on circuitry anatomy and its modification by synaptic plasticity, the second major factor that will influence the neuronal code of a cerebellar neuron is the magnitude of the synaptic responses and how the synaptic responses are encoded into the spike output. This is the subject below.

In general, it is striking how small the individual synaptic responses for intracortical connections in the cerebellar cortex are. This is in contrast to the very large amplitudes of the synaptic responses in the two types of synapses formed by the external afferents, the climbing fiber, and mossy fiber synapses. The climbing fiber synapse is of course outstanding, even within the central nervous system as a whole, but as described above the climbing fibers will not be dealt with in this chapter, as they are assumed to provide some very specific functions in plasticity and overall activity regulation. Instead, we will begin the account with the mossy fiber-to-granule cell synapses, when the information first arrives to the cerebellar cortex. We will then proceed by the intracortical synaptic connections.

The Mossy Fiber-to-Granule Cell Synapse

The mossy fiber-to-granule cell synapse is exceptionally powerful and typically generates excitatory postsynaptic potentials (EPSPs) with amplitudes on the order of 4–8 mV individually (Jorntell & Ekerot, 2006). Nevertheless, the activation of one such synapse is not sufficient to trigger the spike output of the granule cell, even when activated at up to 1000 Hz (Jorntell & Ekerot, 2006). Instead, summation of at least two or three, in some cases possibly four, of the mossy fiber synapses is required to trigger the spike output (D'Angelo, De, Rossi, & Taglietti, 1995). Nevertheless, granule cells have been shown to respond to information very similar to that carried by single mossy fibers both for cutaneous and for joint-related information (Bengtsson & Jorntell, 2009; Jorntell & Ekerot, 2006). The reflection in the individual granule cells of the information carried by single mossy fibers can be explained by the fact that the majority or all of the four mossy fiber synapses that converge onto a single granule cell carry functionally equivalent information (Dean et al., 2010; Jorntell, 2014). This has so far been shown only for cutaneous information. But it is important to remember that the cuneate system, which carried the cutaneously related information in the demonstrated cases, is a special system in which cutaneous information is processed in almost complete isolation (Bengtsson, Brasselet, Johansson, Arleo, & Jorntell, 2013; Jorntell et al., 2014). In many other mossy fiber systems, the integration of various modalities may well occur already at the precerebellar level. In such cases, even if functionally equivalent information is carried by the four mossy fiber synapses mediating the input to the individual granule cell, that cell would naturally still mediate composite or mixed information. But it is clear from both granule and Purkinje cell recordings that the transmission of mossy fiber input from single functional systems is not thresholded or dependent on the simultaneous activation of other functional systems (Ekerot & Jorntell, 2001; Jorntell & Ekerot, 2002; Geborek, Bengtsson, & Jorntell, 2014; Geborek, Spanne, Bengtsson, & Jorntell, 2013), in contrast to the ideas of the original Marr–Albus theory (Albus, 1971; Marr, 1969). Instead, it may be expected that the information carried by single types of mossy fibers is transmitted in a gradable manner. The very large EPSP amplitudes result in individual mossy fibers having a large influence on the cerebellar cortical activity, and the convergence of functionally similar mossy fibers in single granule cells makes it possible to have a detailed reflection of the exact grade of activation of each mossy fiber signal that is provided to the cerebellum.

In contrast to the mossy fiber-to-granule cell synapses, almost all other synapses in the cerebellar cortex have very small unitary amplitudes. This results in the intracortical communication becoming dependent on the concerted activation of larger populations of afferent neurons, to have a profound impression on the firing rate of a targeted neuron. It also means that firing modulations during behavior would be expected to be smooth and without rapid dynamics, in line with the known firing modulations of mossy fibers recorded under behavior.

The Golgi Cell-to-Granule Cell Synapse

Among the main critical determinants of the view of cerebellar processing are the properties of the Golgi cell-to-granule cell inhibitory synapse. Early and more recent theories often assume that the Golgi cell-to-granule cell inhibition is a classical fast inhibitory synapse with a rapid rise time and decay time constant of the inhibitory postsynaptic potential (IPSP) (Schweighofer, Doya, & Lay, 2001). If this were the case, the input layer of the cerebellar cortex would be capable of a relatively complex processing, for example, allowing for sparse coding or a rapid subdivision of a process into a number of time slots where the granular layer is put in different contexts, for example, during a regulated phase of movement. However, this synaptic connection has been found to display a number of unique features in vitro, with the presence of very long-lasting IPSPs and outright tonic modes of inhibition (Duguid, Branco, London, Chadderton, & Hausser, 2012; Jorntell & Ekerot, 2006). In the in vitro setting, typically studies in immature slices, which can sometimes be misleading, a developmental aspect of these tonic components has been discovered and at postnatal day 60 in the rat, an age that is hardly ever explored in in vitro preparations, the pure tonic inhibition was found to be completely dominating and the classical fast inhibition essentially eliminated (Wall & Usowicz, 1997). Interestingly, even in immature rats in vivo, granule cells were indeed found to be dominated by tonic inhibition (Duguid et al., 2012), and in adult cats there is essentially no trace of fast IPSPs in the granule cells (Jorntell & Ekerot, 2006). In the latter case the recordings were also made without anesthesia, which is likely to be important as many known anesthetics potentiate inhibitory synaptic transmission (Bengtsson & Jorntell, 2007). In a 2013 paper with paired Golgi cell–granule cell recordings in vivo this picture of the Golgi cell-to-granule cell inhibitory synaptic communication could be confirmed (Bengtsson, Geborek, & Jorntell, 2013). At a shorter time scale of 100 ms or less the Golgi cell does not influence spontaneous granule cell spiking. However, when Golgi cell spike activity is manipulated and maintained at substantially different rates than at rest, granule cell spiking activity can either be completely depressed or be powerfully potentiated depending on the direction of change of the Golgi cell firing. Hence, the Golgi cell-to-granule cell inhibition can be expected to be almost entirely tonic in the adult cerebellum. This substantially alters the conditions for how the cerebellar cortex can work compared to earlier concepts. Since most movements, or phases of movements, last for one or a few hundred milliseconds only, there is no time to put this synaptic junction into several different levels of inhibition, or states. However, the junction can naturally be put into different states, representing different contexts, between movements or movement phases, which still makes the cerebellar neuronal circuitry versatile or reusable (Spanne & Jorntell, 2013).

The Interneuron-to-Purkinje Cell Synapse

Using a similar technique for dual-neuron recordings in vivo, the interneuron-to-Purkinje cell inhibition was found to be very weak, with individual interneurons having no detectable effect on Purkinje cell spike firing (Bengtsson, Geborek, et al., 2013). Similar weak effects of individual interneurons on Purkinje cells have also been found in juvenile slices in vitro (Hausser & Clark, 1997). The weakness of the inhibitory synapses can be expected to increase as the animal develops into adulthood when the Purkinje cells grow in size and their input resistance is expected to decrease. Using the amplitude values of unitary IPSPs recorded in the juvenile slice and estimated changes in membrane resistance toward adulthood, the expected unitary IPSP amplitudes could be as low as a few microvolts

(Bengtsson, Geborek, et al., 2013). Naturally, assuming plasticity to differentiate the unitary IPSP amplitudes over development, some interneuron-to-Purkinje cell synaptic connections could have more pronounced effects and others much weaker. Nevertheless, among the thousands of interneurons that converge on the single Purkinje cell it seems reasonable to assume that none of them have any detectable effect individually. Hence, in the case of interneuron inhibition in Purkinje cells, sufficient inhibition to have a marked effect on the overall firing of a single Purkinje cell requires a concerted activation of a large number of interneurons.

The Granule Cell-to-Purkinje Cell Synapse

Unitary granule cell-to-Purkinje cell synapses have been more extensively studied in the slice, and a pronounced developmental effect with a gradual decrease in the excitatory postsynaptic current (EPSC) amplitude and a gradually larger number of silent synapses has been observed (Isope & Barbour, 2002; Valera et al., 2012). Using the amplitude values of the effective granule cell-to-Purkinje cell synapses of a few tens of picoamperes and the expected input resistance on the order of $10\,M\Omega$ in the adult Purkinje cell, the individual EPSP amplitudes would be expected to be well below $0.1\,mV$. In addition, because of the size of the Purkinje cell, it may be expected to be electrically compartmentalized in vivo (Jaeger, De Schutter, & Bower, 1997), which would further reduce the somatic amplitudes of the EPSPs produced by synapses out in the dendritic tree. It follows that also the excitatory synapses on Purkinje cells are expected to be exceptionally weak and to have completely negligible effects on the spike output of the Purkinje cell in vivo. A measurable effect on the Purkinje cell spike output hence requires again a concerted activation of a large number of granule cells.

The Synaptic Inputs to Golgi Cells

Similar to Purkinje cells, Golgi cells receive an excitatory synaptic input from granule cells both via parallel fibers and, possibly, via the ascending granule cell axon. Also in the case of Golgi cells, the unitary parallel fiber-to-Golgi cell synaptic response has very small effects electrically (Dieudonne, 1998), and concerted granule cell activation is expected to be required to substantially modulate the Golgi cell ongoing firing activity. In this case, this scenario, of course, makes a lot of sense given the primarily long-term effects of the Golgi cell spike output on the granule cell inhibition. In addition to parallel fiber input, Golgi cells also receive direct mossy fiber excitatory synapses (Holtzman, Cerminara, Edgley, & Apps, 2009). The relative magnitude of the influence of these synapses remains to be elucidated. Golgi cells could also receive inhibitory input from Purkinje cells and/or molecular layer interneurons, which could provide the

Golgi cells with contextual information, that is, if the Purkinje cells are in a high firing state before the onset of movement execution, for example. Golgi cells also receive inhibitory synaptic input from Lugaro cells and in this case it is more clearly contextual information, as the Lugaro cells are powerfully regulated by serotonin (Dieudonne & Dumoulin, 2000).

The Excitatory and Inhibitory Synapses on Molecular Layer Interneurons

Unlike the Purkinje cells and Golgi cells, however, the molecular layer interneurons do exhibit powerful unitary EPSPs, generated by granule cells, and unitary IPSPs, generated by other inhibitory interneurons (Jorntell & Ekerot, 2003). (As discussed in an earlier publication, stellate cells and basket cells are here treated as a uniform group, with essentially the only difference being that the deeper lying interneurons tend to be larger (Jorntell et al., 2010)). Individually, these neurons also have a somewhat larger propensity for firing in small spike bursts, that is, the spiking dynamics seem to match the stronger influence of the unitary synaptic potentials. Nevertheless, as the final target of the interneuron spike output is the Purkinje cell, on which the interneurons have weak effects individually, it is hard to see what the faster dynamics are used for. A possibility is of course that it is just a biological side effect of the interneurons being smaller—the associated faster time constants of the membranes would have this effect. Alternatively, it may be speculated that the faster dynamics is useful for these interneurons to organize dynamically into coherent groups of interneurons that could provide the concerted inhibition required to alter the Purkinje cell spike output.

Summary of the Consequences of the Low-Weight Synaptic Organization

This means that the only real driver of intracortical activity is the mossy fiber-to-granule cell synapse, and the activity of the Purkinje cell can essentially be approximated by the weighted sum of individual mossy fiber inputs. Concerted activation requires redundant representation of information, that is, any single neurons must represent the same or at least similar aspects of the same information. That redundant representation to some extent must apply to the cerebellar neuronal circuitry is supported by the fact that the mossy fiber systems have anatomically distinct regions of termination, which display somatotopical organization representing information related to cutaneous inputs. In cutaneous systems there is a lot of redundancy, with the same receptive field and submodality being represented many times in each individual. In other mossy fiber systems, it may be less straightforward to identify redundant representations. However, the fact that vestibular information has such widespread representations in the cerebellar cortex seems to offer an ideal opportunity to explore the subject. Given that vestibular information is essentially three-dimensional, it would be relatively straightforward to explore the distribution and representation of this information to confirm or reject the idea of redundancy.

SPIKE ENCODING IN THE CEREBELLAR NEURONS

The neuronal integration of synaptic inputs is readily described by the original Hodgkin–Huxley formulations for conductance-based electrical signaling in neurons. In the view portrayed above, concerted activation of dynamic groups of neurons would provide modulations of the intracellular membrane potentials of the neurons. If such concerted synaptic activation is not synchronous but merely more loosely associated with time, these modulations could be relatively smooth and relatively slowly varying over time (i.e., well above 1-ms windows at least). The spike generation process, by which the integrated synaptic signal is converted to a spike output signal, is inevitably subjected to stochasticity (Averbeck, Latham, & Pouget, 2006; Faisal, Selen, & Wolpert, 2008; Spanne et al., 2014b). Stochasticity can arise as a consequence of synaptic input noise, which is inevitable in neuronal networks with spontaneous activity (Vogels, Sprekeler, Zenke, Clopath, & Gerstner, 2011), as a consequence of the intrinsic membrane properties or both.

The stochasticity is difficult to describe without an underlying understanding of the processes involved in its generation. However, one way to show its existence is to simply record the spontaneous activity in stationary states of a neuron and to alter its membrane potential using current injection (Spanne et al., 2014b). The fact that there is a close relationship between the amount of input and the standard deviation of the interspike intervals then strongly suggests that there is an intrinsic component in the stochasticity of spike generation. For the cerebellum in vivo, this type of estimate has been made for Purkinje cells, interneurons, and Golgi cells. Surprisingly, based solely on the relationship between the mean input and the standard deviation of the interspike intervals, these three neuron types are essentially indistinguishable in the sense that the variations between different neurons of the same type are essentially overlapping the variations found between the different types of neurons. This suggests that these spontaneously active neurons have very similar basic spike generation mechanisms, and most of the differences between them arise as a consequence of the relative effectiveness of synaptic inputs in modulating their spike output.

The analysis of the stationary states of spike generation across a range of membrane potentials also makes it possible to model the neurons' responses to time-varying input, that is, the type of input that would be expected to be produced by synaptic activation during behavior (Spanne, Geborek, Bengtsson, & Jorntell, 2014a; Spanne et al., 2014b). As described above, a relatively slowly time-modulated input is what would be expected for the membrane potential of neurons that receive synaptic inputs from a large number of neurons with concerted, but not synchronized, activation. Using a relatively simple model of the variations of spike stochasticity across the stationary states, at least the spike activity of spinocerebellar projection neurons under behavior can be modeled with high accuracy. As long as the membrane potentials of the cerebellar receiving neurons are not more rapidly varied than in spinocerebellar neurons, it is likely that relatively straightforward linear models of spike generation suffice to capture the spike output of these three major types of cerebellar cortical neurons. In this case, the main challenge would be to understand how the intracellular signals are generated. As discussed above, the cerebellar cortical network in itself does probably impose a lot of transformation on the mossy fiber input signals. However, the variety of mossy fiber signals in the cerebellar subsystem must be grasped, and so far this seems to be the main shortcoming in our understanding of the cerebellar neuronal codes.

The spike generation of the granule cells has so far not been described at the same level of detail as the other cerebellar cortical neuron types. In contrast to these cells, and as also discussed above, granule cells differ from other types of cerebellar cortical neurons by having a few massively powerful synaptic inputs with potentially a major direct influence on the spike output of the neuron. This is similar to the situation that can be obtained also in the other cerebellar cortical neurons by applying an artificially synchronous activation of afferent inputs, a method used in many studies in vitro and in vivo that has perhaps contributed to a misunderstanding that cerebellar neurons generate the spike output with a high temporal precision. (In addition, in vitro neurons are hyperpolarized and/or do not receive their pattern of background synaptic noise, which would further tend to exaggerate their spike time precision.) Under such very rapidly time-varying inputs, the stochasticity in the spike generation is put out of play, as the derivative of the membrane potential when it reaches the spike threshold region is very high. Therefore, in granule cells, the spike output may be somewhat more difficult to describe in simpler linear terms, at least if the mossy fiber input is not smoothly time-varying. But relatively slow time modulations have so far been shown to be the primary mode of activation in mossy fibers from a variety of systems, including the vestibular, oculomotor, and limb-controlling subareas of the cerebellar cortex. Hence, until examples of the contrary have been found, it seems reasonable to assume that also granule cells can be expected to behave as linear integrators with essentially no transformation of the mossy fiber signal.

In summary, spike time stochasticity is an inevitable factor that will confuse any analysis of an individual neuron's contribution to behavior. It speaks against the meaningfulness of analyzing any individual neuron's contribution to behavior at too high a level of temporal detail using spike time recordings. A more reasonable approach is to look at, for example, the kernel density estimation of a neuron's spike output to understand its relationship to behavior. A problem in this type of approach is to set the time window over which a neuron's spike can be expected to vary in relation to a given input.

Stochasticity is likely to be a factor that needs to be compensated for in the cerebellar cortical circuitry. One way to compensate for spike stochasticity is by neuronal redundancy, that is, to have several neurons forming part of the same representation in a given context. Hence, not only are neuronal redundancy and concerted neuronal activation required to provide a critical mass of synaptic excitation/inhibition to accomplish detectable changes in a neuron's spike output in the face of weak intracortical synaptic connections, but neuronal redundancy is also a useful approach to compensate for the relatively unreliable information provided by the single neuron owing to stochasticity. Hence, an effective biological strategy to handle stochasticity is to simply distribute the representation of a given function to be monitored across a large number of neurons.

DISTRIBUTED NEURONAL REPRESENTATIONS

As argued for in this chapter, cerebellar processing is to a large degree centered on redundant neuronal representations, in which the Purkinje cell with the aid of its afferent interneurons can form a large associative element where functions represented in the mossy fiber afferents through learning and synaptic plasticity can be given either positive or negative weight (Spanne & Jorntell, 2013). From a neurophysiologist point of view, this is somewhat of a nightmare since a large number of neurons can be expected to participate in the representation of any simple function. This makes it very difficult to capture what is coded using single-neuron or multiple-neuron recordings, which is the typical form of analysis for finding the behavioral correlates of the neuronal codes. In addition, it is possible that there is also a context-dependent assignment of neuronal representations; that is, a group of neurons that represent the same function in one context participate in complementary or even opposite representations in another context.

In the case of the mossy fibers, which carry the functions that the cerebellar cortex can monitor, they typically have widely divergent terminations in the cerebellar cortex (although according to certain organizational patterns) (Gebre, Reeber, & Sillitoe, 2012; Sultan, 2001; Wu, Sugihara, &

Shinoda, 1999). This arrangement is well in line with the idea that mossy fiber functions have widespread representations in the cerebellar cortex, distributed across a vast population of cerebellar neurons that partake in the information processing in any given task for which the function is used. Hence, when looking at the behavioral correlations of the spiking activity of a single neuron, or a small set of neurons, we are looking only at bits and pieces of the representations of several separate functions, which makes it very difficult to interpret precisely what the individual neurons code for.

The workaround for this problem for the cerebellum is to start taking a detailed look at the signals carried by the mossy fibers. The mossy fiber system targeting the cerebellum is probably the most diverse afferent system of the entire central nervous system, as they originate from almost all structures/functional systems of the brain stem and the spinal cord (Ito, 1984). In addition, essentially all parts of the cerebral cortex are represented as mossy fiber inputs via the pontine nuclei (Brodal, 1981). Hence, we may expect a vast array of functions and coding represented in the mossy fiber systems. Once these functions and variations in coding are known, and ideally which parts of the cerebellar cortex each mossy fiber system targets, it starts to become feasible to recognize the functions and their representations within the cerebellar cortex.

There is one additional complication, however. Learning from the example of the spinocerebellar systems, which represent a substantial proportion of the mossy fiber systems, it is clear that each mossy fiber can partake in many different functions. The spinocerebellar neurons monitor the function in the spinal sensorimotor circuitry, which is an integral part of the motor command chain (Alstermark & Isa, 2012; Bengtsson & Jorntell, 2014; Jankowska, 1992; Spanne & Jorntell, 2013). If, for example, the motor cortex initiates locomotion or a more isolated fine movement in a single limb, most of the spinal motor circuitry can be expected to be activated in each case. However, the state of the spinal circuitry can be set differently by the corticospinal system so that the end result becomes different in the two cases. The neurons activated at the spinal level are at least partly the same, and the regions (mossy fiber termination areas) of the cerebellar cortex will naturally also be at least partly the same, even though two completely different motor functions are involved.

Hence, it is necessary to know the functional properties of individual mossy fibers, not only in a given context, but in a range of contexts that they could be expected to be involved in. Ideally, the function of each mossy fiber would be described at the level of the minimal common denominator, which in the case of a spinal neuron comprises the afferents it receives and the synaptic route by which it receives them (many connections at the level of the spinal cord are indirectly mediated, via other spinal neurons). By describing the afferent connectivity of each spinocerebellar neuron, it can be possible to understand also how it will respond in a variety of motor contexts. Since the afferents are activated by cutaneous, muscular, or joint movements, it can be possible to calculate how the spinocerebellar neuron would become activated across a range of movement types. For mossy fiber systems originating in the brain stem, the types of movements or the conditions of activation will in many cases be completely different from those in the spinocerebellar neurons, but a corresponding type of characterization across the range of all possible contexts that it is engaged in is required to fully understand the properties of its activation.

CONCLUSIONS

Given the low-weight synaptic connections between the cerebellar cortical neurons and the rate-modulated character of all mossy fiber systems recorded so far, mossy fiber information is expected to be represented as linear signals widespread across the cerebellar cortex. The Purkinje cells can integrate and find associations between these signals, which can be given an either positive or negative sign depending on whether the signal is transmitted through the interneurons or not. The cerebellar neuronal codes can be expected to be reflections of the integration of these linear signals. It follows that to understand the cerebellar neuronal codes, one first needs to have a thorough understanding of what is signaled by the afferent mossy fiber systems. Our current understanding indicates that the range of mossy fiber signaling will be vast and their input will be widely distributed across the cerebellar cortex. But more details are urgently needed, as this is possibly the final remaining frontier before we can start making predictions of how individual neurons can be modulated under different types of behavior.

References

Albus, J. S. (1971). A theory of cerebellar function. *Mathematical Biosciences, 10,* 25–61.

Alstermark, B., & Isa, T. (2012). Circuits for skilled reaching and grasping. *Annual Review of Neuroscience, 35,* 559–578.

Andersson, G., & Oscarsson, O. (1978). Climbing fiber microzones in cerebellar vermis and their projection to different groups of cells in the lateral vestibular nucleus. *Experimental Brain Research, 32,* 565–579.

Apps, R., & Garwicz, M. (2005). Anatomical and physiological foundations of cerebellar information processing. *Nature Reviews: Neuroscience, 6,* 297–311.

Apps, R., & Hawkes, R. (2009). Cerebellar cortical organization: a one-map hypothesis. *Nature Reviews: Neuroscience, 10,* 670–681.

Armstrong, D. M., Harvey, R. J., & Schild, R. F. (1973). Spino-olivocerebellar pathways to the posterior lobe of the cat cerebellum. *Experimental Brain Research, 18,* 1–18.

Averbeck, B. B., Latham, P. E., & Pouget, A. (2006). Neural correlations, population coding and computation. *Nature Reviews: Neuroscience, 7,* 358–366.

Bengtsson, F., Brasselet, R., Johansson, R. S., Arleo, A., & Jorntell, H. (2013). Integration of sensory quanta in cuneate nucleus neurons in vivo. *PLoS One, 8*, e56630.

Bengtsson, F., Ekerot, C. F., & Jorntell, H. (2011). In vivo analysis of inhibitory synaptic inputs and rebounds in deep cerebellar nuclear neurons. *PLoS One, 6*, e18822.

Bengtsson, F., Geborek, P., & Jorntell, H. (2013). Cross-correlations between pairs of neurons in cerebellar cortex in vivo. *Neural Networks: The Official Journal of the International Neural Network Society, 47*, 88–94.

Bengtsson, F., & Jorntell, H. (2007). Ketamine and xylazine depress sensory-evoked parallel fiber and climbing fiber responses. *Journal of Neurophysiology, 98*, 1697–1705.

Bengtsson, F., & Jorntell, H. (2009). Sensory transmission in cerebellar granule cells relies on similarly coded mossy fiber inputs. *Proceedings of the National Academy of Sciences of the United States of America, 106*, 2389–2394.

Bengtsson, F., & Jorntell, H. (2014). Specific relationship between excitatory inputs and climbing fiber receptive fields in deep cerebellar nuclear neurons. *PLoS One, 9*, e84616.

Blot, A., & Barbour, B. (2014). Ultra-rapid axon-axon ephaptic inhibition of cerebellar Purkinje cells by the pinceau. *Nature Neuroscience, 17*, 289–295.

Brickley, S. G., Cull-Candy, S. G., & Farrant, M. (1996). Development of a tonic form of synaptic inhibition in rat cerebellar granule cells resulting from persistent activation of GABAA receptors. *The Journal of Physiology, 497*(Pt 3), 753–759.

Brodal, A. (1981). The cerebellum. In *Neurological anatomy in relation to clinical medicine* (Vol. 3). New York: Oxford University Press.

D'Angelo, E., De, F. G., Rossi, P., & Taglietti, V. (1995). Synaptic excitation of individual rat cerebellar granule cells in situ: evidence for the role of NMDA receptors. *The Journal of Physiology, 484*(Pt 2), 397–413.

Dean, P., Porrill, J., Ekerot, C. F., & Jorntell, H. (2010). The cerebellar microcircuit as an adaptive filter: experimental and computational evidence. *Nature Reviews: Neuroscience, 11*, 30–43.

Dieudonne, S. (1998). Submillisecond kinetics and low efficacy of parallel fibre-Golgi cell synaptic currents in the rat cerebellum. *The Journal of Physiology, 510*(Pt 3), 845–866.

Dieudonne, S., & Dumoulin, A. (2000). Serotonin-driven long-range inhibitory connections in the cerebellar cortex. *The Journal of Neuroscience, 20*, 1837–1848.

Duguid, I., Branco, T., London, M., Chadderton, P., & Hausser, M. (2012). Tonic inhibition enhances fidelity of sensory information transmission in the cerebellar cortex. *The Journal of Neuroscience: The Official Journal of the Society for Neuroscience, 32*, 11132–11143.

Eccles, J. C., Ito, M., & Szentágothai, J. (1967). *The cerebellum as a neuronal machine.* Berlin: Springer-Verlag.

Ekerot, C. F., Garwicz, M., & Schouenborg, J. (1991). Topography and nociceptive receptive fields of climbing fibres projecting to the cerebellar anterior lobe in the cat. *Journal of Physiology (London), 441*, 257–274.

Ekerot, C. F., & Jorntell, H. (2001). Parallel fibre receptive fields of Purkinje cells and interneurons are climbing fibre-specific. *The European Journal of Neuroscience, 13*, 1303–1310.

Faisal, A. A., Selen, L. P., & Wolpert, D. M. (2008). Noise in the nervous system. *Nature Reviews: Neuroscience, 9*, 292–303.

Geborek, P., Bengtsson, F., & Jorntell, H. (2014). Properties of bilateral spinocerebellar activation of cerebellar cortical neurons. *Frontiers in Neural Circuits, 8*, 128–137.

Geborek, P., Spanne, A., Bengtsson, F., & Jorntell, H. (2013). Cerebellar cortical neuron responses evoked from the spinal border cell tract. *Frontiers in Neural Circuits, 7*, 157.

Gebre, S. A., Reeber, S. L., & Sillitoe, R. V. (2012). Parasagittal compartmentation of cerebellar mossy fibers as revealed by the patterned expression of vesicular glutamate transporters VGLUT1 and VGLUT2. *Brain Structure & Function, 217*, 165–180.

Groenewegen, H. J., Voogd, J., & Freedman, S. L. (1979). The parasagittal zonation within the olivocerebellar projection. II. Climbing fiber distribution in the intermediate and hemispheric parts of cat cerebellum. *Journal of Comparative Neurology, 183*, 551–601.

Hausser, M., & Clark, B. A. (1997). Tonic synaptic inhibition modulates neuronal output pattern and spatiotemporal synaptic integration. *Neuron, 19*, 665–678.

Holtzman, T., Cerminara, N. L., Edgley, S. A., & Apps, R. (2009). Characterization in vivo of bilaterally branching pontocerebellar mossy fibre to Golgi cell inputs in the rat cerebellum. *The European Journal of Neuroscience, 29*, 328–339.

Isope, P., & Barbour, B. (2002). Properties of unitary granule cell-->Purkinje cell synapses in adult rat cerebellar slices. *The Journal of Neuroscience: The Official Journal of the Society for Neuroscience, 22*, 9668–9678.

Ito, M. (1984). *The cerebellum and neural control.* New York: Raven Press.

Ito, M. (2006). Cerebellar circuitry as a neuronal machine. *Progress in Neurobiology, 78*, 272–303.

Jaeger, D., De Schutter, E., & Bower, J. M. (1997). The role of synaptic and voltage-gated currents in the control of Purkinje cell spiking: a modeling study. *The Journal of Neuroscience, 17*, 91–106.

Jankowska, E. (1992). Interneuronal relay in spinal pathways from proprioceptors. *Progress in Neurobiology, 38*, 335–378.

Jorntell, H. (2014). Cerebellar synaptic plasticity and the credit assignment problem. *Cerebellum.* In press.

Jorntell, H., Bengtsson, F., Geborek, P., Spanne, A., Terekhov, A. V., & Hayward, V. (2014). Segregation of tactile input features in neurons of the cuneate nucleus. *Neuron, 83*, 1444–1452.

Jorntell, H., Bengtsson, F., Schonewille, M., & De Zeeuw, C. I. (2010). Cerebellar molecular layer interneurons - computational properties and roles in learning. *Trends in Neurosciences, 33*, 524–532.

Jorntell, H., & Ekerot, C. F. (2002). Reciprocal bidirectional plasticity of parallel fiber receptive fields in cerebellar Purkinje cells and their afferent interneurons. *Neuron, 34*, 797–806.

Jorntell, H., & Ekerot, C. F. (2003). Receptive field plasticity profoundly alters the cutaneous parallel fiber synaptic input to cerebellar interneurons in vivo. *The Journal of Neuroscience: The Official Journal of the Society for Neuroscience, 23*, 9620–9631.

Jorntell, H., & Ekerot, C. F. (2006). Properties of somatosensory synaptic integration in cerebellar granule cells in vivo. *The Journal of Neuroscience: The Official Journal of the Society for Neuroscience, 26*, 11786–11797.

Marr, D. (1969). A theory of cerebellar cortex. *The Journal of Physiology, 202*, 437–470.

Oscarsson, O. (1979). Functional units of the cerebellum - sagittal zones and microzones. *Trends in Neurosciences, 2*, 144–145.

Oscarsson, O., & Sjolund, B. (1974). Identification of 5 spino-olivocerebellar paths ascending through the ventral funiculus of the cord. *Brain Research, 69*, 331–335.

Oscarsson, O., & Uddenberg, N. (1966). Somatotopic termination of spino-olivocerebellar path. *Brain Research, 3*, 204–207.

Reeber, S. L., Loeschel, C. A., Franklin, A., & Sillitoe, R. V. (2013). Establishment of topographic circuit zones in the cerebellum of scrambler mutant mice. *Frontiers in Neural Circuits, 7*, 122.

Schweighofer, N., Doya, K., & Lay, F. (2001). Unsupervised learning of granule cell sparse codes enhances cerebellar adaptive control. *Neuroscience, 103*, 35–50.

Spanne, A., Geborek, P., Bengtsson, F., & Jorntell, H. (2014a). Simulating spinal border cells and cerebellar granule cells under locomotion - a case study of spinocerebellar information processing. *PLoS One, 9*, e107793.

Spanne, A., Geborek, P., Bengtsson, F., & Jorntell, H. (2014b). Spike generation estimated from stationary spike trains in a variety of neurons in vivo. *Frontiers in Cellular Neuroscience, 8*, 199.

Spanne, A., & Jorntell, H. (2013). Processing of multi-dimensional sensorimotor information in the spinal and cerebellar neuronal circuitry: a new hypothesis. *PLoS Computational Biology, 9*, e1002979.

Sugihara, I., & Shinoda, Y. (2004). Molecular, topographic, and functional organization of the cerebellar cortex: a study with combined aldolase C and olivocerebellar labeling. *Journal of Neuroscience, 24*, 8771–8785.

Sultan, F. (2001). Distribution of mossy fibre rosettes in the cerebellum of cat and mice: evidence for a parasagittal organization at the single fibre level. *The European Journal of Neuroscience, 13,* 2123–2130.

Trott, J. R., & Armstrong, D. M. (1987). The cerebellar corticonuclear projection from lobule Vb/c of the cat anterior lobe: a combined electrophysiological and autoradiographic study. I. Projections from the intermediate region. *Experimental Brain Research, 66,* 318–338.

Valera, A. M., Doussau, F., Poulain, B., Barbour, B., & Isope, P. (2012). Adaptation of granule cell to Purkinje cell synapses to high-frequency transmission. *The Journal of Neuroscience: The Official Journal of the Society for Neuroscience, 32,* 3267–3280.

Vogels, T. P., Sprekeler, H., Zenke, F., Clopath, C., & Gerstner, W. (2011). Inhibitory plasticity balances excitation and inhibition in sensory pathways and memory networks. *Science, 334,* 1569–1573.

Wall, M. J., & Usowicz, M. M. (1997). Development of action potential-dependent and independent spontaneous GABAA receptor-mediated currents in granule cells of postnatal rat cerebellum. *The European Journal of Neuroscience, 9,* 533–548.

Wang, S. S., Denk, W., & Hausser, M. (2000). Coincidence detection in single dendritic spines mediated by calcium release. *Nature Neuroscience, 3,* 1266–1273.

Wu, H. S., Sugihara, I., & Shinoda, Y. (1999). Projection patterns of single mossy fibers originating from the lateral reticular nucleus in the rat cerebellar cortex and nuclei. *The Journal of Comparative Neurology, 411,* 97–118.

The Role of the Cerebellum in Optimizing Saccades

Zong-Peng Sun[1,3], Shabtai Barash[2], Peter Thier[1]

[1]Department of Cognitive Neurology, Hertie Institute for Clinical Brain Research, University of Tübingen, Tübingen, Germany; [2]Department of Neurobiology, Weizmann Institute, Rehovot, Israel; [3]Graduate School of Neural and Behavioural Sciences and International Max Planck Research School, University of Tübingen, Tübingen, Germany

Eye movements made by primates fall into two broad categories, goal-directed eye movements and image-stabilizing eye movements. The latter use vestibular as well as visual information to generate eye movements that stabilize the eye axis relative to the outer world ("gaze stabilization"), thereby eliminating or at least reducing the retinal image slip that would otherwise result from head or body movements. Goal-directed eye movements consist of two types that complement each other: **saccades** are fast eye movements that move the eyes from one visual object of interest to the next, taking just a few dozens of milliseconds, while **smooth-pursuit eye movements** (SPEMs) try to stabilize the image of an object of interest on the retina. It has long been recognized that the cerebellum is involved in controlling all of these eye movements. Several distinct regions are relevant for the cerebellar control of eye movements (Fig. 1) and, moreover, these regions seem to have distinct and complementary functions in the control of eye movements.

The major cerebellar substrates of gaze stabilization and its context-dependent manipulation are the **flocculus**; the adjoining **ventral paraflocculus** (together often referred to as the floccular complex (FC)), located in the ventrolateral cerebellum; and lobuli VI and VII of the posterior vermis, the so-called **oculomotor vermis**. The flocculus proper consists of four or five distinct lobuli and is located posterior to the ventral paraflocculus, which comprises another six lobuli. Actually, the FC does not seem to be

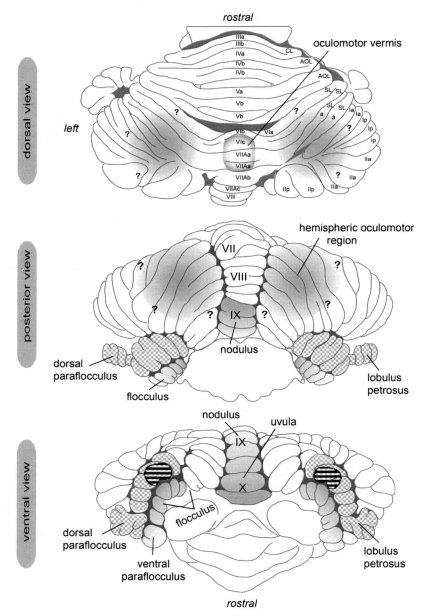

FIGURE 1   Illustration of eye movement-related areas in the primate cerebellum. *(Adapted from Thier (2011).)* The boundaries of the *hemispheric oculomotor region* are ill-defined. The region in the dorsal paraflocculus distinguished by horizontal stripes represents the oculomotor "hot spot" in the dorsal paraflocculus identified by Noda and Mikami (1986). *Views of the cerebellum modified from Madigan and Carpenter (1971).*

confined to controlling gaze stabilization but to make a contribution to SPEMs as well, a dual role that may reflect the need to coordinate different forms of slow eye movements for gaze stabilization, the optokinetic and vestibulo-ocular reflexes and SPEMs (Kahlon & Lisberger, 2000; Medina & Lisberger, 2008, 2009; Rambold, Churchland, Selig, Jasmin, & Lisberger, 2002; Zee, Yamazaki, Butler, & Gucer, 1981). Also the dorsal paraflocculus, located dorsal to the FC, does not seem to be confined to one type of eye movement. The evidence available suggests contributions to the control of saccades and SPEMs (Hiramatsu et al., 2008; Noda & Mikami, 1986), whose specific roles, however, still await characterization. The same has to be said with respect to the hemispheric oculomotor representation in the cerebellum, a fairly large bilateral region with ill-defined boundaries, involving the cerebellar cortex in lobulus simplex, crus I, and crus II, adjoining vermal lobuli VII, and therefore often referred to as **HVII** for hemispheric (region) VII. We know that HVII houses saccade as well as smooth-pursuit-related information (Mano, Ito, & Shibutani, 1991; Ron & Robinson, 1973) and, moreover, that lesions of the HVII cause both saccade and smooth-pursuit deficits (Barash et al., 1999; Ohki et al., 2009). Yet, it remains to be clarified what the specific contributions of HVII to these two types of goal-directed eye movements are and how they differ from those of the posterolateral cerebellum and, in particular, those of the third oculomotor area, the posterior or oculomotor vermis (OV). The OV is a well-defined oculomotor region, comprising the caudal part of vermal lobulus VI and the anterior part of lobulus VII that projects to the caudal pole of the **fastigial nuclei** (caudal fastigial nuclei, cFN), the innermost pair of deep cerebellar nuclei, serving as a gateway to a number of brain-stem centers for eye movements. This chapter discusses the role of the OV and the cFN in controlling saccades with occasional excursions to SPEMs and argue that they help to maintain the precision of these eye movements despite the ever-changing physical and cognitive boundary conditions under which they unfold.

THE OCULOMOTOR VERMIS: THE MAJOR CEREBELLAR SITE OF SACCADES AND SACCADIC ADAPTATION

The OV can be identified physiologically most easily and reliably in the monkey by electrical microstimulation. In contrast to stimulation of its neighborhood, OV stimulation with currents of only a few microamperes suffices to evoke saccades, probably by activating Purkinje cell (PC) axons aiming at the cFN close to their soma (Noda & Fujikado, 1987). In recording experiments, the same region exhibits dense saccade-related background when the microelectrode traverses the granule cell layer. Saccade-related

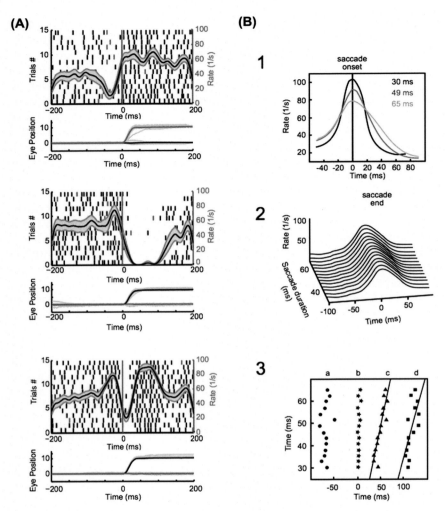

FIGURE 2   (A) Three examples of saccade-related PCs recorded from the oculomotor vermis, documenting the heterogeneity of response types. The monkey was asked to make visually guided saccades into various directions. The individual panels show peristimulus time histograms (spike density functions, 10-ms kernel) of the SSs for particular saccade directions aligned with respect to the saccade onset (time 0, vertical red line). In the raster plots, SS and CS are indicated by black and red dots, respectively. Individual spike density functions are based on a minimum of 15 trials. The traces below the spike density functions show the X (black) and Y (red) components of eye position. (B1) SS population burst profiles based on a group of 94 saccade-related vermal PCs studied during normal, unadapted visually guided saccades for three saccade durations of 30, 49, and 65 ms. The population signal starts, independent of saccade duration, about 20 ms before saccade onset, peaks right at saccade onset, again independent of saccade duration, and then declines. This decline takes longer the longer the saccade lasts (see also (B3)). (B2) The dependence of the duration of the population burst on saccade duration is not confined to the three durations shown in (B1).

responses are also exhibited by mossy fiber afferents, mainly originating from the dorsal and medial pontine nuclei, the reticular nucleus of the pontine tegmentum (NRTP), and the paramedian pontine reticular formation (PPRF) (Fries, 1990; Gerrits & Voogd, 1986; Giolli et al., 2001; Nagao, 2004; Thielert & Thier, 1993), by Golgi cells as well as by PC simple spikes (SSs) and complex spikes (CSs) (Catz, Dicke, & Thier, 2005, 2008; Kase, Miller, & Noda, 1980; Prsa, Dash, Catz, Dicke, & Thier, 2009; Thier, Dicke, Haas, & Barash, 2000). CSs in the OV reflect climbing fiber input from the caudal parts of the medial accessory inferior olivary nucleus (Ikeda, Noda, & Sugita, 1989). Both the CSs and the SSs make it to the terminals of PC axons that contact target neurons in the deep cerebellar nuclei, with the former being converted into a small group of conventional sodium spikes, indistinguishable from those triggered by SSs. The small number of CS-dependent spikes at the level of PC–axon terminals makes it very unlikely that they will significantly modify the information encoded in the stream of the much more numerous SSs. CSs should be seen as a reflection of the impact of climbing fiber activity at the level of the PC, where it may influence the PC-output code, arguably in an attempt to modify the behavior at stake. We will later return to the role of the climbing fiber input. On the other hand, if we want to understand what the OV tells premotor circuits for goal-directed eye movements, we should try to understand the SS code.

The saccade-related SS responses of PCs are very heterogeneous. Some PCs fire saccade-related SS bursts, others saccade-related pauses or more complex saccade-related response patterns consisting of sequences of bursts and pauses (see Fig. 2(A) for examples), characterized by a substantial degree of variability. Numbers on the relative shares of these various response types differ between studies. While this is to some extent an inevitable consequence of the stochastic nature of drawing small samples of neurons from a large population, differences between individual monkeys may matter as well. For instance, in our own work, we have seen

◀ (B2) shows a pseudo-three-dimensional plot of the population burst as a function of saccade duration for a larger number of saccade durations. The x-axis plots the time relative to saccade onset at 0 ms, the y-axis saccade duration, and the z-axis the mean instantaneous discharge rate of a population of 94 PCs. (B3) Regression plots relating various parameters characterizing the population burst timing relative to the saccade. We measured the times of the onset (a), peak (b), and end (c) of the population burst relative to saccade onset for each saccade duration. Curve (d) is the population burst duration given by (c–a). We determined the population onset and offset times as the times when the population burst reached four times the baseline firing rate when building up and when declining from the peak. The figure plots time t as a function of (a–d), respectively. The plots are fitted by linear regressions. Both (c) and (d) increased significantly with the time of saccade termination and saccade duration, respectively, whereas neither (a) nor (b) depended significantly on saccade duration. The end of the population burst (c) as predicted by the regression corresponds very closely to the end of the saccades. *From Thier et al. (2000).*

monkeys in which more than 90% of the PCs exhibited saccade-related SS bursts (Catz et al., 2008; Thier et al., 2000), whereas in others, the numbers of pause and burst units were more or less balanced, as in the most recent study by Arnstein, Junker, Smilgin, Dicke, and Thier (2015). Moreover, we have seen unquestionable transitions from one response category to another in the context of saccadic adaptation (Catz et al., 2008) (see Fig. 1 for an example). The observation that responses vary widely between individual cells is not compatible with the notion that individual cells predict behavior, unless we assume that qualitatively different response types reflect specific functional roles in the network, based on different connections. However, rather than supporting functionally distinct output channels, the anatomical data are more suggestive of mixing of individual response types. This is a consequence of the profound convergence of the terminals of a few dozens to hundreds of PCs on individual target neurons in the deep cerebellar nuclei (Palkovits, Mezey, Hamori, & Szentagothai, 1977; Person & Raman, 2012). While we cannot exclude that a developmental principle may select axons according to response types, ensuring that convergence of axons is restricted to particular response types, our own findings strongly argue against selection.

We simulated unrestricted, nonselective convergence of information on target neurons by calculating PC SS population responses based on larger samples of PCs of any type (Thier et al., 2000). We found that these SS population responses were able to precisely predict the duration of visually guided saccades (Fig. 2(B)). As duration and saccade length are linearly related, with large saccades taking longer, a prediction of duration is tantamount to predicting saccade amplitude. Not even the individual unit with the highest precision in reflecting saccade timing that had contributed to the population signal was able to yield roughly comparably reliable predictions of saccade duration and length. Actually, a representation of saccade duration in the population signal is a consequence of the fact that the signal starts reliably at the same time, tens of milliseconds before saccade onset, while ending precisely at the time the saccade ends. Acute lesions of the OV lead to saccades that are too short (hypometric), that is, saccades whose duration is too short (Barash et al., 1999). This suggests that the cerebellar output based on a saccade-related population signal expands the duration of a hypometric default saccade, programmed by the brain stem so as to allow the eyes to hit the target. In other words, the eyes keep moving as long as the PC population signal is up, and they stop—due to the transition of the population signal to baseline—at a point in time that corresponds to a normometric saccade amplitude.

A critical test of this interpretation is offered by short-term saccadic plasticity or adaptation, a form of saccadic learning in which consistent performance errors prompt changes in saccade amplitude and duration. Performance errors can be introduced by shifting the peripheral target to a new location while the eyes are on their way to the target (McLaughlin, 1967). Saccadic suppression prevents the target shift from being noticed. The eyes arrive at where the target used to be before the onset of the shift and a corrective saccade is then added to finally fovealize the target image. If these shifts are carried out repetitively and consistently, one observes that the amplitude of the primary saccades changes in a way allowing the eyes to get closer to the target at its new location after the shift. After several dozen trials in humans and several hundred trials in monkeys, the eyes may finally manage to hit the target in one go, rendering a second, corrective saccade unnecessary. If the target is shifted further out during the first saccade, saccade amplitude will grow (gain-increase adaptation) and this increase in saccade length is associated with an increase in saccade duration (Catz et al., 2008).

This increase in saccade duration is accurately predicted by the PC population signal as the population signal ends at the same later point in time as the adapted saccade. However, as the population signal associated with the adapted saccade also starts later relative to saccade onset, the overall duration of the population signal does not change significantly. These observations are in accordance with the notion that the major function of the OV is the adjustment of the later parts of a saccade by fine-tuning its duration. At a first glance, this conclusion seems to be challenged by the fact that gain-decrease-adapted saccades—a consequence of stepping the target a little bit back during the saccade—do not exhibit a correspondingly close relationship between the end of the population signal and the saccade end (Catz et al., 2008). Actually, in this case, the population signal ends much earlier than the adapted saccade, whose smaller amplitude is a consequence of reduced saccade velocity but unchanged duration, compared with unadapted saccades. A similar decline of velocity characterizes saccades affected by fatigue. However, in this case an upregulation of movement duration ensures that the amplitude remains normal (Prsa, Dicke, & Thier, 2010). The comparison of gain-decrease-adapted saccades and saccades affected by fatigue suggests that gain-decrease adaptation is a consequence of fatigue, not compensated for by an upregulation of movement duration. Arguably, this upregulation is missing because the PC population signal may end too early to have a significant influence on "default" saccades determined by the brain stem. This hypothesis is perfectly in line with the fact that—as mentioned earlier—acute lesions of the OV, eliminating the population signal, cause hypometric saccades. We used the term saccadic fatigue before to allude to changes in saccade kinematics observed when long sequences of stereotypic saccades are carried out. The majority of observations suggest that saccadic fatigue is a consequence of a drop in motivation and arousal rather than of changes in the orbital plant (Prsa et al., 2010; Xu-Wilson, Zee, & Shadmehr, 2009). However, the question concerning the specific nature of saccadic fatigue is actually irrelevant for the proposed cerebellar mechanism stabilizing the amplitudes of fatigued saccades by choosing a movement duration that takes changes of saccade velocity into account. The increase in saccade duration characterizing the maintenance of normometric amplitudes of fatigued saccades is of the same order as the duration increase in gain-increase-adapted saccades. This suggests that the two actually rely on the same mechanism or, to put it differently, that the gain-increase variant of short-term saccadic adaptation taps a mechanism normally used for the compensation for fatigue. Given the fact that the first signs of fatigue can be observed after just a few saccades, this compensation mechanism must operate on a very short time scale. Here we argue that the neuronal basis of this compensation mechanism is the appropriate adjustment of an OV PC SS population signal.

Short-term saccadic adaptation and, arguably, also fatigue compensation are driven by the performance error, that is, the difference between the ideal saccade, needed to fovealize the peripheral target, and the actually executed saccade. If the two do not match, the target image lands on a location outside the fovea. Soetedjo, Fuchs, and Kojima (2009) have suggested that the vector connecting the locations with the fovea, that is, the retinal (target) error, is represented by the superior colliculus (SC) by activating specific SC locations in a topographically specific manner. Activation of a particular location of the SC right after a saccade to a peripheral target should signal that the saccade missed the target, reflecting a particular error vector. They reasoned that electrical microstimulation of this SC location after a saccade should mimic this scenario. Indeed they could successfully induce gradual changes in saccade amplitude when using microstimulation to simulate constant retinal errors after saccades. The direction of the changes induced depended on the direction of the simulated constant errors. The SC is known to project to the inferior olive (Harting, 1977) and, arguably, also to the medial accessory nucleus of the inferior olive, the major source of climbing fibers reaching the OV (Saint-Cyr & Courville, 1982). Hence, the microstimulation results seemed to be in line with the notion that the climbing fiber system supports saccadic learning—and in general motor learning—by providing an error signal as posited by the Marr–Albus hypothesis (Albus, 1971; Marr, 1969). However, the SC projects not only to the inferior olive but also to a couple of precerebellar nuclei that send mossy fiber input to the OV, among them the dorsal pontine nuclei and the NRTP (Altman & Carpenter, 1961; Benevento & Fallon, 1975; Graham, 1977; Harting, 1977; Scudder, Moschovakis, Karabelas, & Highstein, 1996), and there is no reason to assume that SC microstimulation would selectively activate only the output to the inferior olive. The argument would become much more conclusive if selective stimulation of the SC–inferior olive–climbing fiber pathway, for example, by directly activating the medial accessory nucleus of the inferior olive (MAO), had the same effect as stimulation of the SC.

Unfortunately, as of this writing, this experiment has not been carried out. Also, the pattern of climbing fiber firing is much more complicated than predicted by a simple "error signal" hypothesis.

In an earlier experiment (Catz et al., 2005), we studied the CS, the hallmark of the climbing fiber input, of a large sample of more than 170 OV PCs during and following saccadic adaptation. In separate experiments we considered both gain-decrease and gain-increase adaptation. In clear contradiction to the "error signal" concept we found that CSs occurred at random before adaptation onset, that is, when the error was maximal and built up gradually to a specific saccade-related discharge profile during the course of adaptation. This profile, whose specific shape depended on the direction of adaptation, became most pronounced at the end of adaptation, that is, when the error had reached near zero. This result clearly suggested that the CS firing may underlie the stabilization of a learned motor behavior, rather than serving as an electrophysiological correlate of an error. Also attempts to use functional magnetic resonance imaging to study the processing of saccadic errors in the human OV have failed to reveal any significant activity (van Broekhoven et al., 2009). On the other hand, Soetedjo and Fuchs recorded a small sample of 14 PCs in the OV during simultaneous adaptation of saccades in two opposite directions but having the same direction of error (Soetedjo & Fuchs, 2006). The same cells were then tested once more with the same adaptation sequence but with the error occurring in the opposite direction compared to before. Regardless of the direction of the primary saccades, CS discharges during the error interval showed an unambiguous preference for one of the two opposite error directions in 10 of the 14 neurons. However, as the error progressively decreased during adaptation, no significant changes in the CS discharges modulating the size of the error could be observed. Independent of the question of whether the CSs of individual PCs might be influenced by saccadic errors, it is very clear that the collective activity of CSs from many PCs in the OV exhibits a specific pattern of behavior-related modulation that can be seen with the naked eye, without resorting to subtle statistics (Catz et al., 2005). And the same pattern is observable in the responses of many individual CS units. The modulation builds up in parallel with the development of saccadic adaptation and becomes maximal once the learning is complete (Fig. 3). Actually, a very similar pattern of change in PC CS activity was also observed when monkeys adaptively increased or decreased the velocity of SPEMs (Dash, Catz, Dicke, & Thier, 2010). This observation strongly suggests a generalization to multiple motor learning modalities. Actually, the different findings on the behavior of CSs during saccadic adaptation may not be as incompatible as they seem at first glance. We think that the buildup of CS modulation paralleling the buildup of adaptation may reflect integration of a very tiny yet consistent influence of an error signal on the CS discharge. It is tempting

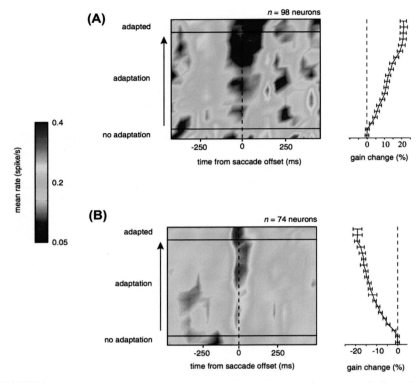

FIGURE 3   Change in complex spike population responses in the course of adaptation. (A) The left side depicts the population response based on 98 posterior vermal PCs studied during outward adaptation, and the right side shows the mean saccadic gain change (±SEM) as a function of adaptation level for the 54 outward adaptation sessions that were necessary to collect the PC contributing to the population data. (B) The left side shows the population response for 74 posterior vermal PCs (not overlapping with the "outward" population depicted in (A)) studied during inward adaptation. The right side depicts saccade gain change (±SEM) as a function of adaptation level based on 42 inward adaptation sessions that were required to collect the sample of PCs. Complex spike population responses are plotted as a function of time relative to saccade offset (x-axis) and normalized adaptation level (y-axis) from no adaptation (horizontal line) to full adaptation (top). The part underneath the horizontal line represents trials prior to the onset of target displacements. The color code represents the mean rate of CS activity in the population for time bins of 25 ms (x-axis) and adaptation bins, corresponding to 1/20 of the range from no to full adaptation. A Gaussian filter (SD 50 ms) was used to smooth the plot along the x-axis. *From Catz et al. (2005).*

to speculate that the known feedback from the OV to the inferior olive via a distinct set of deep cerebellar nuclei (DCN) neurons may actually be the structural basis of the assumed integration. But why should there be a need for a buildup of a consistent CS modulation reaching its maximum at the time the error has reached zero and the new behavior is fully established? An answer is suggested by a comparison of the PC CS and

SS patterns at the end of adaptation. In the case of gain-increase adaptation, the probability of observing CS declines around the time of the saccade. Conversely, in the case of gain-decrease adaptation, the probability increases (Fig. 3) (Catz et al., 2005). Maximal long-term adaptation (LTD) at parallel fiber synapses is observed when a CS occurs within 200 ms after simple spikes (Wang & Linden, 2000). Hence, this CS "burst" during gain-decrease adaptation, reaching its maximum around −20 ms relative to the saccade end might induce LTD if the saccade-related SS burst appeared between −220 and −20 ms relative to saccade offset. SSs, which would normally have appeared in this period, would be suppressed. As a result, the SS population signal would stop earlier. On the other hand, the suppression of CSs during gain-increase adaptation, reaching its maximum at −10 ms, should reduce the LTD of SSs in the 200 ms before, thereby unleashing SSs in this period and consequently extending the SS population signal. In other words, relative to nonadapted saccades, we would expect to see saccade-related SS activity that is longer lasting in the case of gain-increase adaptation, but shorter lasting saccade-related SS activity for gain-decrease adaptation. This is exactly what Catz et al. found in their study of SS discharge during and after saccadic adaptation (Catz et al., 2008). Hence, the pattern of CS determines the SS pattern needed by facilitating the SS responses of those individual PCs whose timing is appropriate and by suppressing the responses of those whose timing is inappropriate. For this mechanism to work, the spectrum of occurrences of individual SS responses should cover the full temporal range by the population signal. As SS responses depend on their parallel fiber input, which in turn reflects the activity of mossy fibers, the expectation is that the temporal dispersion of saccade-related mossy fiber discharges is at least as wide as the temporal extent of the SS PC signal. Actually, this is the case, as the saccade-related mossy fiber signals cover a range of time relative to the saccade that is much wider than the one covered by SSs (Prsa et al., 2009). In other words, as summarized in the conceptual model shown in Fig. 4, we suggest that CSs are a selection tool that carves out an SS population signal optimally suited to drive the behavior needed based on a highly dispersed input. And this selection tool is continuously updated by information on the performance error.

THE CAUDAL FASTIGIAL NUCLEUS: A GATEWAY FOR SACCADE-RELATED SIGNALS ORIGINATING FROM THE OCULOMOTOR VERMIS

The paired fastigial nuclei are the medialmost DCN, lying on either side of the midline. Their caudal poles (the cFN) are the major recipients of fibers originating from the OV. By injecting anterograde tracers into the

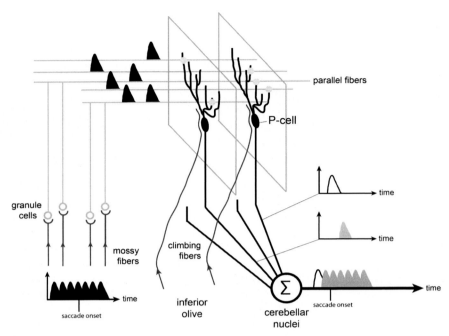

FIGURE 4   Conceptual model of the role of the OV in the adaptation of saccadic eye movements. The shark-fin-like profiles represent the discharge of individual units: black, parallel
fibers; gray, PC simple spike burst stabilized by climbing fiber activity; white, PC simple
spike unit eliminated or weakened by climbing fiber activity. Saccade-related responses in
the mossy fiber input to the OV cover a wide temporal range relative to saccade onset and
end (Prsa et al., 2009). The selection from this wide spectrum of choices brought to PCs by the
parallel fibers is carried out by the CF input and the ensuing CSs (Catz et al., 2005). The end
result is a population signal of PC SSs that ends simultaneously with the end of the saccadic
eye movement. This population output of the OV sent to individual neurons in the DCN
determines the size of saccades by optimizing their duration (Catz et al., 2008; Thier et al.,
2000). *Adapted from Prsa and Thier (2011).*

OV of macaques, Yamada and Noda (1987) could demonstrate that PC
axons terminated ipsilaterally on target neurons in the cFN, which in turn
project contralateral to a number of brain-stem nuclei implicated in saccades such as the PPRF, the dorsomedial medullary reticular formation,
the omnipause neuron region, and the more rostral parts of the superior
colliculus (Batton, Jayaraman, Ruggiero, & Carpenter, 1977; Homma,
Nonaka, Matsuyama, & Mori, 1995; May, Hartwich-Young, Nelson, Sparks, &
Porter, 1990; Noda, Sugita, & Ikeda, 1990; Sato & Noda, 1991; Sugita &
Noda, 1991), as well as the MAO (Dietrichs & Walberg, 1985; Ikeda et al.,
1989; Ruigrok & Voogd, 1990). All the target structures serve saccadic eye
movements in one or another way.

   The apparent lack of specificity of the projection contrasts with
the emphasis occasionally given to particular targets in an attempt to

conceptualize the role of the cFN (see later). The tight link with the contralateral brain-stem premotor system for saccades explains the fact that microstimulation of the cFN can evoke saccades to the contralateral sides with very low currents (usually <10 μA) (Noda et al., 1988). The ipsiversive saccades that are evoked by stimulating the dorsal portion of the cFN are probably not a consequence of activation of cFN neurons or their axons but of activation of PC axon preterminals, mimicking the natural activation of strong GABAergic inhibition of cFN target neurons by PC axon terminals. The view that ipsiversive saccades are indeed a result of an artificial activation of the PC input finds support from the observation that blockade of PC synapses by injecting the GABA antagonist bicuculline is able to veto the stimulation effect (Noda et al., 1988). Natural saccades made while bicuculline blocks the PC input on cFN target neurons are hypometric in the ipsilateral and hypermetric in the contralateral direction (Sato & Noda, 1992), an observation that is compatible with the notion that each cFN generates a tonic saccade drive to the contralateral side. Correspondingly, unilateral injection of the GABA agonist muscimol into the cFN, thought to boost the inhibition of cFN target neurons, induces faster hypermetric ipsilateral saccades and slower hypometric contralateral saccades (Fuchs, Robinson, & Straube, 1993; Goffart, Chen, & Sparks, 2004), whereas bilateral injections of muscimol make saccades slower and hypermetric to both sides (Fuchs et al., 1993). Finally, vertical saccades are horizontally bent toward the inactivated side, an observation that can be explained by a release of the ipsiversive horizontal drive.

While the stimulation results and the pharmacological manipulations have allowed us to understand the consequences of changing the tonic level of activity in one of the cFNs with interesting implications for the interpretation of natural lesions of the human cFN, they have been of little value in an attempt to understand how OV signals for the control of saccade duration and other aspects of saccade kinematics are processed for their final targets in the brain-stem premotor circuitry for saccades. This understanding requires knowledge of the discharge properties of cFN neurons and ideally causal manipulations with sufficient spatial and temporal specificity as offered by optogenetic manipulations. While these studies are still a long time in the coming, we have at least some knowledge on eye-movement-related discharges of neurons in the cFN.

Previous work has emphasized the existence of saccade-related burst responses, which are thought to reflect an excitatory saccade-related mossy fiber input originating from the NRTP, the PPRF, and the dorsomedial pontine nuclei (Noda et al., 1990; Ohtsuka & Noda, 1992) able to override the inhibition provided by PC terminals (Thier et al., 2000). There is consensus between the studies available that these saccade-related bursts start in general earlier for contralateral saccades than for ipsilateral saccades (see Fig. 5(B) for an example from our own material) (Fuchs et al., 1993; Helmchen, Straube, & Büttner, 1994; Kleine, Guan, & Büttner, 2003; Ohtsuka & Noda, 1990, 1991; Sun, Junker, Dicke, & Thier, 2013). Moreover, the burst accompanying ipsiversive saccades often exhibits a preceding pause. It is of course tempting to try to relate this pause–burst sequence back to a putatively earlier onset of PC inhibition relative to a somewhat later mossy excitation. Yet, in contradiction to this simple scenario saccade-related mossy fiber bursts start earlier and last longer than saccade-related PC activity (Catz et al., 2008; Prsa et al., 2009; Thier et al., 2000). In any case, the onset of bursts associated with contralateral saccades precedes saccade onset by 7.9–18.5 ms, whereas the onset of bursts for ipsilateral saccades follows saccade onset by an amount that increases with saccade amplitude (from −10.3 ms relative to saccade onset for small saccades up to a few milliseconds after saccade onset for large saccades) (Fuchs et al., 1993). Actually, burst onset for ipsiversive saccades seems to be much more precisely correlated with saccade offset than with saccade onset, with the burst onset preceding saccade end by 23–28 ms (Fuchs et al., 1993).

Fuchs and colleagues have proposed a conceptual model that tries to use the conspicuous difference between the timing of bursts for ipsi- and contraversive bursts to explain the tonic contralateral saccade drive exerted by the cFN, suggested by the lesion experiments discussed earlier (Fuchs et al., 1993). The conceptual model builds on the assumption that the cFN exerts control on saccades based on projections to excitatory (EBN) and inhibitory (IBN) burst neurons in the contralateral PPRF. According to this scheme, the left cFN is assumed to excite EBNs as well as IBNs on the right, whereas the right cFN would exhibit the corresponding mirror pattern. Based on the activation of EBNs on the right, the early burst fired by the left cFN for contraversive saccades would cause an activation of right-sided abducens motoneurons and left-sided medial rectus motoneurons (the latter is a consequence of an activation of internuclear neurons in the abducens nucleus, projecting to contralateral rectus medialis motoneurons). The resulting rightward saccade would be facilitated by concurrent reduction in the tone of the respective antagonist muscles due to the activation of the IBNs on the right, maintaining a projection to the left abducens nucleus. The late burst fired by the left cFN in the case of ipsiversive saccades is assumed to help stop the saccade by increasing the tone of the antagonists by way of the projection to the EBNs and IBNs on the right. While this conceptual model is meritorious, as it offers an explanation of the metric and kinematic consequences of cFN lesions at least on a qualitative level, it is not able to explain the subtle adjustments of saccades based on short-term saccadic adaptation or fatigue. Moreover, the anatomical and functional assumptions made reflect a degree of simplification that may question the validity of this "standard" cFN

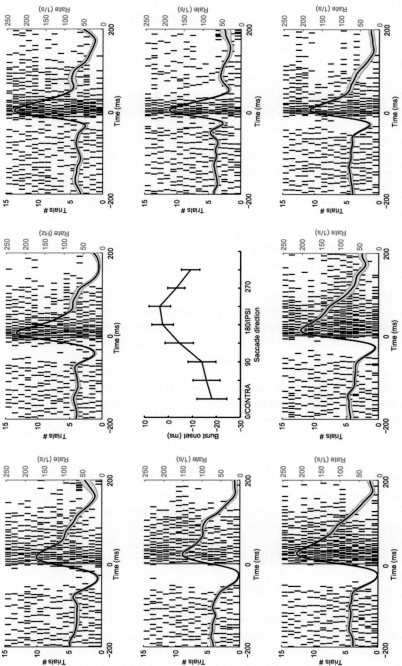

FIGURE 5 Example of a saccade-related burst neuron recorded from the cFN. The monkey was asked to make visually guided saccades in eight different directions (0°/rightward, 45°/upward, 90°/upward, 135°/leftward, 180°/IPSI, 215°/downward, 270°/downward, and 315°) in the frontoparallel plane, starting from straight ahead. The eight outer panels show the peristimulus time histograms (spike density functions, 10-ms kernel) of discharge aligned with respect to saccade onset (time 0, vertical red line). The central panel plots burst onset time relative to saccade onset as a function of direction, documenting the typical difference between ipsiversive and contraversive saccades.

model. (1) As said earlier, cFN neurons contact many targets apart from brain-stem EBNs and IBNs, singled out in the model as the only targets of importance. And some of the projections (e.g., the one to the SC) not considered are actually stronger than the ones emphasized. (2) cFN neurons are not the assumed homogeneous entity. Neurons in the cFN and the DCN in general exhibit distinct morphologies and transmitters (Bagnall et al., 2009; Chen & Hillman, 1993; Sultan, Konig, Mock, & Thier, 2002; Uusisaari, Obata, & Knopfel, 2007), most probably maintaining distinct connections and arguably hardly conveying the same signals to their respective targets. For instance, the cFN neurons projecting to the inferior olive are GABAergic and significantly smaller than the glutamatergic projection neurons contacting the many other brain-stem centers such as the PPRF, the SC, and the NRTP. While the neurons that make up the latter pool look similar, this certainly does not exclude the possibility that the signals they convey may differ.

Our recent observations on saccade-related neurons in the monkey cFN challenge the prevailing assumption of homogeneous response types. In a sample of 96 units recorded from the cFN of three monkeys, 74 responded to visually guided saccades. Actually, only 56 of them showed the typical saccade-related bursts emphasized by previous work. The others exhibited pause responses or more complex patterns such as sequences of bursts and pauses or tonic eye position-dependent responses and, in some cases, without exhibiting the clear differences between the onset latencies for contra- and ipsiversive saccades emphasized by previous work on the cFN (see Fig. 5 for an example of the last). Unfortunately, we lack pertinent information that would allow us to figure out if particular response patterns are associated with distinct cell-type morphologies and/or projection targets. In any case, the response patterns deviating from the burst pattern, thought to be prototypic for cFN neurons, would hardly fit into the model of cFN–brain-stem interactions, sketched before.

As this model sees excitatory and inhibitory burst neurons as the sole targets of cFN output, it is also not able to easily accommodate another result of our work on the cFN, namely the fact that cFN neurons are not specific for saccades. Already earlier work had described smooth-pursuit-related signals in the cFN (Büttner, Fuchs, Markert-Schwab, & Buckmaster, 1991; Fuchs et al., 1993; Fuchs, Robinson, & Straube, 1994). However, until recently it was assumed that they form an entity different from the saccade-related neurons. Yet, in a 2015 study (Sun, Smilgin, Dicke, & Thier, in preparation) we could obtain first evidence that this is probably not the case. Of 16 saccade-related cFN neurons tested, 13 turned out to be responsive to SPEMs as well. Actually, sensitivity to SPEMs exhibited by cFN neurons responding to saccades is not that unexpected in view of a similar integration of sensitivities to smooth pursuit and to saccades at the level of the OV output. Of 80 PCs with saccade-related discharge,

76 also responded to SPEMs (Smilgin, Dicke, & Thier, 2012; Sun et al., in preparation). Actually, shared sensitivities for SPEMs and for saccades also hold for many neurons in one of the major sources of mossy fibers for the OV, the dorsal pontine nuclei. There, about 20% of the eye-movement-related neurons studied by Dicke, Barash, Ilg, and Thier (2004) exhibited responses to saccades and to SPEMs. On the other hand, it is usually held that the brain-stem pathways for saccades and SPEMs are largely separated, with EBNs and IBNs thought to be largely committed to saccades (Thier & Ilg, 2005). If these brain-stem neurons were indeed major targets of cerebellar input, we should also expect them to exhibit smooth-pursuit-related responses. While PPRF burst neurons have been described that discharge spikes for saccades as well as for smooth-pursuit (Keller & Missal, 2003), it is not clear if this subgroup is representative for classical EBNs and IBNs. However, independent of the question if EBNs and IBNs serve as the major target of a shared cFN–OV pathway for saccades and for SPEMs, the existence of such a shared pathway seems puzzling in view of the well-established role of the OV in both saccadic and smooth-pursuit adaptation. As the adaptation is a consequence of changes at the level of the OV PC, one might expect that adjustments due to adaptation of saccades should affect not only their contribution to saccades but also that to SPEMs, if the required oculomotor behavior were changed. Conversely, smooth-pursuit adaptation should transfer to saccades. It is hard to see why such transfer between kinematically and dynamically very different types of eye movements should be useful.

Our behavioral studies do not support the existence of a significant transfer of learning between these two forms of goal-directed eye movements (Smilgin, Sun, Telgen, Dicke, & Thier, in preparation). If we assume that saccadic as well as smooth-pursuit adaptation is a consequence of changes in the efficacy of parallel fiber synapses induced and maintained by climbing fiber input, the absence of learning transfer would be compatible with two largely separated pools of synapses, one accommodating saccades, the other one SPEMs. In other words, we suggest an economical computational scheme in which the same set of OV PCs is able to make fully independent contributions to two very different oculomotor behaviors. Given the uniformity of the cerebellar cortex, it would be surprising if this multiplexing scheme were specific to the OV and its contribution to goal-directed eye movements. Although certainly attractive, this scheme is most certainly incomplete as it is not able to deal with two major problems. The first is that it leads behavioral specificity of PC output back to the existence of separate pools of synapses, one for saccades, a second one for SPEMs. However, the mossy fiber input to the OV may not be as clearly divided into separate streams for saccades and for SPEMs. As discussed in conjunction with the role of brain-stem EBNs and IBNs, do we have to assume separate premotor circuits for saccades and SPEMs?

The very different kinematic and dynamic demands of these two types of eye movements allow us to expect at least a certain degree of separation. But then a mechanism for demultiplexing the cerebellar input would be indispensable. Using information on the type of eye movement at stake, only the input to the appropriate target would be gated and the input to the inappropriate one would be blocked. Actually, all these speculations are based on the implicit assumption that learning-related signals offered by the OV are indeed faithfully transmitted by the cFN. This is certainly a very plausible assumption. At least with respect to saccadic learning it is fully supported by the effects of pharmacological lesions reported by Robinson, Fuchs, and Noto (2002). They carried out unilateral and bilateral injections of muscimol into the cFN and found that standard saccadic adaptation protocols were unable to evoke adaptation as long as the muscimol could be expected to shut fastigial neurons down. If the monkeys were given time to recover from the muscimol injections in darkness, thereby preventing the annihilation of the experience of the preceding adaptation protocol, a significant amount of saccadic adaptation could be observed. This result is fully compatible with the notion that saccadic adaptation occurred upstream of the cFN, namely at the level of OV PCs, with muscimol only temporarily blocking the transmission of the adaptation effects to the brain stem. This view is also in line with the finding of a long-lasting abolition of short-term saccadic adaptation due to pure OV lesions (Barash et al., 1999) that likewise argues against a relevant role for structures downstream of the OV in short-term saccadic adaptation.

The cFN, however, is clearly a candidate structure that may be involved in adjustments of saccade metrics that take place on a much longer time scale. An example of such long-term saccadic learning is the slow recovery from the initial saccadic hypometria after acute OV lesions, taking weeks (Barash et al., 1999). Another one is long-term saccadic adaptation as described by Robinson and co-workers (Mueller, Davis, & Robinson, 2012; Robinson, Soetedjo, & Noto, 2006). In these experiments, monkeys were exposed to intrasaccade target steps in daily experiments over many subsequent days, combined with an intervention preventing normal visual experiences between sessions. In the course of 2–3 weeks, this treatment led to changes in saccade amplitudes (depending on the direction of the intrasaccadic step amplitude either decreases or increases), which were much larger than the one achieved by standard short-term saccadic adaptation sessions. The fact that, even at the end of the long procedure, a standard short-term saccadic adaptation experiment could evoke additional changes seemed to argue for independent mechanisms for short-term and long-term saccadic adaptation.

A role of the cFN in the pathway subserving short-term saccadic adaptation is also supported by single-unit recording studies (Inaba, Iwamoto, & Yoshida, 2003; Scudder & McGee, 2003). The few reports available concur that neurons in the cFN exhibit changes in their discharge during adaptation, although the results reported are too diverse to allow a fully conclusive interpretation. Scudder and McGee studied adaptation to surgically weakened medial and lateral rectus muscles of one eye (Scudder & McGee, 2003). When the paretic eye is covered by a patch, the saccades of the operated eye remain too small, whereas the intact eye exhibits saccades that are normal in size (Kommerell, Olivier, & Theopold, 1976). However, if the intact eye is patched, the amplitude of the operated eye saccades grows slowly and may eventually become normal, whereas those of the intact eye become hypermetric, changes that are reversible if the patch is reversed. Scudder and McGee could record from a small group of cFN neurons to changes in saccade size due to patching one eye and found changes in a couple of discharge parameters. One of these changes was a somewhat earlier onset of the saccade-related burst for ipsiversive gain decrease adaptation, a finding that was also reported by Inaba et al. (2003) for gain-decrease adaptation based on intrasaccadic target steps. Against the backdrop of the standard cFN model, Scudder and McGee (2003) suggested that the earlier ipsiversive burst might lead to an earlier activation of the antagonists, thereby stopping the saccade earlier than normal. In the case of contraversive gain-increase adaptation, they observed that, among others, bursts started later and ended later. The fact that cFN neurons show clear adaptation-related changes in the timing of their responses is, in principle, in accordance with the work on OV PCs, which has also emphasized changes in discharge timing as the major mechanism.

SUMMARY

Our work on the role of the oculomotor vermis in the control of saccades and their continuous optimization has led to a number of conclusions with relevance to our thinking about the working of the cerebellum at large: the idea that the major function of cerebellum-based learning is the rapid correction of inevitable performance inaccuracies due to fatigue, probably independent of whether fatigue is cognitive, muscular, or eventually even neuronal; the notion that the climbing fiber system not only initiates learning but is intimately involved in stabilizing the new behavior; and finally the idea that the cerebellar output is based on a simple spike population signal whose shape is determined by the climbing fiber signals.

Acknowledgments

Parts of our own work discussed in this review were supported by grants from the German Ministry of Education, Science, Research, and Technology through the Bernstein Center for Computational Neuroscience (Grant FKZ 01GQ1002) and the Deutsche Forschungsgemeinschaft (Grant FOR 1847-A3 TH425/13-1) to P.T.

References

Albus, J. S. (1971). A theory of cerebellar function. *Mathematical Biosciences, 10,* 25–26.

Altman, J., & Carpenter, M. B. (1961). Fiber projections of the superior colliculus in the cat. *Journal of Comparative Neurology, 116,* 157–177.

Arnstein, D., Junker, M., Smilgin, A., Dicke, P. W., & Thier, P. (2015). Microsaccade control signals in the cerebellum. *Journal of Neuroscience, 35*(8), 3403–3411. http://dx.doi.org/10.1523/jneurosci.2458-14.2015.

Bagnall, M. W., Zingg, B., Sakatos, A., Moghadam, S. H., Zeilhofer, H. U., & du Lac, S. (2009). Glycinergic projection neurons of the cerebellum. *Journal of Neuroscience, 29*(32), 10104–10110. http://dx.doi.org/10.1523/jneurosci.2087-09.2009.

Barash, S., Melikyan, A., Sivakov, A., Zhang, M., Glickstein, M., & Thier, P. (1999). Saccadic dysmetria and adaptation after lesions of the cerebellar cortex. *Journal of Neuroscience, 19*(24), 10931–10939.

Batton, R. R., Jayaraman, A., Ruggiero, D., & Carpenter, M. B. (1977). Fastigial efferent projections in the monkey: an autoradiographic study. *Journal of Comparative Neurology, 174*(2), 281–305. http://dx.doi.org/10.1002/cne.901740206.

Benevento, L. A., & Fallon, J. H. (1975). The ascending projections of the superior colliculus in the rhesus monkey (*Macaca mulatta*). *Journal of Comparative Neurology, 160*(3), 339–361. http://dx.doi.org/10.1002/cne.901600306.

van Broekhoven, P. C., Schraa-Tam, C. K., van der Lugt, A., Smits, M., Frens, M. A., & van der Geest, J. N. (2009). Cerebellar contributions to the processing of saccadic errors. *Cerebellum, 8*(3), 403–415. http://dx.doi.org/10.1007/s12311-009-0116-6.

Büttner, U., Fuchs, A. F., Markert-Schwab, G., & Buckmaster, P. (1991). Fastigial nucleus activity in the alert monkey during slow eye and head movements. *Journal of Neurophysiology, 65*(6), 1360–1371.

Catz, N., Dicke, P. W., & Thier, P. (2005). Cerebellar complex spike firing is suitable to induce as well as to stabilize motor learning. *Current Biology, 15*(24), 2179–2189. http://dx.doi.org/10.1016/j.cub.2005.11.037.

Catz, N., Dicke, P. W., & Thier, P. (2008). Cerebellar-dependent motor learning is based on pruning a Purkinje cell population response. *Proceedings of the National Academy of Sciences, 105*(20), 7309–7314. http://dx.doi.org/10.1073/pnas.0706032105.

Chen, S., & Hillman, D. E. (1993). Colocalization of neurotransmitters in the deep cerebellar nuclei. *Journal of Neurocytology, 22*(2), 81–91.

Dash, S., Catz, N., Dicke, P. W., & Thier, P. (2010). Specific vermal complex spike responses build up during the course of smooth-pursuit adaptation, paralleling the decrease of performance error. *Experimental Brain Research, 205*(1), 41–55. http://dx.doi.org/10.1007/s00221-010-2331-2.

Dicke, P. W., Barash, S., Ilg, U. J., & Thier, P. (2004). Single-neuron evidence for a contribution of the dorsal pontine nuclei to both types of target-directed eye movements, saccades and smooth-pursuit. *European Journal of Neuroscience, 19*(3), 609–624.

Dietrichs, E., & Walberg, F. (1985). The cerebellar nucleo-olivary and olivo-cerebellar nuclear projections in the cat as studied with anterograde and retrograde transport in the same animal after implantation of crystalline WGA-HRP. II. The fastigial nucleus. *Anatomy and Embryology (Berl), 173*(2), 253–261.

Fries, W. (1990). Pontine projection from striate and prestriate visual cortex in the macaque monkey: an anterograde study. *Visual Neuroscience, 4*(3), 205–216.

Fuchs, A. F., Robinson, F. R., & Straube, A. (1993). Role of the caudal fastigial nucleus in saccade generation. I. Neuronal discharge pattern. *Journal of Neurophysiology, 70*(5), 1723–1740.

Fuchs, A. F., Robinson, F. R., & Straube, A. (1994). Participation of the caudal fastigial nucleus in smooth-pursuit eye movements. I. Neuronal activity. *Journal of Neurophysiology, 72*(6), 2714–2728.

Gerrits, N. M., & Voogd, J. (1986). The nucleus reticularis tegmenti pontis and the adjacent rostral paramedian reticular formation: differential projections to the cerebellum and the caudal brain stem. *Experimental Brain Research, 62*(1), 29–45.

Giolli, R. A., Gregory, K. M., Suzuki, D. A., Blanks, R. H., Lui, F., & Betelak, K. F. (2001). Cortical and subcortical afferents to the nucleus reticularis tegmenti pontis and basal pontine nuclei in the macaque monkey. *Visual Neuroscience, 18*(5), 725–740.

Goffart, L., Chen, L. L., & Sparks, D. L. (2004). Deficits in saccades and fixation during muscimol inactivation of the caudal fastigial nucleus in the rhesus monkey. *Journal of Neurophysiology, 92*(6), 3351–3367. http://dx.doi.org/10.1152/jn.01199.2003.

Graham, J. (1977). An autoradiographic study of the efferent connections of the superior colliculus in the cat. *Journal of Comparative Neurology, 173*(4), 629–654. http://dx.doi.org/10.1002/cne.901730403.

Harting, J. K. (1977). Descending pathways from the superior collicullus: an autoradiographic analysis in the rhesus monkey (*Macaca mulatta*). *Journal of Comparative Neurology, 173*(3), 583–612. http://dx.doi.org/10.1002/cne.901730311.

Helmchen, C., Straube, A., & Büttner, U. (1994). Saccade-related activity in the fastigial oculomotor region of the macaque monkey during spontaneous eye movements in light and darkness. *Experimental Brain Research, 98*(3), 474–482.

Hiramatsu, T., Ohki, M., Kitazawa, H., Xiong, G., Kitamura, T., Yamada, J., et al. (2008). Role of primate cerebellar lobulus petrosus of paraflocculus in smooth pursuit eye movement control revealed by chemical lesion. *Neuroscience Research, 60*(3), 250–258. http://dx.doi.org/10.1016/j.neures.2007.11.004.

Homma, Y., Nonaka, S., Matsuyama, K., & Mori, S. (1995). Fastigiofugal projection to the brainstem nuclei in the cat: an anterograde PHA-L tracing study. *Neuroscience Research, 23*(1), 89–102.

Ikeda, Y., Noda, H., & Sugita, S. (1989). Olivocerebellar and cerebelloolivary connections of the oculomotor region of the fastigial nucleus in the macaque monkey. *Journal of Comparative Neurology, 284*(3), 463–488. http://dx.doi.org/10.1002/cne.902840311.

Inaba, N., Iwamoto, Y., & Yoshida, K. (2003). Changes in cerebellar fastigial burst activity related to saccadic gain adaptation in the monkey. *Neuroscience Research, 46*(3), 359–368.

Kahlon, M., & Lisberger, S. G. (2000). Changes in the responses of Purkinje cells in the floccular complex of monkeys after motor learning in smooth pursuit eye movements. *Journal of Neurophysiology, 84*(6), 2945–2960.

Kase, M., Miller, D. C., & Noda, H. (1980). Discharges of Purkinje cells and mossy fibres in the cerebellar vermis of the monkey during saccadic eye movements and fixation. *The Journal of Physiology, 300*, 539–555.

Keller, E. L., & Missal, M. (2003). Shared brainstem pathways for saccades and smooth-pursuit eye movements. *Annals of the New York Academy of Sciences, 1004*, 29–39.

Kleine, J. F., Guan, Y., & Büttner, U. (2003). Saccade-related neurons in the primate fastigial nucleus: what do they encode? *Journal of Neurophysiology, 90*(5), 3137–3154. http://dx.doi.org/10.1152/jn.00021.2003.

Kommerell, G., Olivier, D., & Theopold, H. (1976). Adaptive programming of phasic and tonic components in saccadic eye movements. Investigations of patients with abducens palsy. *Investigative Ophthalmology, 15*(8), 657–660.

Madigan, J. C., & Carpenter, M. B. (1971). *Cerebellum of the rhesus monkey: atlas of lobules, laminae, and folia, in sections*. Baltimore: University Park Press.

Mano, N., Ito, Y., & Shibutani, H. (1991). Saccade-related Purkinje cells in the cerebellar hemispheres of the monkey. *Experimental Brain Research, 84*(3), 465–470.

Marr, D. (1969). A theory of cerebellar cortex. *The Journal of Physiology, 202*(2), 437–470.

May, P. J., Hartwich-Young, R., Nelson, J., Sparks, D. L., & Porter, J. D. (1990). Cerebellotectal pathways in the macaque: implications for collicular generation of saccades. *Neuroscience, 36*(2), 305–324.

McLaughlin, S. C. (1967). Parametric adjustment in saccadic eye movements. *Perception and Psychophysics, 2*(8), 359–362.

Medina, J. F., & Lisberger, S. G. (2008). Links from complex spikes to local plasticity and motor learning in the cerebellum of awake-behaving monkeys. *Nature Neuroscience, 11*(10), 1185–1192. http://dx.doi.org/10.1038/nn.2197.

Medina, J. F., & Lisberger, S. G. (2009). Encoding and decoding of learned smooth-pursuit eye movements in the floccular complex of the monkey cerebellum. *Journal of Neurophysiology, 102*(4), 2039–2054. http://dx.doi.org/10.1152/jn.00075.2009.

Mueller, A. L., Davis, A. J., & Robinson, F. R. (2012). Long-term size-increasing adaptation of saccades in macaques. *Neuroscience, 224*, 38–47. http://dx.doi.org/10.1016/j.neuroscience.2012.08.012.

Nagao, S. (2004). Pontine nuclei-mediated cerebello-cerebral interactions and its functional role. *Cerebellum, 3*(1), 11–15. http://dx.doi.org/10.1080/14734220310012181.

Noda, H., & Fujikado, T. (1987). Involvement of Purkinje cells in evoking saccadic eye movements by microstimulation of the posterior cerebellar vermis of monkeys. *Journal of Neurophysiology, 57*(5), 1247–1261.

Noda, H., & Mikami, A. (1986). Discharges of neurons in the dorsal paraflocculus of monkeys during eye movements and visual stimulation. *Journal of Neurophysiology, 56*(4), 1129–1146.

Noda, H., Murakami, S., Yamada, J., Tamada, J., Tamaki, Y., & Aso, T. (1988). Saccadic eye movements evoked by microstimulation of the fastigial nucleus of macaque monkeys. *Journal of Neurophysiology, 60*(3), 1036–1052.

Noda, H., Sugita, S., & Ikeda, Y. (1990). Afferent and efferent connections of the oculomotor region of the fastigial nucleus in the macaque monkey. *Journal of Comparative Neurology, 302*(2), 330–348. http://dx.doi.org/10.1002/cne.903020211.

Ohki, M., Kitazawa, H., Hiramatsu, T., Kaga, K., Kitamura, T., Yamada, J., et al. (2009). Role of primate cerebellar hemisphere in voluntary eye movement control revealed by lesion effects. *Journal of Neurophysiology, 101*(2), 934–947. http://dx.doi.org/10.1152/jn.90440.2009.

Ohtsuka, K., & Noda, H. (1990). Direction-selective saccadic-burst neurons in the fastigial oculomotor region of the macaque. *Experimental Brain Research, 81*(3), 659–662.

Ohtsuka, K., & Noda, H. (1991). Saccadic burst neurons in the oculomotor region of the fastigial nucleus of macaque monkeys. *Journal of Neurophysiology, 65*(6), 1422–1434.

Ohtsuka, K., & Noda, H. (1992). Burst discharges of mossy fibers in the oculomotor vermis of macaque monkeys during saccadic eye movements. *Neuroscience Research, 15*(1–2), 102–114.

Palkovits, M., Mezey, E., Hamori, J., & Szentagothai, J. (1977). Quantitative histological analysis of the cerebellar nuclei in the cat. I. Numerical data on cells and on synapses. *Experimental Brain Research, 28*(1–2), 189–209.

Person, A. L., & Raman, I. M. (2012). Purkinje neuron synchrony elicits time-locked spiking in the cerebellar nuclei. *Nature, 481*(7382), 502–505. http://dx.doi.org/10.1038/nature10732.

Prsa, M., Dash, S., Catz, N., Dicke, P. W., & Thier, P. (2009). Characteristics of responses of Golgi cells and mossy fibers to eye saccades and saccadic adaptation recorded from the posterior vermis of the cerebellum. *Journal of Neuroscience, 29*(1), 250–262. http://dx.doi.org/10.1523/jneurosci.4791-08.2009.

Prsa, M., Dicke, P. W., & Thier, P. (2010). The absence of eye muscle fatigue indicates that the nervous system compensates for non-motor disturbances of oculomotor function. *Journal of Neuroscience, 30*(47), 15834–15842. http://dx.doi.org/10.1523/jneurosci.3901-10.2010.

Prsa, M., & Thier, P. (2011). The role of the cerebellum in saccadic adaptation as a window into neural mechanisms of motor learning. *European Journal of Neuroscience, 33*(11), 2114–2128. http://dx.doi.org/10.1111/j.1460-9568.2011.07693.x.

Rambold, H., Churchland, A., Selig, Y., Jasmin, L., & Lisberger, S. G. (2002). Partial ablations of the flocculus and ventral paraflocculus in monkeys cause linked deficits in smooth pursuit eye movements and adaptive modification of the VOR. *Journal of Neurophysiology, 87*(2), 912–924.

Robinson, F. R., Fuchs, A. F., & Noto, C. T. (2002). Cerebellar influences on saccade plasticity. *Annals of the New York Academy of Sciences, 956,* 155–163.

Robinson, F. R., Soetedjo, R., & Noto, C. (2006). Distinct short-term and long-term adaptation to reduce saccade size in monkey. *Journal of Neurophysiology, 96*(3), 1030–1041. http://dx.doi.org/10.1152/jn.01151.2005.

Ron, S., & Robinson, D. A. (1973). Eye movements evoked by cerebellar stimulation in the alert monkey. *Journal of Neurophysiology, 36*(6), 1004–1022.

Ruigrok, T. J., & Voogd, J. (1990). Cerebellar nucleo-olivary projections in the rat: an anterograde tracing study with Phaseolus vulgaris-leucoagglutinin (PHA-L). *Journal of Comparative Neurology, 298*(3), 315–333. http://dx.doi.org/10.1002/cne.902980305.

Saint-Cyr, J. A., & Courville, J. (1982). Descending projections to the inferior olive from the mesencephalon and superior colliculus in the cat. An autoradiographic study. *Experimental Brain Research, 45*(3), 333–348.

Sato, H., & Noda, H. (1991). Divergent axon collaterals from fastigial oculomotor region to mesodiencephalic junction and paramedian pontine reticular formation in macaques. *Neuroscience Research, 11*(1), 41–54.

Sato, H., & Noda, H. (1992). Saccadic dysmetria induced by transient functional decortication of the cerebellar vermis [corrected]. *Experimental Brain Research, 88*(2), 455–458.

Scudder, C. A., & McGee, D. M. (2003). Adaptive modification of saccade size produces correlated changes in the discharges of fastigial nucleus neurons. *Journal of Neurophysiology, 90*(2), 1011–1026. http://dx.doi.org/10.1152/jn.00193.2002.

Scudder, C. A., Moschovakis, A. K., Karabelas, A. B., & Highstein, S. M. (1996). Anatomy and physiology of saccadic long-lead burst neurons recorded in the alert squirrel monkey. I. Descending projections from the mesencephalon. *Journal of Neurophysiology, 76*(1), 332–352.

Smilgin, A., Dicke, P. W., & Thier, P. (2012). Purkinje cells of the monkey oculomotor vermis respond to saccades as well as to smooth pursuit initiation. *Society for Neuroscience Abstract, 580,* 01.

Smilgin, A., Sun, Z. P., Telgen, S., Dicke, P. W., & Thier, P. Short term saccadic adaption spills over to smooth pursuit initiation?, in preparation.

Soetedjo, R., & Fuchs, A. F. (2006). Complex spike activity of purkinje cells in the oculomotor vermis during behavioral adaptation of monkey saccades. *Journal of Neuroscience, 26*(29), 7741–7755. http://dx.doi.org/10.1523/jneurosci.4658-05.2006.

Soetedjo, R., Fuchs, A. F., & Kojima, Y. (2009). Subthreshold activation of the superior colliculus drives saccade motor learning. *Journal of Neuroscience, 29*(48), 15213–15222. http://dx.doi.org/10.1523/jneurosci.4296-09.2009.

Sugita, S., & Noda, H. (1991). Pathways and terminations of axons arising in the fastigial oculomotor region of macaque monkeys. *Neuroscience Research, 10*(2), 118–136.

Sultan, F., Konig, T., Mock, M., & Thier, P. (2002). Quantitative organization of neurotransmitters in the deep cerebellar nuclei of the Lurcher mutant. *Journal of Comparative Neurology, 452*(4), 311–323. http://dx.doi.org/10.1002/cne.10365.

Sun, Z. P., Junker, M., Dicke, P. W., & Thier, P. (2013). Saccade-related neurons in the caudal fastigial nucleus are more diverse than hitherto assumed. *Society of Neuroscience Abstract, 647,* 04.

Sun, Z. P., Smilgin, A., Dicke, P. W., & Thier, P. Cerebellar vermis and cFN responses during smooth pursuit eye movement, in preparation.

Thielert, C. D., & Thier, P. (1993). Patterns of projections from the pontine nuclei and the nucleus reticularis tegmenti pontis to the posterior vermis in the rhesus monkey: a study using retrograde tracers. *Journal of Comparative Neurology, 337*(1), 113–126. http://dx.doi.org/10.1002/cne.903370108.

Thier, P. (2011). The oculomotor cerebellum. In S. Liversedge, L. Gilchrist, & S. Everling (Eds.), *The Oxford handbook of eye movements.* Oxford Library of Psychology (p. 173).

Thier, P., Dicke, P. W., Haas, R., & Barash, S. (2000). Encoding of movement time by populations of cerebellar Purkinje cells. *Nature, 405*(6782), 72–76. http://dx.doi.org/10.1038/35011062.

Thier, P., & Ilg, U. J. (2005). The neural basis of smooth-pursuit eye movements. *Current Opinion in Neurobiology, 15*(6), 645–652. http://dx.doi.org/10.1016/j.conb.2005.10.013.

Uusisaari, M., Obata, K., & Knopfel, T. (2007). Morphological and electrophysiological properties of GABAergic and non-gabaergic cells in the deep cerebellar nuclei. *Journal of Neurophysiology, 97*(1), 901–911. http://dx.doi.org/10.1152/jn.00974.2006.

Wang, Y. T., & Linden, D. J. (2000). Expression of cerebellar long-term depression requires postsynaptic clathrin-mediated endocytosis. *Neuron, 25*(3), 635–647.

Xu-Wilson, M., Zee, D. S., & Shadmehr, R. (2009). The intrinsic value of visual information affects saccade velocities. *Experimental Brain Research, 196*(4), 475–481. http://dx.doi.org/10.1007/s00221-009-1879-1.

Yamada, J., & Noda, H. (1987). Afferent and efferent connections of the oculomotor cerebellar vermis in the macaque monkey. *Journal of Comparative Neurology, 265*(2), 224–241. http://dx.doi.org/10.1002/cne.902650207.

Zee, D. S., Yamazaki, A., Butler, P. H., & Gucer, G. (1981). Effects of ablation of flocculus and paraflocculus of eye movements in primate. *Journal of Neurophysiology, 46*(4), 878–899.

Coordination of Reaching Movements: Cerebellar Interactions with Motor Cortex

Eric J. Lang

Department of Neuroscience & Physiology, New York University School of Medicine, New York, NY, USA

The importance of the motor cortex and cerebellum in generating normal movements has been known for well over a century. For example, the association of the cerebellum with motor function dates back at least to the studies of Rolando in the early 1800s (for a review, see Dow & Moruzzi, 1958), and the major motor deficits caused by cerebellar damage were already characterized in detail about a century ago (Holmes, 1917). Similarly, recognition of the importance of the motor cortex for motor function dates back to the studies of Hughlings Jackson, Fritsch and Hitzig, and Ferrier in the mid- to late 1800s (Bennett & Hacker, 2002; Humphrey, 1986).

Since these early reports, many studies have investigated the specific roles of these two brain regions in motor control. The goal of this chapter, however, is not simply to review the individual contributions of the motor cortex and cerebellum to motor control. Instead, the focus will be on the interaction of these two areas, because brain functions are not performed by single regions in isolation. Rather, they are implemented by networks of interconnected regions, and therefore, to understand how the brain performs any particular function requires knowledge not only of the individual areas involved, but also of their interactions, and of the information flowing between them.

The motor cortex and cerebellum are an excellent pair of brain regions for addressing the issue of interaction of brain areas in motor control, as they are highly interconnected anatomically, and both play important roles in the control of voluntary movements. Cerebral cortical influence on the cerebellum is mediated via both of the major types of cerebellar afferents: mossy fibers and olivocerebellar axons (climbing fibers). In particular, the cerebral cortex projects to a number of brain-stem nuclei that give rise to mossy fibers, the largest set of these nuclei being those of the basilar pons, whereas the cortical input to the inferior olive, the origin of the climbing fibers, is primarily via disynaptic pathways that relay in midbrain nuclei. Conversely, cerebellar pathways to the motor cortex largely originate in the deep cerebellar nuclei (DCN), the major output stations of the cerebellum. The DCN project to many targets throughout the neuraxis (a point we will return to later); however, the most direct pathway from the DCN to the motor cortex is via a disynaptic pathway that arises mainly from the dentate and interposed nuclei and relays in the ventrolateral portion of the thalamus.

Although the cerebellum and motor cortex are reciprocally connected, the main focus here is on the question of what movement-related signals are sent from the cerebellum to the motor cortex. Moreover, although the cerebellum and motor cortex are involved in the control of a variety of movements, ranging from reflexive to fully voluntary, this review is limited to cerebellar–motor cortex interactions during voluntary movements and, especially, to interactions during reaching and/or prehensile movements of the forelimb. These movements have been extensively studied, form a particularly important group of voluntary movements, and are dependent on both motor cortex and cerebellum.

To address the issue of how the cerebellum influences the motor cortex during reaching movements, we will focus on single-unit recording studies from the interpositus and dentate nuclei in animals performing various forelimb movement tasks. However, before describing the results of these studies in detail, it is worth putting them in the context of how the cerebellum and cerebrum were thought to interact when studies recording their activity during voluntary movements first started being performed, namely during the 1960s. The theories at the time were heavily based on what was then known about the anatomical connectivity of various cerebellar regions with the periphery and the cerebrum. Much of this is still thought to be correct today; however, some significant changes in our understanding of this connectivity have occurred and will be discussed later.

ANATOMICAL CONNECTIVITY SUGGESTS DISTINCT ROLES FOR THE DENTATE AND INTERPOSITUS NUCLEI IN THE MOTOR SYSTEM HIERARCHY

The cerebellum has been divided into longitudinal zones or compartments based on various criteria, including myeloarchitectonics, sensory responses, and molecular markers (Apps & Hawkes, 2009; Voogd & Ruigrok, 1997). As of this writing, more than 20 distinct longitudinal

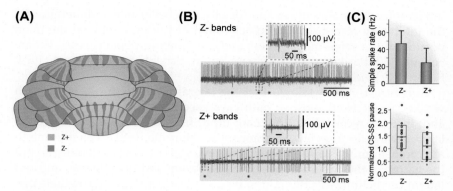

FIGURE 1   Differences in simple spike activity between zebrin-positive (Z+) and -negative (Z–) Purkinje cells. (A) Schematic of zebrin staining of rat cerebellum. (B) Recordings of Z– and Z+ Purkinje cells. Asterisks and insets show complex spikes. Note the higher firing rates and more regular activity for the Z– Purkinje cell. Also note the shorter absolute pause in simple spikes after a complex spike. (C) Bar graphs show differences in simple spike firing rate and normalized pause in simple spikes following a complex spike. Note that when normalized for average firing rate. Z– Purkinje cells show a longer pause, indicating a stronger active suppression mechanism. Dotted line at 0.5 is the expected pause length (half the interspike interval) if there is no active suppression of simple spikes. *Adapted from figures from Cerminara et al. (2015)* Nature Reviews Neuroscience *16, 79–93.* http://dx.doi.org/10.1038/nrn3886. *See Xiao et al. (2014) for further details on these results.*

compartments are recognized in all mammalian cerebella, based on zebrin staining (Fig. 1(A); Sugihara & Shinoda, 2004); however, at the time when recordings of DCN activity in behaving animals were first performed much simpler schemes were used to compartmentalize the cerebellum. For example, a tripartite scheme, which is still used, divided the cerebellum into three broad longitudinally running regions, medial (vermis), intermediate (paravermis), and lateral (hemisphere), each region comprising a part of the cortex along with a corresponding member (or members) of the DCN (fastigial, interposed, and dentate, respectively). The medial region was thought to be primarily involved in the control of posture and balance and with eye movements, whereas the intermediate and lateral areas (with the primary exception of the flocculus) were thought to have roles in controlling limb movements. Thus, the latter two areas are the focus here.

The intermediate cerebellum was known to receive significant input from ascending somatosensory pathways, conveying both tactile and proprioceptive information. This had been shown both anatomically and physiologically (for a review, see Bloedel & Courville, 1981). In particular, activation of tactile receptors and muscle spindle afferents had been shown to evoke a series of excitatory and inhibitory responses in interpositus neurons, with the excitatory phases due to direct excitation of the interpositus by mossy fibers and/or olivocerebellar fiber collaterals, and the inhibitory responses due to activation of Purkinje cells by the main portion of the same mossy fibers and/or climbing fibers (Eccles, Rosen, Scheid, & Taborikova, 1972; Eccles, Rosén, Scheid, & Táboríková, 1974; Rosén & Scheid, 1972).

In contrast, it was known that the lateral cerebellum received much weaker input from sensory pathways ascending from the spinal cord and, instead, received its dominant input from the cerebropontocerebellar pathway (for a review, see Bloedel & Courville, 1981). The intermediate cerebellum was also known to receive input from the cerebrum, but the nature of the circuits between the cerebrum and the intermediate and lateral cerebellum was thought to be quite distinct. The intermediate cerebellum was thought to form an essentially closed-loop circuit with the motor cortex, both receiving input, via the pons, from the motor cortex and projecting back to it, via the thalamus. In contrast, the cerebropontocerebellar pathway to the lateral cerebellum was thought to have a more widespread origin, including contributions from the association cortex in the frontal and parietal lobes, but the projection back to the cortex from the thalamus was thought to target primarily the motor cortex (for review, see Allen & Tsukahara, 1974). Thus, rather than a closed-loop configuration, the circuit between the lateral cerebellum and the cerebrum was thought of as one involving a major convergence from the higher order association areas to the motor cortex.

In sum, at the time that recordings from the DCN in behaving animals were first being made, hierarchical views of the motor system, which were largely based on the connectivity patterns just described, placed the dentate early in the chain and the interpositus at or near the end (Allen & Tsukahara, 1974; Eccles, 1967; Evarts & Thach, 1969). These views guided much of the research and the specific analyses and interpretations of the data. In particular, the lateral cerebellum was assigned a role in the planning and initiation of voluntary movements, and thus, the signals leaving the dentate nucleus were hypothesized to encode abstract parameters related to the early stages of planning a movement. In contrast, the interpositus's proposed function was to help correct errors in the execution of a movement by using sensory feedback signals generated by the ongoing movement itself.

Finally, two major changes in our understanding of the anatomy of motor circuits should be mentioned, because they bear on how the findings to be reviewed are interpreted. First, the circuits connecting the lateral cerebellum and the cerebrum are now thought to have a closed-loop configuration, because the cortical areas targeted by the dentate are now known to be much more widespread (Dum & Strick, 2003; Strick, Dum, & Fiez, 2009). Second, it is now known that multiple cortical areas, rather than just the motor cortex, contribute to the descending motor pathways (for a review, see Dum & Strick, 2002; Graziano, Taylor, Moore, & Cooke, 2002). Both of these changes suggest that the motor system is organized in a more parallel distributed fashion than is conceived by the strictly hierarchical models.

With this context in mind, we now review the results of extracellular recording studies from the DCN in behaving animals. Such recordings should provide the most direct information about the signals being sent from the cerebellum to the motor cortex. Although a number of investigators have performed such recordings, the studies of Thach were among the first, and they remain among the most extensive. The ensuing discussion is largely organized around them because they provided many of the key findings that have framed the debate on what information is encoded in DCN activity and thus on the content of the motor-related output of the cerebellum.

DEEP CEREBELLAR NUCLEI NEURONS HAVE HIGH SPONTANEOUS FIRING RATES ABOUT WHICH MOVEMENT-RELATED MODULATION OCCURS

Baseline activity varies significantly between central nervous system structures, and even among neurons within a single area, with potentially significant consequences for signal transmission to the efferent targets of an area. Interpositus and dentate cells were both found to have high spontaneous firing rates (on average, 37 Hz) (Thach, 1968). Such high levels of activity were (and perhaps still are) surprising, given the synaptic input that DCN cells receive. Purkinje cells are the numerically dominant input to the nuclear cells, as they give rise to 70–80% of the total synapses onto a DCN cell (De Zeeuw & Berrebi, 1995; Palkovits, Mezey, Hamori, & Szentagothai, 1977). Moreover, Purkinje cells are inhibitory (Ito & Yoshida, 1966; Ito, Yoshida, & Obata, 1964; Ito, Yoshida, Obata, Kawai, & Udo, 1970) and fire simple spikes at high frequencies, an average of 70 Hz in the same study by Thach (1968). Of course it is possible that the DCN cells recorded by Thach (and others subsequently) are unrepresentative of the DCN population as a whole, because extracellular recording techniques are biased to detect spontaneously active cells (e.g., cells of the lateral amygdala, which have very low firing rates, generally failed to be detected in single-unit studies until they were specifically searched for (Gaudreau & Pare, 1996)). Similarly, DCN cells that have little or no spontaneous activity could have been missed, shifting the reported firing rate distributions to the right. In fact, in one study search stimuli were generated by an electrode in the ascending limb of the superior cerebellar peduncle, and antidromic responses were observed in otherwise silent cells, providing evidence for a small population of DCN neurons with essentially no spontaneous activity (Harvey, Porter, & Rawson, 1979). This population, however, accounts for only about 15% of the total DCN population.

Thus, the large majority of DCN projection neurons (at least those whose axons enter the ascending limb of the superior peduncle and thus potentially project to the motor cortex) maintain relatively high levels of spontaneous activity in the face of tonic inhibition from their major synaptic input, the Purkinje cells. Thach suggested that this spontaneous activity reflected either an intrinsic drive to generate spikes or a powerful excitatory synaptic input that overrode the Purkinje cell inhibition (Thach, 1968). Subsequent evidence suggests that, in fact, both of these factors contribute to the high baseline firing of DCN cells. For example, it is now known that most DCN cells are intrinsically active. Recordings from slice preparations show that the large majority of DCN cells fire spontaneously at firing rates similar to those seen in vivo, even when glutamate receptors are blocked (Aizenman & Linden, 1999; Jahnsen, 1986). This activity is driven by a variety of intrinsic currents (Uusisaari & Knopfel, 2011).

Interestingly, a small subpopulation of DCN neurons, comprising large glycinergic cells, has been shown to not display spontaneous activity; however, it is unlikely that these neurons correspond to the silent cells found with searching stimuli in vivo, as the glycinergic neurons appear to project to the cerebellar cortex rather than to extracerebellar sites (Uusisaari & Knopfel, 2010). Thus, the 15% figure given above is likely to be an underestimate of the fraction of silent cells in the DCN population; however, given the numbers of DCN neurons that project to extracerebellar targets (McCrea, Bishop, & Kitai, 1978), and the fact that these projection cells generally have spontaneous activity (Najac & Raman, 2015; Uusisaari & Knopfel, 2011), the conclusion that the large majority of the DCN neurons have spontaneous activity is still valid.

Finally, that most nuclear cells are spontaneously active does not necessarily exclude the alternative possibility that they receive a strong excitatory drive to counter what should be a massive tonic inhibition from the Purkinje cells. Indeed, the close similarity of the firing rates in the slice preparation to those in the intact animal suggests that there must be some balancing of synaptic input and either that the collaterals of the afferent fibers produce an excitatory drive that is greater than expected based on the anatomy or that tonic simple spike activity has a much weaker than expected action. Evidence for the relative importance of the excitatory collaterals driving activity is that movement-related bursts in DCN cells persist following local injection of $GABA_A$ antagonists into the DCN, which would block Purkinje cell inhibition (Holdefer, Houk, & Miller, 2005).

In sum, the DCN provide a significant tonic, primarily excitatory drive to their targets (except the inferior olive). An obvious use for such baseline activity would be to allow bidirectional modulation of activity during behavior, and this does happen. However, as detailed below, increases in activity during movement are far more common, and so the reasons for DCN neurons having high firing rates are not fully clear.

RELATIVE TIMING OF DENTATE AND INTERPOSITUS ACTIVITY WITH RESPECT TO MOVEMENT ONSET

The timing of changes in neuronal activity relative to that of the motor act is fundamental to establishing causal links between the two. Beyond that, information about the relative timing can provide clues as to what aspect of the movement (e.g., initiation or termination) the activity of a particular brain region is related to and, as such, can test specific hypotheses concerning the overall organization of the motor system. For example, the serial hierarchical view of the motor system assigned the dentate a role in the planning and initiation of movements, whereas the interpositus was supposed to help modify or correct an ongoing movement and perhaps help with its termination (Allen & Tsukahara, 1974; Eccles, 1967; Evarts & Thach, 1969). If this hierarchical scheme were correct, the timing of activity changes in the dentate and interpositus should reflect their positions in the hierarchy. That is, the dentate should show changes in activity well before the onset of a movement and thus well before the onset of changes in interpositus activity, which should occur after the start of the movement.

Many studies have measured the time of onset for modulation of dentate and interpositus activity using a variety of motor tasks. Overall, they are in general agreement with the relative timing of the onset of activity modulation between the dentate and the interpositus with respect to movement, but less so on the absolute timing of this modulation. Studies consistently find that some cells in both the interpositus and the dentate start modulating their activity before the onset of the movement (and generally before the onset of electromyographic (EMG) activity), but that there are also cells whose activity starts being modulated well after movement onset (Burton & Onoda, 1977, 1978; Chapman, Spidalieri, & Lamarre, 1986; Fortier, Kalaska, & Smith, 1989; van Kan, Houk, & Gibson, 1993; Thach, 1970; Wetts, Kalaska, & Smith, 1985). Thus, the population distributions for modulation onset times for the two nuclei are widespread and overlapping.

A precise comparison of the timing of dentate and interpositus activity across studies is difficult because the absolute times at which such changes in activity start in each nucleus vary significantly between studies. (Parenthetically, this variability suggests that the specifics of the behavioral task greatly influence when the DCN are engaged and thus that these nuclei may be engaged for distinct operations depending on the particulars of the task at hand. Therefore, they cannot be assigned one specific role in motor function, nor would the signals they send to the motor cortex generally contain equivalent information.)

In a few studies, however, direct quantitative comparisons across nuclei were made for the same tasks (Chapman et al., 1986; MacKay, 1988; Thach, 1970). In all of these studies, the onset of modulation started earlier in the dentate than in the interpositus, both on average, and in terms of the limits of their distributions. However, the absolute times of these changes vary significantly even between these studies. For example, in the study by Thach, the time of modulation onset for each neuron was defined as the earlier of the times at which it started showing modulation for flexion or extension movements (Thach, 1970). Using this method and the data in Tables 1 and 2 of Thach (1970), one can calculate average latencies with respect to movement onset of −36 and −2 ms for dentate and interpositus neurons, respectively. In contrast, in the study by Chapman et al., the relative timing of dentate and interpositus activity modulations was the same, but in absolute latency, both dentate and interpositus neurons changed activity levels much earlier with respect to movement onset (dentate, −154 ms; interpositus, −84 ms) (Chapman et al., 1986).

The questions then are what to make of the difference in the onset of activity modulation between the dentate and the interpositus, and does it support the traditionally assigned roles of the dentate and the interpositus? Perhaps because of the dominance of the hierarchical viewpoint at the times these studies were performed, the small shifts in the time of modulation onset of the dentate and interpositus were indeed interpreted as fitting with the proposed places of these nuclei in the motor hierarchy; nevertheless, in retrospect, with the additional studies that have been performed and the changing view of the motor system organization that has resulted, the interpretation now seems less than clear cut, given the degree of overlap in onset latencies and that both dentate and interpositus cells can modulate their activity before movement onset and continue to do so throughout the movement until its termination. Moreover, the wide variation shown between studies further clouds the issue. Indeed, even at the time, Thach remarked, "But the more obvious fact is the overlap, and in this study it can be questioned whether there is any demonstrated timing difference ..." (Thach, 1978).

The premovement onset of modulation of activity is particularly significant with regard to questioning the proposed role of the interpositus to regulate the ongoing movement on the basis of sensory feedback generated by the movement, which obviously cannot exist prior to movement onset. Indeed, while in some of the initial studies interpositus activity changed only shortly before movement onset (e.g., Burton & Onoda, 1977, 1978), and possibly could be ascribed to the earlier contraction in axial muscles, in other studies changes in interpositus activity preceded movement onset by hundreds of milliseconds (e.g., in one study the onset of modulation preceded movement onset by 107 ms, on average, and by more than 200 ms in some neurons (van Kan et al., 1993)).

In sum, while there may be other reasons for assigning the dentate and interpositus roles in distinct stages of motor control, the timing of their activity changes provides less than compelling evidence for such a division. Rather it would seem that both dentate and interpositus are involved in multiple stages of generating a movement, even if their specific contributions may differ.

TEMPORAL CORRELATION WITH SENSORY CUES OR MOTOR RESPONSES

To investigate the relationship of brain activity with movement, animals are often conditioned to make movements either in response to a sensory cue or to track a target. In such experiments the question arises as to whether the changes in neuronal activity reflect sensory processing or computing of the motor response. This question is of particular relevance here, as somatosensory, auditory, and visual stimuli all evoke activity in the DCN (e.g., Mortimer, 1973, 1975). Determining the answer to this question could therefore provide information about the specific roles of each DCN in the generation of movements. Thus, to investigate whether dentate and interpositus activity is more closely tied to the sensory cue or the actual motor response, correlations between these events and the onset of neuronal activity were calculated in several studies.

In one study monkeys were trained to grasp a lever and hold it in one of two positions until a light came on (Thach, 1970). The light signaled the animal to move the lever to the second position by rotating its wrist, where it then had to hold the lever until the light signaled the animal to move again. The reaction time to the light cue varied among trials, allowing determination of whether the changes in neuronal activity began at a fixed latency with respect to the light cue or whether their onset varied with the latency of the movement. In fact, for both dentate and interpositus cells, the onset of task-related changes in activity was not time-locked to the occurrence of the cue, but was instead correlated with the reaction time of the movement, suggesting that the activity of both nuclei was more closely tied to the motor aspects of the task. The same results were found in another task, in which the animal had to generate wrist flexion or extension torques isometrically (Thach, 1975).

Somewhat different results, however, were found in a subsequent study (Chapman et al., 1986). In this case auditory, visual, and somatosensory cues were used as simple "go" signals for the monkey to make a flexion or extension movement about the elbow. Note that the cues did not specify the direction of movement, as this was kept constant for a block of trials and then switched to the opposing direction for the next trial block. Thus, despite the multiple modalities of the cues in this task, they were playing a role equivalent to those in the studies of Thach (1970, 1975). The onset of the change in DCN activity was again measured with respect to the timing of the cue and to the onset of movement. For interpositus neurons, the large majority (89%) were classified as movement-related based on a significant correlation between the onset of a change in neuronal activity and the movement initiation, consistent with the earlier studies of Thach (1970, 1975). In contrast, in the dentate, 79% of the cells were classified as having stimulus-related activity based on the onset of activity occurring at a fixed latency from the stimulus, disagreeing with the previous studies of Thach and highlighting a potential functional difference between the dentate and the interpositus nuclei.

It is important to note that this "stimulus-related" activity was not simply being driven by the stimuli themselves, as its presence depended on the subsequent occurrence of a movement on the trial (Chapman et al., 1986). That is, if the monkey made no movement on a particular trial, no response to the sensory stimulus was seen in the neuronal activity. Moreover, later parts of the responses of both movement-related and so-called stimulus-related cells showed evidence of being closely tied to the movement. In sum, these results still point to the dentate playing a role in motor function, but perhaps at an earlier stage than the interpositus.

DEEP CEREBELLAR NUCLEI NEURONS TEND TO SHOW INCREASED ACTIVITY DURING MOVEMENT

High spontaneous baseline activity of DCN neurons that was described earlier suggests that these neurons could encode information by modulating their activity in both positive and negative directions. However, the predominant modulation that has been observed in most studies is an increase (Chapman et al., 1986; Fortier et al., 1989; Harvey et al., 1979; van Kan et al., 1993; MacKay, 1988; Schieber & Thach, 1985; Thach, 1970). It is noteworthy that this finding has been observed for all of the DCN across multiple paradigms, including single-joint and whole-arm movements, trained movements using apparatuses, free-form unpracticed movements, and slow and fast movements. Thus, this asymmetry may be a fundamental aspect of the signals the DCN sends to the rest of the nervous system.

This is not to say that DCN neurons do not show inhibitory responses during movement. Indeed, both excitatory and inhibitory modulation are seen during movement; however, the excitatory modulations dominate. The task-related activity of most DCN neurons can be categorized as showing one of the following distinct modulation patterns. *Reciprocal patterns* are defined as those in which activity increases for movements in one direction and decreases for movements in the other. *Unidirectional patterns* refer to when activity changes (usually increases) for movement in one direction and does not change from baseline for movements in the opposite direction. Finally, *bidirectional patterns* are those in which activity changes in the same direction (though not necessarily to the same extent) for all movement directions.

The study of Harvey et al. (1979) describes what is probably the closest to a symmetric distribution of excitatory and inhibitory modulation. In this study, reciprocal changes in neuronal activity were found for about 50% of dentate and interpositus cells, but almost all other cells showed the unidirectional increase pattern of activity. In all other studies the bias toward excitatory responses is even stronger. For example, in one study in which rapid wrist flexion and extension movements were made in response to a light cue, only 16 and 20% of dentate and interpositus neurons, respectively, showed reciprocal activity, while most of the other cells showed bi- or unidirectional patterns, of which most were of the bi- or unidirectional increase type (dentate, 48 and 16%; interpositus, 51 and 17%) (Thach, 1970). In another task, in which slow ramp-type movements of the wrist were made to track a visual target, even larger percentages of cells showing bidirectional increases in activity were found (dentate, 67%; interpositus, 68%) (Schieber & Thach, 1985). Similarly, in a task involving elbow movements most (64%) dentate neurons were found to have initial increases in activity with movement, and of cells that showed directional tuning of activity, almost none had reciprocal-type activity for flexion and extension movements (Chapman et al., 1986). Finally, in the experiments of van Kan et al. (1993), all but one of 134 neurons showed increased discharge as the primary (largest amplitude) modulation. Thus, essentially, inhibitory modulation occurred in only 28% of cells as a smaller amplitude modulation relative to their primary modulation, and the remaining cells showed purely excitatory-type responses (uni- or bidirectional excitation) (van Kan et al., 1993).

Many of the studies described in this section used tasks that involved movements in only two directions (e.g., flexion and extension about the wrist). In such tasks it is possible that the preferred and anti-preferred directions of a recorded cell (the directions generating maximal positive and negative modulations in activity) might not correspond to the movement directions being performed, and this could potentially lead to misclassification of reciprocal cells as bidirectional, or of any type of directional cell as nondirectional (e.g., this could occur if the directions of movement were approximately orthogonal to the preferred direction of the cell). To address this possibility, DCN cells were studied in a center–out task, in which reaching movements were made from a point at the center of a circle to one of eight points equally spaced along the circumference of the circle (Fortier et al., 1989). However, similar to the tasks that involved movements in only two directions, excitatory responses predominated, with only a minority of cells showing reciprocal responses (dentate, 20%; interpositus, 37%). Most of the remaining cells showed either graded (the multidirectional equivalent of bi- and unidirectional categories) or nondirectional-type responses (Fortier et al., 1989).

In sum, the evidence suggests that DCN cells predominantly show excitatory responses during limb movement. The reason for the asymmetry between excitatory and inhibitory responses, however, is not clear and could simply relate to asymmetries in the pattern of muscle activation underlying movements (e.g., reciprocal activation of prime movers and their antagonists, but coactivation of axial muscles and of muscles acting about more proximal joints to stabilize the joint about which rotations are occurring). The preferential involvement of the DCN with proximal musculature was argued for by some investigators (Harvey et al., 1979; MacKay, 1988); however, others have argued against this explanation and for alternative, more functional reasons (Schieber & Thach, 1985; van Kan et al., 1993).

THE CODING OF MOVEMENT-RELATED PARAMETERS IN THE DEEP CEREBELLAR NUCLEI

To know what detailed movement-related information the cerebellum could provide to the motor cortex, it is necessary to determine the correlates of DCN activity with specific parameters of the movement. Such studies have been undertaken with respect to both the dentate and the interpositus nuclei. In fact, many of these studies recorded from both of these nuclei to facilitate comparisons between them in the hope of providing evidence to distinguish their functional roles in motor control. Thus, we next review the major findings of these studies to better define the specific roles of these two nuclei in motor control and, in particular, to understand what information may be flowing to the motor cortex from each nucleus.

DCN activity has been correlated with essentially all parameters of movement, including direction (i.e., the reciprocal, bidirectional and unidirectional firing patterns described in the previous section), duration (Harvey et al., 1979; van Kan et al., 1993), joint position (Chapman et al., 1986; Thach, 1978), amplitude (van Kan et al., 1993), velocity (Burton & Onoda, 1977, 1978; Chapman et al., 1986; van Kan et al., 1993; Soechting, Burton, & Onoda, 1978; Wetts et al., 1985), force/EMG activity (Thach, 1978; Wetts et al., 1985), dF/dt (Wetts et al., 1985), and preparatory set (Strick, 1983; Thach, 1978). However, at the same time, some studies, particularly those of dentate neurons, have found little correlation between DCN activity and specific movement parameters, reporting just general increases in activity or bursts of activity during movement (MacKay, 1988; Robertson & Grimm, 1975; Schieber & Thach, 1985). Moreover, the percentages of cells showing significant correlations with a particular parameter vary widely between studies. The divergent, and sometimes contradictory, results raise the question of what information is actually being conveyed from cerebellum to motor cortex.

DOES SPECIFIC INFORMATION ABOUT MOVEMENT PARAMETERS GET SENT TO MOTOR CORTEX FROM THE DEEP CEREBELLAR NUCLEI?

Although DCN activity can be correlated with a number of movement parameters, it is not certain that this information is forwarded to the motor cortex or that it is an important factor in shaping the relationship of motor cortical activity to specific movement parameters. First, the percentages of DCN cells whose activity correlated with a specific movement parameter were far from 100% in most of the studies reviewed above, and the DCN project to many extracerebellar sites other than the motor cortex. Thus, the percentage of DCN cells that project to the motor cortex (via the thalamus) that encode information about any particular movement parameter is not known. In fact, the study by Harvey et al. (1979) is the only study to identify DCN cells that specifically send their axons into the ascending portion of the superior cerebellar peduncle, which contains the axons heading to the thalamus. In this study, the main parameter with which DCN activity correlated with was movement duration, and in particular, no clear relation of neuronal activity to limb position was found. However, a detailed assessment of the relationship of DCN activity to other movement parameters was not reported. In sum, very little is known about whether the DCN directs different types of information to each of its targets, and in particular, little is known about what information the DCN send to the motor cortex.

This issue can also be viewed from the motor cortex perspective by asking whether the cerebellum could be an important source of its information about specific movement parameters. In particular, the directional tuning of DCN neurons is relatively poor compared to that found for motor cortex cells. For example, in one study comparing cerebellar and motor cortex cells on the same task (the center–out reaching task described earlier), motor cortex cells had sharper directional tuning curves, were more likely to show reciprocal firing patterns, and showed more trial-to-trial variation for repetitions of the same movement (Fortier, Smith, & Kalaska, 1993).

We can address this question further by looking at the response properties of the nuclei of the ventrolateral thalamus that receive input from the DCN, although we should note that these nuclei also receive major projections from the motor cortex itself, which could drive their activity. Anderson and Turner (1991) recorded from thalamic neurons that were shown to receive input from the cerebellum while animals performed a visually guided reaching task (Anderson & Turner, 1991). Most of these neurons (81%) were found to increase their firing rate in relation to movement, which is consistent with the predominance of increased activity in the DCN and the excitatory nature of the DCN cells that project to the thalamus. Moreover, thalamic neurons had a wide distribution of times for the onset of the modulation in their activity, ranging from −200 to 400 ms relative to movement onset, with the mode being 100–150 ms before movement onset. This timing is again consistent with DCN activity driving thalamic activity during movements. In another study recordings from cerebellar receiving areas in the thalamus showed similar results, with most neurons showing increases in their activity with movement (van Donkelaar, Stein, Passingham, & Miall, 1999). The exact timing of the onset differed between visually triggered and internally generated movement tasks, but in both cases, modulation of activity started well before movement onset (100–200 and 200–300 ms).

These studies unfortunately did not investigate the relationship of the thalamic activity to various parameters of the movements being performed. However, a study by Butler, Horne, and Hawkins (1992) did investigate the relationship of activity in the cerebellar thalamus to specific movement parameters. Monkeys were trained to make rapid flexion and extension wrist movements to capture a visual target. While the animals performed this task, neurons were recorded from the ventroposterolateral pars oralis nucleus in the thalamus. Most of these neurons had phasic activity that showed a reciprocal modulation pattern for the flexion and extension movements. The onset of the thalamic activity preceded EMG activity on average, consistent with the two studies just described (Anderson & Turner, 1991; van Donkelaar et al., 1999), but, significantly, occurred after the onset of movement-related activity in the motor cortex (which was also recorded from in this study).

In terms of specific movement parameters, a significant correlation was found for most cells between the duration of the change in neuronal activity and the movement duration (Butler et al., 1992; Ivanusic, Bourke, Xu, Butler, & Horne, 2005). Other than movement duration, the activity of thalamic cells generally was not well correlated with other movement parameters, including force and joint position (Butler et al., 1992; Ivanusic et al., 2005); however, a minority (23%) of cells did have activity correlated with movement velocity.

In sum, these results suggest that the motor parameters generally coded by motor cortex activity largely do not reflect (or are not specifically determined by) activity arising in the cerebellum. Rather, cerebellar thalamic neurons primarily seem to encode information about the duration of a movement (Butler et al., 1992; Ivanusic et al., 2005), which may help time the motor commands being sent from the motor cortex. Such a timing role actually matches with much classical (and recent) thinking and experimental results about the importance of the cerebellum for timing, in both motor and nonmotor tasks (Braitenberg, 1967; Hallett, Shahani, & Young, 1975; Holmes, 1922; Hore, Timmann, & Watts, 2002; Ivry, 1997; Ivry & Keele, 1989; Llinás, 1991; Perrett, 1998).

FUTURE DIRECTIONS AND CONCLUDING THOUGHTS

Although the studies of the DCN reviewed above have revealed important information about their activity during movement, many questions remain as to the specific role(s) of the DCN in motor control and, in particular, regarding information they provide to the motor cortex. Most previous studies have made the assumption that the individual nuclei that comprise the DCN represent the functional units of cerebellar output. This assumption probably originated from the simple fact that the nuclei appear as discrete anatomical entities, but it certainly grew in strength from the differences in connectivity that were found between the various nuclei. Indeed, many of the recording studies reviewed here were certainly undertaken with the assumption in mind that the DCN, the interpositus and dentate specifically had distinct functional roles in motor control, and the results of these studies clearly show that these nuclei do not behave identically during movement. And yet, in trying to interpret the results of these studies one is also struck by the degree of overlap in characteristics that was often seen, including overlap in the timing of the modulation of their activity, the types of activity patterns observed, and the relationship of the activity to various movement parameters. All of this suggests that whatever functions are carried out by the DCN, they may each be distributed across nuclear boundaries. Thus, functional divisions of the DCN may not respect the traditional nuclear boundaries.

A second pattern that requires some explanation is the variability in the findings across studies. Some of this variability certainly reflects the differences in the tasks used in the different studies and, more specifically, the constraints and requirements for solving these tasks. Indeed, the encoding of information by a particular neuron/nucleus can change depending on what is needed to solve a particular task. For example, in the motor cortex the coding of force has been shown to be context-dependent (Hepp-Reymond, Kirkpatrick-Tanner, Gabernet, Qi, & Weber, 1999). Yet, intertask variability is unlikely to be the full explanation for the variations in cell activity reviewed here, because even within one and the same study DCN activity suggested the presence of multiple functionally distinct populations (e.g., the three-cell populations in the study of Thach whose activity was either muscle-like, coded for joint position, or related to the upcoming movement direction (Thach, 1978)).

Part of the answer to the issues just raised may be related to the idea that the cerebellum comprises a series of modules or microcircuits (Apps & Hawkes, 2009). This idea arises from the fact that the cerebellar cortex can be divided into zones or compartments based on the expression of a variety of molecular markers, the best studied of which is zebrin (Apps & Hawkes, 2009; Hawkes, Brochu, Doré, Gravel, & LeClerc, 1992; Hawkes & Gravel, 1991; Voogd & Ruigrok, 1997). As already mentioned, based on zebrin expression, more than 20 distinct compartments can be defined in the cerebellar cortex (Fig. 1(A)) (Sugihara & Shinoda, 2004). Furthermore, many of the afferent and efferent connections of the cerebellum, as well as connections from the cerebellar cortex to the DCN, align with the zebrin compartments, giving rise to the concept that the cerebellum consists of a series of distinct modules, each of which contains a cortical compartment and a corresponding region of the DCN that is targeted exclusively by Purkinje cells of that module's cortical compartment.

Traditional views of the cerebellum generally assume that differences in function between modules primarily reflect differences in their afferent and efferent connectivity, as the near uniformity of the cerebellar cortical circuitry has generally been taken to mean that the cerebellum performs essentially equivalent computational operations on all of its inputs (Albus, 1971; Bloedel, 1992; Braitenberg, 2002; D'Angelo & Casali, 2012; Eccles, 1973; Eccles, Ito, & Szentágothai, 1967; Marr, 1969). However, much evidence now indicates that zebrin-positive and -negative compartments have very different intrinsic physiology (Fig. 1(B) and (C)) (reviewed in Cerminara, Lang, Sillitoe, & Apps, 2015). In particular, work indicates that zebrin-positive and -negative Purkinje cell firing rates and firing patterns are very different (e.g., simple spike rates of zebrin-negative cells are almost double those of zebrin-positive cells) (Xiao et al., 2014; Zhou et al., 2014). These differences become of interest in the present context because zebrin-positive and -negative Purkinje cells target different regions of the DCN (Chung, Marzban, & Hawkes, 2009; Sugihara, 2011; Sugihara & Shinoda, 2007). Thus, the DCN are subdivided into zebrin-positive and -negative territories that are likely to have distinctive operational and functional properties as a result of systematic variations in the intrinsic physiology of the cerebellar cortex.

In addition to this zebrin-related variation in Purkinje cell physiology, studies of the DCN neurons have shown that these cells are also quite diverse (Aizenman, Huang, & Linden, 2003; Aizenman & Linden, 1999; Czubayko, Sultan, Thier, & Schwarz, 2001; Husson, Rousseau, Broll, Zeilhofer, & Dieudonne, 2014; Molineux et al., 2006; Najac & Raman, 2015; Uusisaari & Knopfel, 2010, 2011; Uusisaari, Obata, & Knopfel, 2007).

If these functional variations in DCN intrinsic physiology are combined with the differing actions of the zebrin-positive and -negative Purkinje cells, a complex and heterogeneous substrate is formed that plausibly could underlie the varied responses seen by DCN neurons during movements.

Finally, it is striking that in all the DCN recording studies reviewed in this chapter, only one sought to identify the target of the DCN cells being recorded (Harvey et al., 1979). Probably this was because of the added complexity and potential complications of inserting stimulation electrodes into the brain stem in chronic recording preparations. However, given the many targets of the DCN, the consequence is that it is hard to know with any certainty from the published studies what signals are actually being sent to the motor cortex via the thalamus and what signals are being sent to other brain-stem targets, most notably, the inferior olive and basilar pontine nuclei. Indeed, it is possible that the reason for the lack of much kinematic information in the cerebellar thalamic cells is that many of the DCN cells that do code such information may project to other sites.

Looking forward, the previous work has provided an intriguing set of results that clearly establish that cerebellar activity is correlated with various stages of the motor control process by which coordinated movements are generated. Moreover, some aspects of how the cerebellum and motor cortex interact in this process have been suggested. Experiments using the powerful new molecular and optogenetic techniques that have been developed in recent years will allow selective manipulation and recording from distinct DCN cell types, which, in combination with accounting for the systematic variations of cerebellar cortical physiology, could provide answers to the question of what information the cerebellum provides to the motor cortex.

Acknowledgments

This work was supported by a grant from the NSF (IOS-1051858).

References

Aizenman, C. D., Huang, E. J., & Linden, D. J. (2003). Morphological correlates of intrinsic excitability in neurons of the deep cerebellar nuclei. *Journal of Neurophysiology, 89,* 1738–1747.

Aizenman, C. D., & Linden, D. J. (1999). Regulation of the rebound depolarization and spontaneous firing patterns of deep nuclear neurons in slices of rat cerebellum. *Journal of Neurophysiology, 82,* 1697–1709.

Albus, J. S. (1971). A theory of cerebellar function. *Mathematical Biosciences, 10,* 25–61.

Allen, G. I., & Tsukahara, N. (1974). Cerebrocerebellar communication systems. *Physiological Reviews, 54,* 957–1006.

Anderson, M. E., & Turner, R. S. (1991). Activity of neurons in cerebellar-receiving and pallidal-receiving areas of the thalamus of the behaving monkey. *Journal of Neurophysiology, 66,* 879–893.

Apps, R., & Hawkes, R. (2009). Cerebellar cortical organization: a one-map hypothesis. *Nature Reviews. Neuroscience, 10,* 670–681.

Bennett, M. R., & Hacker, P. M. S. (2002). The motor system in neuroscience: a history and analysis of conceptual developments. *Progress in Neurobiology, 67,* 1–52.

Bloedel, J. R. (1992). Functional heterogeneity with structural homogeneity: how does the cerebellum operate? *Behavioral and Brain Science, 15,* 666–678.

Bloedel, J. R., & Courville, J. (1981). Cerebellar afferent systems. In J. M. Brookhart, & V. B. Mountcastle (Eds.), *Handbook of physiology. Section 1 the nervous system Motor control: Vol. II.* (pp. 735–764). Bethesda, Md: American Physiological Society.

Braitenberg, V. (1967). Is the cerebellar cortex a biological clock in the millisecond range? *Progress in Brain Research, 25,* 334–346.

Braitenberg, V. (2002). In defense of the cerebellum. *Annals of the New York Academy of Sciences, 978,* 175–183.

Burton, J. E., & Onoda, N. (1977). Interpositus neuron discharge in relation to a voluntary movement. *Brain Research, 121,* 167–172.

Burton, J. E., & Onoda, N. (1978). Dependence of the activity of interpositus and red nucleus neurons on sensory input data generated by movement. *Brain Research, 152,* 41–63.

Butler, E. G., Horne, M. K., & Hawkins, N. J. (1992). The activity of monkey thalamic and motor cortical neurones in a skilled, ballistic movement. *The Journal of Physiology (London), 445,* 25–48.

Cerminara, N. L., Lang, E. J., Sillitoe, R. V., & Apps, R. (2015). Redefining the cerebellar cortex as an assembly of non-uniform Purkinje cell microcircuits. *Nature Reviews Neuroscience, 16,* 79–93.

Chapman, C. E., Spidalieri, G., & Lamarre, Y. (1986). Activity of dentate neurons during arm movements triggered by visual, auditory, and somesthetic stimuli in the monkey. *Journal of Neurophysiology, 55,* 203–226.

Chung, S. H., Marzban, H., & Hawkes, R. (2009). Compartmentation of the cerebellar nuclei of the mouse. *Neuroscience, 161,* 123–138.

Czubayko, U., Sultan, F., Thier, P., & Schwarz, C. (2001). Two types of neurons in the rat cerebellar nuclei as distinguished by membrane potentials and intracellular fillings. *Journal of Neurophysiology, 85,* 2017–2029.

D'Angelo, E., & Casali, S. (2012). Seeking a unified framework for cerebellar function and dysfunction: from circuit operations to cognition. *Frontiers in Neural Circuits, 6,* 116.

De Zeeuw, C. I., & Berrebi, A. S. (1995). Postsynaptic targets of Purkinje cell terminals in the cerebellar and vestibular nuclei of the rat. *The European Journal of Neuroscience, 7,* 2322–2333.

van Donkelaar, P., Stein, J. F., Passingham, R. E., & Miall, R. C. (1999). Neuronal activity in the primate motor thalamus during visually triggered and internally generated limb movements. *Journal of Neurophysiology, 82,* 934–945.

Dow, R. S., & Moruzzi, G. (1958). Historical introduction. In *The physiology and pathology of the cerebellum* (pp. 3–7). Minneapolis: University of Minnesota Press.

Dum, R. P., & Strick, P. L. (2002). Motor areas in the frontal lobe of the primate. *Physiology and Behavior, 77,* 677–682.

Dum, R. P., & Strick, P. L. (2003). An unfolded map of the cerebellar dentate nucleus and its projections to the cerebral cortex. *Journal of Neurophysiology, 89,* 634–639.

Eccles, J. C. (1967). Circuits in the cerebellar control of movement. *Procedings of the National Academy of Sciences of the United States of America, 58,* 336–343.

Eccles, J. C. (1973). The cerebellum as a computer: patterns in space and time. *Journal of Physiology (London), 229,* 1–32.

Eccles, J. C., Ito, M., & Szentágothai, J. (1967). *The cerebellum as a neuronal machine.* Berlin: Springer-Verlag.

Eccles, J. C., Rosen, I., Scheid, P., & Taborikova, H. (1972). Cutaneous afferent responses in interpositus neurones of the cat. *Brain Research, 42,* 207–211.

Eccles, J. C., Rosén, I., Scheid, P., & Táboríková, H. (1974). Temporal patterns of responses of interpositus neurons to peripheral afferent stimulation. *Journal of Neurophysiology, 37,* 1424–1437.

Evarts, E. V., & Thach, W. T. (1969). Motor mechanisms of the CNS: cerebrocerebellar interrelations. *Annual Review of Physiology, 31,* 451–498.

Fortier, P. A., Kalaska, J. F., & Smith, A. M. (1989). Cerebellar neuronal activity related to whole-arm reaching movements in the monkey. *Journal of Neurophysiology, 62,* 198–211.

Fortier, P. A., Smith, A. M., & Kalaska, J. F. (1993). Comparison of cerebellar and motor cortex activity during reaching: directional tuning and response variability. *Journal of Neurophysiology, 69,* 1136–1149.

Gaudreau, H., & Pare, D. (1996). Projection neurons of the lateral amygdaloid nucleus are virtually silent throughout the sleep–waking cycle. *Journal of Neurophysiology, 75,* 1301–1305.

Graziano, M. S. A., Taylor, C. S. R., Moore, T., & Cooke, D. F. (2002). The cortical control of movement revisited. *Neuron, 36,* 349–362.

Hallett, M., Shahani, B. T., & Young, R. R. (1975). EMG analysis of patients with cerebellar deficits. *Journal of Neurology, Neurosurgery and Psychiatry, 38,* 1163–1169.

Harvey, R. J., Porter, R., & Rawson, J. A. (1979). Discharges of intracerebellar nuclear cells in monkeys. *Journal of Physiology (London), 297,* 559–580.

Hawkes, R., Brochu, G., Doré, L., Gravel, C., & LeClerc, N. (1992). Zebrins: molecular markers of compartmentation in the cerebellum. In R. Llinás, & C. Sotelo (Eds.), *The cerebellum revisited* (pp. 22–55). New york: Springer-Verlag.

Hawkes, R., & Gravel, C. (1991). The modular cerebellum. *Progress in Neurobiology, 36,* 309–327.

Hepp-Reymond, M. C., Kirkpatrick-Tanner, M., Gabernet, L., Qi, H.-X., & Weber, B. (1999). Context-dependent force coding in motor and premotor cortical areas. *Experimental Brain Research, 128,* 123–133.

Holdefer, R. N., Houk, J. C., & Miller, L. E. (2005). Movement-related discharge in the cerebellar nuclei persists after local injections of $GABA_A$ antagonists. *Journal of Neurophysiology, 93,* 35–43.

Holmes, G. (1917). The symptoms of acute cerebellar injuries due to gunshot injuries. *Brain, 40,* 461–535.

Holmes, G. (1922). Clinical symptoms of cerebellar disease and their interpretation. Lecture 1. *Lancet,* 142–147.

Hore, J., Timmann, D., & Watts, S. (2002). Disorders in timing and force of finger opening in overarm throws made by cerebellar subjects. *Annuals of the New York Academy of Sciences, 978,* 1–15.

Humphrey, D. R. (1986). Representation of movements and muscles within the primate precentral motor cortex: historical and current perspectives. *Federation Proceedings, 45,* 2687–2699.

Husson, Z., Rousseau, C. V., Broll, I., Zeilhofer, H. U., & Dieudonne, S. (2014). Differential GABAergic and glycinergic inputs of inhibitory interneurons and Purkinje cells to principal cells of the cerebellar nuclei. *The Journals of Neuroscience, 34,* 9418–9431.

Ito, M., & Yoshida, M. (1966). The origin of cerebellar-induced inhibition of deiters neurones. I. Monosynaptic initiation of the inhibitory postsynaptic potentials. *Experimental Brain Research, 2,* 330–349.

Ito, M., Yoshida, M., & Obata, K. (1964). Monosynaptic inhibition of the intracerebellar nuclei induced from the cerebellar cortex. *Experientia (Basel), 20,* 575–576.

Ito, M., Yoshida, M., Obata, K., Kawai, N., & Udo, M. (1970). Inhibitory control of intracerebellar nuclei by the Purkinje cell axons. *Experimental Brain Research, 10,* 64–80.

Ivanusic, J. J., Bourke, D. W., Xu, Z. M., Butler, E. G., & Horne, M. K. (2005). Cerebellar thalamic activity in the macaque monkey encodes the duration but not the force or velocity of wrist movement. *Brain Research, 1041,* 181–197.

Ivry, R. (1997). Cerebellar timing systems. *International Review of Neurobiology, 41,* 555–573.

Ivry, R. B., & Keele, S. W. (1989). Timing functions of the cerebellum. *Journal of Cognitive Neuroscience, 1,* 136–152.

Jahnsen, H. (1986). Electrophysiological characteristics of neurones in the Guinea-pig deep cerebellar nuclei *in vitro. Journal of Physiology (London), 372,* 129–147.

van Kan, P. L., Houk, J. C., & Gibson, A. R. (1993). Output organization of intermediate cerebellum of the monkey. *Journal of Neurophysiology, 69,* 57–73.

Llinás, R. (1991). The noncontinuous nature of movement execution. In D. .R. Humphrey, & H.-J. Freund (Eds.), *Motor control: Concepts and issues* (pp. 223–242). New York: John Wiley & Sons.

MacKay, W. A. (1988). Cerebellar nuclear activity in relation to simple movements. *Experimental Brain Research, 71,* 47–58.

Marr, D. (1969). A theory of cerebellar cortex. *Journal of Physiology (London), 202,* 437–470.

McCrea, R. A., Bishop, G. A., & Kitai, S. T. (1978). Morphological and electrophysiological characteristics of projection neurons in the nucleus interpositus of the cat cerebellum. *The Journal of Comparative Neurology, 181,* 397–420.

Molineux, M. L., McRory, J. E., McKay, B. E., Hamid, J., Mehaffey, W. H., Rehak, R., et al. (2006). Specific T-type calcium channel isoforms are associated with distinct burst phenotypes in deep cerebellar nuclear neurons. *Proceedings of the National Academy of Sciences in United States of America, 103,* 5555–5560.

Mortimer, J. A. (1973). Temporal sequence of cerebellar Purkinje and nuclear activity in relation to the acoustic startle response. *Brain Research, 50,* 457–462.

Mortimer, J. A. (1975). Cerebellar responses to teleceptive stimuli in alert monkeys. *Brain Research, 83,* 369–390.

Najac, M., & Raman, I. M. (2015). Integration of purkinje cell inhibition by cerebellar nucleo-olivary neurons. *The Journal of Neuroscience, 35,* 544–549.

Palkovits, M., Mezey, E., Hamori, J., & Szentagothai, J. (1977). Quantitative histological analysis of the cerebellar nuclei in the cat. I. Numerical data on cells and on synapses. *Experimental Brain Research, 28,* 189–209.

Perrett, S. P. (1998). Temporal discrimination in the cerebellar cortex during conditioned eyelid responses. *Experimental Brain Research, 121,* 115–124.

Robertson, L. T., & Grimm, R. J. (1975). Responses of primate dentate neurons to different trajectories of the limb. *Experimental Brain Research, 23,* 447–462.

Rosén, I., & Scheid, P. (1972). Cerebellar surface cooling influencing evoked activity in cortex and in interpositus nucleus. *Brain Research, 45,* 580–584.

Schieber, M. H., & Thach, W. T. (1985). Trained slow tracking. II. Bidirectional discharge patterns of cerebellar nuclear, motor cortex, and spindle afferent neurons. *The Journal of Neurophysiology, 54,* 1228–1270.

Soechting, J. F., Burton, J. E., & Onoda, N. (1978). Relationships between sensory input, motor output and unit activity in interpositus and red nuclei during intentional movement. *Brain Research, 152,* 65–79.

Strick, P. L. (1983). The influence of motor preparation on the response of cerebellar neurons to limb displacements. *The Journal of Neuroscience, 3,* 2007–2020.

Strick, P. L., Dum, R. P., & Fiez, J. A. (2009). Cerebellum and nonmotor function. *Annual Review of Neuroscience, 32,* 413–434.

Sugihara, I. (2011). Compartmentalization of the deep cerebellar nuclei based on afferent projections and aldolase C expression. *Cerebellum, 10,* 449–463.

Sugihara, I., & Shinoda, Y. (2004). Molecular, topographic, and functional organization of the cerebellar cortex: a study with combined aldolase C and olivocerebellar tracing. *The Journal of Neuroscience, 24,* 8771–8785.

Sugihara, I., & Shinoda, Y. (2007). Molecular, topographic, and functional organization of the cerebellar nuclei: analysis by three-dimensional mapping of the olivonuclear projection and aldolase C labeling. *The Journal of Neuroscience, 27,* 9696–9710.

Thach, W. T. (1968). Discharge of Purkinje and cerebellar nuclear neurons during rapidly alternating arm movements in the monkey. *The Journal of Neurophysiology, 31,* 785–797.

Thach, W. T. (1970). Discharge of cerebellar neurons related to two maintained postures and two prompt movements. I. Nuclear cell output. *The Journal of Physiology (London), 33,* 527–536.

Thach, W. T. (1975). Timing of activity in cerebellar dentate nucleus and cerebral motor cortex during prompt volitional movement. *Brain Research, 88,* 233–241.

Thach, W. T. (1978). Correlation of neural discharge with pattern and force of muscular activity, joint position, and direction of intended next movement in motor cortex and cerebellum. *The Journal of Neurophysiology, 41,* 654–676.

Uusisaari, M., & Knopfel, T. (2010). GlyT2+ neurons in the lateral cerebellar nucleus. *Cerebellum, 9,* 42–55.

Uusisaari, M., & Knopfel, T. (2011). Functional classification of neurons in the mouse lateral cerebellar nuclei. *Cerebellum, 10,* 637–646.

Uusisaari, M., Obata, K., & Knopfel, T. (2007). Morphological and electrophysiological properties of GABAergic and non-GABAergic cells in the deep cerebellar nuclei. *The Journal of Neurophysiology, 97,* 901–911.

Voogd, J., & Ruigrok, T. J. H. (1997). Transverse and longitudinal patterns in the mammalian cerebellum. *Progress in Brain Research, 114,* 21–37.

Wetts, R., Kalaska, J. F., & Smith, A. M. (1985). Cerebellar nuclear cell activity during antagonist cocontraction and reciprocal inhibition of forearm muscles. *The Journal of Neurophysiology, 54,* 231–244.

Xiao, J., Cerminara, N. L., Kotsurovskyy, Y., Aoki, H., Burroughs, A., Wise, A. K., et al. (2014). Systematic regional variations in Purkinje cell spiking patterns. *PLoS One, 9,* e105633.

Zhou, H., Lin, Z., Voges, K., Ju, C., Gao, Z., Bosman, L. W., et al. (2014). Cerebellar modules operate at different frequencies. *eLife, 3,* e02536.

A Spatiotemporal Hypothesis on the Role of 4- to 25-Hz Field Potential Oscillations in Cerebellar Cortex

Richard Courtemanche[1,2,4], Ariana Frederick[1,3]

[1]FRQS Groupe de Recherche en Neurobiologie Comportementale (CSBN), Concordia University, Montréal, QC, Canada; [2]Department of Exercise Science, Concordia University, Montréal, QC, Canada; [3]Department of Biology, Concordia University, Montréal, QC, Canada; [4]PERFORM Centre, Concordia University, Montréal, QC, Canada

INTRODUCTION

We are about to witness an amazing feat of sensorimotor performance, the one-timer ice hockey slap shot. The Montreal Canadiens are on a 5 versus 4 power play, and this is an optimal time to break the 2–2 tie. They have two minutes with probably more puck possession. Now in the opposing zone, the two Canadiens' defensemen are exchanging the puck at the opposing blue line, and both are very well skilled, as well as possessing potent slap shots. More often than not, a privileged option will have star defenseman P.K. Subban receive one of Andrei Markov's slick puck passes, delivered at the optimal speed and location, so that P.K. can unleash a ferocious slap shot. This consists in one swift movement, to catapult the puck, aimed at a small target (say over the goalie's shoulder, in a top corner of the net): a demonstration of both power and precision. Using all of the biomechanical energy P.K. can store in his body and hockey stick, he will accurately hit the puck with a violent but precise ballistic movement. This is P.K.'s already established motor plan, and he has practiced this motor act thousands of times, hitting a "one-timer" slap shot.

He is now simply waiting for the cue, the incoming puck stimulus, from Markov, to execute. In this context, P.K. even has a mental image of the incoming puck, the slap-shot execution, and the result. One important brain area in this sensorimotor act, among, of course, a group of others, is the cerebellum (Lisberger and Thach, 2013). The movement initiation and movement execution are regulated by precise control of the motor output and monitoring of the sensory input. Many studies have established that the cerebellum will be involved in the internal representation of this skill.

In the period during which P.K. waits for the puck, a number of brain areas contribute to the sensorimotor preparedness. An important component is to have participating brain areas synchronized, poised to communicate information from their respective domains of specialization (Buzsaki, 2004, 2006; Moser et al., 2010; Traub & Whittington, 2010). When all works well, P.K. has his brain networks optimized to provide the best sensorimotor response. How are all areas pooled together? More precisely, how are all cerebellar subareas pooled together? In this chapter, we explore the role of cerebellar oscillations in the timing of cerebellar information processing, potentially leading to the production of a movement; we also address the potential advantage of oscillatory control in networks involved in prediction and preparation.

In the context of this review, spatiotemporal aspects of the flow of activity through the cerebellum will be important. For the temporal aspect and oscillations, the flow will depend on the coordination between signals coming from putative oscillators, which in fact implicate a spatiotemporal analysis. The other premise of this review is to focus on how the cerebellum could use rhythmicity and synchrony to predict future events or coordinate actions. Indeed, the cerebellum provides accurate computations about the state of the world around us and provides us with an enhanced capacity to further influence this world, quite probably in predicting our, and its, future state (Bell, Bodznick, Montgomery, & Bastian, 1997; Bell, Han, & Sawtell, 2008; Courchesne & Allen, 1997; Paulin, 1993). Oscillations in cerebellar circuits can certainly contribute to this time-dependent process and help relate its activity to other structures of the sensorimotor systems. What role could these oscillations have in prediction? First, they could form a temporal predictability metric. This is based on the simple temporal capacity of oscillatory circuits to shape the timing of spiking activity with temporally predictable loops. In addition, it would be interesting to speculate as to why the information does propagate through those loops. Considering the location in the cerebellum, the afferent input, and the temporal properties of those oscillations, one possibility is that the predictive capacity of these networks of neurons would reside in the signal interplay between two sides: a corollary discharge and the sensory afferent input. P.K.'s cerebellum, in the movement initiation for the slap shot, might use those cerebellar oscillations to time the neural activity and to integrate the proper information to transmit to further nodes in the sensorimotor system. We briefly review some of the oscillatory phenomena in the cerebellum and then describe a specific hypothesis below.

SYNCHRONIZATION AND OSCILLATIONS IN CEREBELLAR CIRCUITS

There have been a few reviews that have addressed cerebellar oscillations and synchrony (Courtemanche, Robinson, & Aponte, 2013; D'Angelo et al., 2009; De Zeeuw et al., 2011; de Zeeuw, Hoebeek, & Schonewille, 2008). Synchronization of neural activity would serve to group together the information coming from various local circuits. With its peculiar organization (Voogd & Glickstein, 1998), the flow of information across the circuits of the cerebellar cortex has been an interesting question. An inspiration for researchers and engineers is that it has led many to try to figure out the interrelations between its distinctive elements (Eccles, Ito, & Szentágothai, 1967; Ito, 2006). For instance, for the defenseman about to hit a one-timer slap shot, how do all the different subareas of the cerebellum, modules likely to be corresponding to the various body parts, converge? The question of the "holding" of activity, in-between events or in expectancy of future events, is one that has been approached from the standpoint of oscillatory activity. An interesting question is how the cerebellar circuits deal with sensorimotor preparation, and how the cerebellum switches between modes of operation. These modes can include specific input–output fast operations, but also the capacity to generate or reverberate oscillatory activity, during expectancy periods. We isolate here a situation in which expectancy can develop.

How do cerebellar cortex neurons shape into a population forming one of its many coherent representations, at a given moment in time? What is the time-specific signature of cerebellar populations? It would just make sense that a large structure such as the cerebellum, with its massive cortex, should be able to communicate effectively with the other sensorimotor oscillatory networks. The temporal patterning of cerebellar activity should coordinate its participation in sensorimotor transformations. Since the recording of olivocerebellar activity in the context of harmaline administration (De Montigny & Lamarre, 1973; Llinás & Volkind, 1973), and the subsequent explorations of population coding in olivocerebellar circuits, Bullock (1997) had noted a widely silent echo in the rest of the cerebellar circuitry to the perimovement oscillatory manifestations seen in the cerebral cortex. In this chapter, we will not fully address the olivocerebellar oscillations, interesting in their own right (Llinás, 2009; Welsh, Lang, Sugihara, & Llinás, 1995), or the faster oscillations—probably related to the Purkinje cell connectivity (Cheron, Servais, & Dan, 2008; Middleton et al., 2008;

de Solages et al., 2008), or slower oscillations (Chen et al., 2009; Ros, Sachdev, Yu, Sestan, & McCormick, 2009). We have reviewed those elsewhere (Courtemanche et al., 2013). We will focus on the cerebellar cortex population 4- to 25-Hz oscillations, forming multiple oscillation patterns in the cerebellar cortex circuitry (Courtemanche et al., 2013; D'Angelo et al., 2009; de Zeeuw et al., 2008). We review here potential influences these mechanisms could have on predictive information processing.

CEREBELLAR CORTEX 4- TO 25-Hz OSCILLATIONS

Among the oscillations at less than 30 Hz in the cerebellum that have received the greatest attention is the ~10-Hz oscillatory activity in the olivocerebellar system. This has been studied in vivo and in vitro, and a quick overview will be given here, having been well reviewed by other authors (e.g., Jacobson, Rokni, & Yarom, 2008; Llinás, 2009; Llinás, Brookhart, & Mountcastle, 1981, Llinás, Humphrey, & Freund, 1991; Llinás & Sugimori, 1992; Welsh & Llinas, 1997). Furthermore, in the past few years, additional rhythmic phenomena have appeared in vivo in the cerebellar cortex granule cell layer (GCL), which have subsequently been investigated in vitro.

Olivocerebellar activity. Under systemic harmaline, rhythmic olivocerebellar climbing fiber spikes are produced (De Montigny & Lamarre, 1973; Lamarre, De Montigny, Dumont, & Weiss, 1971; Llinás & Volkind, 1973). Instead of complex spikes discharge at ~1 Hz, this harmaline model produced massive coherent firing at ~10 Hz. The discrepancy between the ~1-Hz firing under normal conditions and the 10-Hz firing under harmaline is explained by the cells firing on every oscillatory cycle; 10-Hz oscillations appear as subthreshold oscillations in vitro (Devor & Yarom, 2002), and in vivo (Chorev, Yarom, & Lampl, 2007). Networks of Purkinje cells exhibit complex spike synchrony patterns (Sasaki, Bower, & Llinás, 1989), and olivocerebellar afferent inputs could serve to coordinate the Purkinje cell population code (Blenkinsop & Lang, 2006; Lang, 2002; Lang, Sugihara, & Llinás, 1996). In the awake behaving animal, these olivocerebellar networks show heightened oscillatory anteroposterior synchrony (Lang, Sugihara, Welsh, & Llinás, 1999). These networks also form task-specific network mosaics, relying on olivocerebellar oscillatory activity, while the animal performs rhythmic movements (Welsh et al., 1995). The inferior olive could thus work as a motor clock (Welsh, Ahn, & Placantonakis, 2005). A nucleus such as the inferior olive could indeed temporally influence the cerebellar cortex neural sheet. While clock rhythmic activity of the olive has been disputed (Keating & Thach, 1995, 1997), the concept that olive rhythmicity could help organize activity in the cerebellar cortex has remained strong (Jacobson et al., 2008; Llinás, 2009). Recent models predict a capacity of these networks to work at an even finer grain than 10 Hz (Jacobson, Lev, Yarom, & Cohen, 2009; Jacobson et al., 2008).

GCL oscillations. Oscillations recorded in the local field potentials (LFPs) of the granule cell layer have permitted the characterization of the other source of afferents to the cerebellar cortex, the mossy fiber system. These have been mostly found in the monkey and the rodent so far; but there are clear indications that such activity can be recorded in the human cerebellum (Dalal, Osipova, Bertrand, & Jerbi, 2013). Important for our one-timer slap-shot example, there is mounting evidence that human rhythmic slow activity is also related to cerebellar sensorimotor processing (Gross et al., 2002).

Monkey. Pellerin and Lamarre (1997) found paramedian lobule rhythmic GCL spindle-like activity at ~14 Hz in the LFPs. These appeared spontaneously, but in a predictable manner, as the rhesus monkey was immobile, but attentive to its environment. This rhythmic activity could be stopped by sensory events and/or motor output. The LFPs were best related to granule cell multiunit activity and partially to Purkinje cell simple spikes; however, there was no relation to complex spikes (Courtemanche, Pellerin, & Lamarre, 2002). The optimal behavior was active expectancy, or "waiting for the proper time to trigger the movement" (Courtemanche et al., 2002). GCL oscillations would also increase if the animal was in a state of passive expectancy, the spindles lasting as long as the waiting period (Courtemanche et al., 2002). Courtemanche and Lamarre (2005) found a dynamic relationship between cerebral LFPs and cerebellar GCL 10- to 25-Hz LFP oscillations. In a lever-press task, paramedian lobule GCL LFPs were synchronized with contralateral primary somatosensory cortex LFPs, primarily in the waiting period in anticipation of the right time to press. Synchronization was better in active expectancy than in passive expectancy or rest, meaning that the synchronization points to a functional role. Primary motor cortex versus paramedian lobule GCL 10- to 25-Hz oscillations seemed less linked in the context of the tasks, though active expectancy also seemed to incite the greatest synchronization.

As important as the timing of the oscillations is the spatial relationship in which they occur. Courtemanche, Chabaud, and Lamarre (2009) found a spatiotemporal organization of cerebellar cortex GCL oscillations in the rhesus cerebellum: they show a primarily parasagittal organization of the GCL oscillations when the animal is at rest. There are many spatial modules in the cerebellar cortex that are strongly parasagittal (Ebner, Wang, Gao, Cramer, & Chen, 2012; Hawkes et al., 1997; Herrup & Kuemerle, 1997). However, during a task, the coronal plane LFP synchronization increases. Thus, the putative sagittal module expands laterally during a sensorimotor task. Such a lateral recruitment mechanism has been seen for task-related Purkinje cell simple spike firing (Heck, Thach, & Keating, 2007).

Rodent. Hartmann and Bower (1998) found similar activity in the crus II GCL of the awake rodent at ~7 Hz, tightly correlated with GCL activity. Oscillations were correlated across the hemisphere, as well as with the other hemisphere. Many similarities with Pellerin and Lamarre (1997) were evident: the LFP oscillations were from the posterior lobe, were GCL unit related, were present during periods of immobility of the animal, and were spindle-shaped. Despite their frequency-band difference, these oscillations were more alike than different. O'Connor et al. (2002) also found ~7-Hz synchronized activity across the crus II cerebellar cortex and addressed the interactions across the somatosensory system. The coherence improved when the rat whisker movements were absent or small. The large-network coherence was thus optimal during immobility. In addition, Dugué et al. (2009) showed that Golgi cells formed a network that could maintain 4- to 25-Hz resonance in the GCL circuitry.

Overall, these studies have shown that GCL 4- to 25-Hz oscillations can serve to organize temporally, and spatiotemporally, the communication (1) within the GCL, through the organization of the cellular networks; (2) from the GCL to the cerebellar cortex output, by influencing the Purkinje cell simple spikes; (3) in the spatial patterns of GCL synchronization in time, as seen in the context of functional units; and (4) between the cerebellum and the cerebral cortex, as seen through LFP synchronization between the two structures during task performance. These GCL oscillations can thus help in the investigation of information flow throughout the cerebellar cortex and communicating units in the sensorimotor system pathways. Important to this idea, the strong GCL resonance in the 4- to 25-Hz frequencies allows the organization of circuits around the cell properties of both the granule cells (D'Angelo et al., 2001) and the Golgi cells (Forti, Cesana, Mapelli, & D'Angelo, 2006). This confers specific time windows for optimal GCL processing of information and for synaptic plasticity (D'Angelo, 2008; D'Angelo et al., 2009; D'Angelo & de Zeeuw, 2009).

SPATIOTEMPORAL ASPECTS OF GRANULE CELL LAYER SYNCHRONIZATION

As shown in primate recordings, the patterns of synchronization in the GCL LFPs, supported by the oscillations, are anisotropic, meaning that they follow a particular direction, in this case favoring a parasagittal organization, despite a prediction that oscillations at this frequency would be patchy (de Zeeuw et al., 2008). This coherence pattern is seen in the GCL in the context of tasks (Courtemanche et al., 2009). As anatomical support, mossy fiber afferents (Heckroth & Eisenman, 1988; Ruigrok, 2011; Scheibel, 1977) and Golgi cell axons follow a sagittal distribution (Sillitoe, Chung, Fritschy, Hoy, & Hawkes, 2008). During a task in which likely sensorimotor binding must occur, a distinct dynamic lateral expansion of the areas of high synchrony is observable, leading to the interpretation of an enhanced active zone during a sensorimotor task. In application, this would mean that for the hockey player, a lateral expansion of the recruitment would occur in the posterior lobe as the player is getting ready to launch a slap shot.

How could this rhythmicity be optimal for the lateral recruitment? Putative sagittal GCL–Purkinje modules could be optimally synchronized at this frequency (Courtemanche et al., 2013). Briefly, in the case of GCL 7- to 25-Hz rhythmicity, loops will present delays of 40–250 ms. This corresponds to "up phases" lasting between 20 and 125 ms, which corresponds to periods of enhanced excitability for local groups of GCL neurons. Combined with the slow conduction velocity of the parallel fibers (0.2–0.3 m/s; Bell & Grimm, 1969; Vranesic, Iijima, Ichikawa, Matsumoto, & Knopfel, 1994), conjoined excitation at two cerebellar cortex sites separated by the length of the parallel fibers (up to 6 mm; Brand, Dahl, & Mugnaini, 1976) would be covered in a period of 20–30 ms. The up states supported by GCL rhythmicity would thus have to last longer than 20–30 ms to provide a rhythmic advantage. From this calculation, a rhythm with a period of more than 20 ms (or frequencies less than 50 Hz) could support a spatiotemporal pattern of synchronization through the parallel fibers. This mechanism could be complemented by the connectivity of Lugaro cells (Dieudonné & Dumoulin, 2000), presumably leading to faster interactions. These cells are inhibitory interneurons transversely connected to Golgi cells (Lainé & Axelrad, 1996). This connection could thus potentially serve as an oscillatory amplifier to the Golgi–granule interactions. The Lugaro cell could form a second mechanism by which a spatially defined, orthogonal network (sagittal for Golgi cell axons and Lugaro dendrites (Geurts, De Schutter, & Dieudonne, 2003), coronal for Lugaro axons), could influence the GCL oscillations.

In the case of our hockey player, from the purely somatosensory perspective, there is a definite passage from a state of postural immobility (balancing on skates) to a whole-body movement requiring very precise interlimb coordination. This interlimb coordination must rely on a specific motor plan, based on the monitoring of sensory input. In this respect, given the mapping parameters in the cerebellum (Voogd & Glickstein, 1998; Lisberger and Thach, 2013), it is very likely that the sensorimotor computations are performed across multiple modules (Ruigrok, 2011; Voogd, Ruigrok, de Zeeuw, & Strata, 1997). These modules have been coactivated in time through repeated practice; the coordinated synchronization brought about by the repeated practice has been repeated many times. In the context of a highly learned behavior, evidence is mounting that patterns of synchronization appear in the modules (microzones) for coordinated information processing (De Gruijl, Hoogland, & De Zeeuw, 2014). It is very likely that repeated coactivations proceeded to change the plasticity of the elements concerned (e.g., mossy fiber to granule cell; Golgi cell to granule cell; granule cell to Purkinje cell), by the very nature of the repeated practice. Like the theta frequency for the hippocampus

(Buzsaki & Moser, 2013), there is building evidence that coordinated activity at slow frequencies in the cerebellum would favor LTP-like plasticity mechanisms (D'Angelo et al., 2011; D'Angelo & de Zeeuw, 2009). In addition to the identified role of climbing fiber long-term adaptation (Ito, 2006; Schweighofer, Lang, & Kawato, 2013), in which the inferior olive also seems to have a preference for ~10-Hz rhythmicity, the overall circuits thus have marked distributed plasticity across many synapses (Gao, van Beugen, & De Zeeuw, 2012), which could optimally be operating or be facilitated by the 4- to 25-Hz rhythmicity. As P.K. Subban practiced his slap shot, repeated olivary cycles of around 10-Hz waves of activity were attempting to steer circuits in the cerebellar cortex, combined with near-10-Hz patterns of mossy fiber input, grouping together the required modules.

CIRCUIT INTERACTIONS—A POTENTIAL EFFERENCE COPY ROLE?

The precise interpretation of the functional role of these cerebellar oscillations is a question that remains outstanding, just as is the role of cerebral cortex oscillations in many instances. Considering the behavioral conditions under which the GCL oscillations appear, potential interpretations would be (1) a general role in attention and readiness, as the animals that had optimal oscillations were either in active monitoring of the environment or involved in a specific task-related premovement information processing; (2) an idling rhythm, which would be less elaborate in information processing, a passive consequence of a lack of specific stimulation; or (3) a monitoring rhythm that would affect the processing of sensory input and motor output. The last interpretation has been more fully established in the case of somatosensory cortex processing (Cardin et al., 2009; Rossiter, Worthen, Witton, Hall, & Furlong, 2013), but those rhythms would certainly apply in the many aspects of cerebellar sensorimotor processing, as this monitoring role is emphasized for areas of massive afferent input (the GCL); oscillatory activity has been an essential element of optimal processing in many systems dealing with a massive entry of information (e.g., visual (Fries, 2009), auditory (Lakatos, Chen, O'Connell, Mills, & Schroeder, 2007), and olfactory (Laurent, 1996; Nikonov, Parker, & Caprio, 2002)). We develop here a particular context for the role of these cerebellar oscillations in sensorimotor processing, in which the sensory information would be compared to the motor command or to the expected feedback. This type of feed-forward and/or feedback comparison has been identified as part of the basic building blocks of internal models. We will attempt to link the 4- to 25-Hz oscillatory process to a rhythmic corollary discharge comparison with the sensory input (Crapse & Sommer, 2008), happening at the level of the GCL. With specific comparisons having been identified in cerebellum-like structures, the relationship could even have the effect of a network-level efference copy.

Corollary discharges have been studied for many years and have been identified in multiple systems (Bell et al., 1997, 2008; Crapse & Sommer, 2008; Duhamel, Colby, & Goldberg, 1992; McCloskey & Brooks, 1981; Requarth, Kaifosh, & Sawtell, 2014; Sperry, 1950). In the case of the role of cerebellar oscillations in this context, we formulate here an interesting hypothesis, but we fully understand that we are using circumstantial evidence. However, the multiple elements do converge on an attractive possibility for a function of cerebellar slow oscillations. The case can thus be made only semiquantitatively. However, this role of oscillations in sampling information coming through the cerebellum applies well to situations of changes of state.

For example, let's come back to our defenseman just about to hit a one-timer slap shot. A reductionist version in the primate or rodent would be when the animal is immobile and attentive to the environment, waiting for the proper time to initiate a simple movement. There is quite likely an optimal level of sensory monitoring and motor matching taking place in the cerebellum; sensory, in assessing the stimulus that will serve as a trigger for movement, but also as to the body state, and motor, in assessing the best movement that will be adapted to the stimulus and the state. Under those conditions, as shown in Courtemanche et al. (2002), the GCL oscillations are optimal and appear in the form of spindles, in waxing-and-waning episodes. These oscillations show a progressive increase in amplitude in the GCL, come to a maximum, only to decrease in amplitude as movement initiation gets nearer. The example is given in Fig. 1(A). Of note is that at the time of movement initiation, oscillations have decreased to minimum amplitude in the GCL. While it might not be the only reason, we could posit that (1) the spindle is terminated because the required computation has taken its course and (2) these oscillations could represent the actual comparison, exchange in alternation between one side of the comparison (the motor command) and the other side of the comparison, the sensory status. These are illustrated with different colors in Fig. 1(B). At the time of the voluntary movement initiation, the comparison would be mature, and the subtraction between sensory and motor aspects would provide a result around zero, confirming that the movement can be initiated. As such, no more oscillations would be required to initiate the movement. This amplitude modulation would provide a readout of the comparison taking place at the GCL site.

As proven experimentally, there are two ways to effectively end GCL oscillatory spindles. The first method is to execute a movement, which is a predictable occurrence, and the GCL spindle shows a progression toward motor execution. The second method, less predictable, concerns with unplanned sensory input. In this case, the oscillatory activity does not

(A)

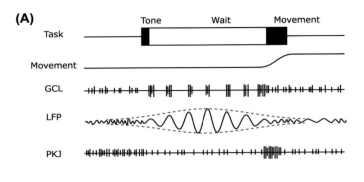

(B)

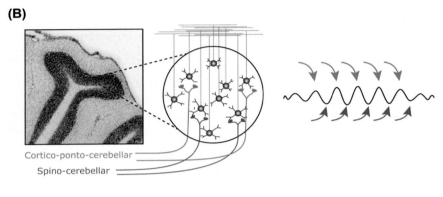

Cortico-ponto-cerebellar
Spino-cerebellar

(C)

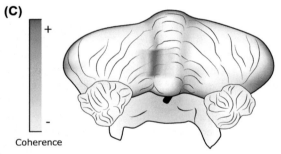

Coherence

FIGURE 1   Schematic diagrams illustrating the hypothesis for a spatiotemporal role of 4- to 25-Hz oscillations in the cerebellar cortex GCL LFPs. (A) Temporal process in which oscillatory activity spindles in the GCL can serve in sensorimotor preparation, for a passage from immobility to movement (trace illustrating elbow flexion, for example), *based on Courtemanche et al. (2002)* PKJ-Purkinje cell firing example. (B) Afferent interactions at the level of the GCL sites, and the effect on LFP oscillations. Input from mossy fiber afferents from cortico-ponto-cerebellar sources (e.g., corollary discharge of motor commands) is compared with the afferents from spinocerebellar sources (e.g., sensory input), at the level of granule cells in the GCL. This comparison, with a decreasing difference with each progressive iteration, could lead to a tightening of the local network involved, leading to a decrease in oscillatory LFP amplitude. A local selection of the neuronal output would then trigger activity in defined Purkinje cells. This comparison would serve to define the involved populations and output. (C) Spatial schematic process of coherence in the primate paramedian lobule, based on electrode locations and synchronization *data from Courtemanche et al. (2009)*. Here, the LFP synchrony was strong in a parasagittal manner at rest, yet showed lateral expansion during a lever-press task. The color code shows the coherence pattern expected if electrodes were placed to record LFPs, with one electrode in the "red" area. Together, the larger scale networks could bind together control modules for different body parts, as the local network performs a corollary discharge comparison.

show this progressive decrease in amplitude—the sensory input appears to reset the oscillatory activity by introducing an unplanned element. As the state change can be anticipated (Scheffer et al., 2012), when motor information comes through the circuits, it will probably serve to reset the comparison to a new state estimation. In the case of phasic unplanned input, the networks will need to perform new computations to establish the next state of environment they will need to match. A motor command or external phasic event thus changes the state and produces a transition and subsequently the search for a new equilibrium state.

We would then argue that the GCL oscillations (here 4–25 Hz) could serve to establish the sensorimotor dialog in the paramedian lobule and posterior lobe of the cerebellar cortex, providing an LFP-level population monitor of computations that are produced within local GCL modules. This sensorimotor dialog is reminiscent of the efference copy mechanism present within cerebellum-like structures (Bell et al., 1997, 2008). In such structures, the corollary discharge and the sensory afferent are compared within determined cells and the sensory afferent is subtracted from the corollary discharge to provide a difference, which, in the case of autostimulation in the electric fish, equals zero. This process has been further identified in the context of somatosensory afferents in individual granule cells (Requarth et al., 2014). We consider that such a process could take place in the GLC of the cerebellar cortex at the population level. As seen in Fig. 1, a possibility would be that sensory feedback and corollary discharges could meet at specific sites of the GCL and offer a cancelation mechanism occurring over multiple cycles. This sampling would best happen and be optimally adapted to the information entry that follows a particular temporal pattern (Ahissar, Haidarliu, & Zacksenhouse, 1997).

CONDITIONS SUPPORTING A PREDICTIVE SENSORIMOTOR DIALOG

The hypothesis presented is based on more than the mere temporal pattern of GCL oscillations. Granted, at this point, the comparison can be identified only as a hypothesis; there are many elements necessary to be tested before establishing this as a process taking place in the GCL for information processing. However, multiple converging pieces of evidence point to a particular alignment of the sensory and motor information comparison being an optimal process.

1. The posterior lobe of the cerebellum (and the paramedian lobule specifically) receives overlapping mossy fibers from the corticopontocerebellar afferent and from the spinocerebellar afferents (Allen & Tsukahara, 1974; King, Armstrong, Apps, & Trott, 1998; Voogd & Glickstein, 1998). This emphasizes that the paramedian lobule receives appropriate information to accomplish this comparison.

2. Electrophysiological activity in the posterior lobe of the cerebellum shows that this region responds to both sensory and motor afferent inputs (Sasaki, Oka, Matsuda, Shimono, & Mizuno, 1975; Sasaki & Massion, 1979).

3. GCL activity in the cerebellar cortex of the posterior lobe shows responses to somatosensory stimulation (Bower, Beerman, Gibson, Shambes, & Welker, 1981; Hartmann & Bower, 2001) in regions that also correspond to common input from the primary somatosensory cortex (Morissette & Bower, 1996). From this end, some considerations are that those circuits correspond to the comparison of the sensory input with the expected input (Bower & Schmahmann, 1997; Bower, de Zeeuw, Strata, & Voogd, 1997; Gao, Parsons, Bower, Xiong, & Fox, 1996).

4. In cerebellum-like structures in mildly electric fish, the corollary discharge activity and proprioceptive activity are mixed at the level of the GCL of the mossy fibers. This would set the stage for local comparisons occurring at the level of single GCL sites (Requarth et al., 2014). Such information is present at individual local GCL sites (Huang et al., 2013; Requarth et al., 2014). In this case, the interpretation is not only that the corollary discharge and sensory input interact, but that they truly cancel each other, hence the concept of efference copy (Bell et al., 1997).

5. In the case of the sensorimotor local oscillations, the local network around the electrode goes from an oscillatory mode, in which a larger group of neurons are likely to be synchronized to form a larger LFP amplitude, to a less rhythmic local network, which would then give more control to command neurons sending the information out of the modules. This could mean that the local computation of the comparison first requires multiple synchronized neurons in order to be effective, but then requires fewer synchronized neurons. This could be controlled by Golgi cells (D'Angelo et al., 2013). Of course, a caveat is that the oscillations at 4–25 Hz are probably covering large expanses of lobules, and so many GCL sites, simultaneously.

6. In a period preceding movement initiation, oscillations coordinate across sensorimotor systems. These ensure a capacity to functionally bind the information, including sensory and motor, from multiple sites (Buzsaki, Logothetis, & Singer, 2013; Engel et al., 2010; Frederick, Bourget-Murray, & Courtemanche, 2013). In the cerebellar cortex, as seen in the LFP synchrony, multiple modules (microzones) could be brought together during the computation of the sensorimotor matching. This is illustrated in Fig. 1(C), using data from primate LFP GCL synchronization in or close to the paramedian lobule, with a wider lateral recruitment during a lever-press task (Courtemanche et al., 2009).

7. Coordinated modular activity probably takes place in the cerebellum to process according to sensorimotor modules, recruiting up to the Purkinje cells (Ito, 2006, 2010), and probably ends up forming patterns of inhibition to the deep cerebellar nuclei (Person & Raman, 2012).

Such elements support that the local comparison occurs between a corollary discharge and the actual sensory input. While the main example that is given here is for a comparison between sensory and motor elements, it is also possible that somatosensory input is compared to the sensory expectation for certain sites. Somatosensory cerebral cortical processing and somatosensory cerebellar processing show many modes of interaction (Morissette & Bower, 1996), and the local oscillations from each site can synchronize (Courtemanche & Lamarre, 2005; O'Connor, Berg, & Kleinfeld, 2002). However, our basic comparison between sensory input and motor commands remains a strong candidate, as the cerebellum is a key site for sensory and motor interactions at the cellular level (Proville et al., 2014).

GRANULE CELL LAYER OSCILLATIONS AND INTERNAL MODELS

The particular role for this GCL comparison is optimal in the context of an internal model representation (Bastian, 2006; Bhanpuri, Okamura, & Bastian, 2013, 2014; Imamizu, Kuroda, Miyauchi, Yoshioka, & Kawato, 2003; Schweighofer, Arbib, & Kawato, 1998; Wolpert, Miall, & Kawato, 1998). At its simplest, in an internal model, the neurons are tasked with predicting the future state of the action, based on an internal representation of this action. What we propose here, in particular, is that this process could be partially done via synaptic plasticity at the level of the GCL. On each iteration at 4–25 Hz, the correspondence between the intended conditions and the sensory afference would be computed. This would reinforce plasticity elements with LTP-like mechanisms, building this internal model. When the internal model image and the sensory expectations are equal, then movement would be produced. In the case of immobility prior to movement, the state estimation could be of the proprioceptive or teleceptive information available, waiting to reach an optimal value to initiate movement. It would be unwise here to discuss which type of internal model is being implemented in the GCL. Both the forward type of model (causal, sensory consequences) and the inverse model (desired state) could coexist in the cerebellum (Cullen & Brooks, 2015; Wolpert et al., 1998). In the case of the GCL, it appears as if both types of coordinate systems could be present. To add to the variety, the Golgi cells can act as both feed-forward and feedback elements in the GCL (Bell & Dow, 1967; D'Angelo et al., 2013; Galliano, Mazzarello, & D'Angelo, 2010), sculpting the firing out of the GCL in a rhythmic manner (Dugué et al., 2009). With its capacity to use mixed feed-forward and feedback quickly, the general framework of optimal feedback control might prove useful (Yarrow, Brown, & Krakauer, 2009). However, the establishment of the role of the GCL connectivity in the establishment of those models should be clear. It is also important to note that the mode of operation will also need to satisfy nonmotor functions (Popa, Hewitt, & Ebner, 2014).

CONCLUSION—AND BACK TO THE HOCKEY ...

The framework shown here aims to address some questions we would have on the potential advantage of oscillations in the cerebellar GCL circuits. Of course this particular hypothesis is mainly based on converging evidence that would require controlled experiments to verify the particular nature of the error computed at the population level. Particularly interesting approaches would rely on tasks and models that can control the sensory input or the planning of motor output. There would also be an advantage to addressing certain ataxic models, in terms of the presence or absence of oscillations (Bares et al., 2011; Bhanpuri et al., 2013, 2014; Peterburs et al., 2015).

Oscillations at 4–25 Hz should have a role in regulating the traffic of signals and plasticity across the cerebellar cortex. Interactions at many nodes of the cerebellar circuitry at those frequencies can lead to spatiotemporal control of information flow. In the GCL, coding by granule cells, Golgi cells, and Lugaro cells is only beginning to be explored. In addition, interactions with the olivocerebellar system at these frequencies can be predicted (Courtemanche et al., 2013). These interactions will also determine the memory capacities of those circuits. With its capacity to influence the other structures, the cerebellum certainly participates in the overall coding of behavior and also synchronizes its activity with cerebral cortical areas; the variety of oscillatory phenomena that have been identified in cerebral cortical circuits will have to be explored in its relation to cerebellar circuitry.

What we have addressed here is mostly a single context that is optimal for 4- to 25-Hz oscillations, the passage from immobility to movement, with a waiting period. In the case of our hockey player, this waiting period allows the comparison of his intended movement with the current state of his body and the speed, weight, and direction of the incoming puck in order to meet his target. There are of course many situations in which the waiting period is not offered or available. Take, for instance, the super-quick reaction time that the goaltender must display in trying to prevent the one-timer slap shot from P.K. Subban from entering the net—no time for oscillations then. In such a case, more phasic coding strategies will take place. However, there is also strong conceptual support for the role of the cerebellum in general prediction and preparation, for perceiving sensory events or in cognitive planning (Allen, Buxton, Wong, & Courchesne, 1997; Courchesne & Allen, 1997; Paulin, 1993).

It must be evident by now—P.K.'s execution was outstanding ... he shot a laser beam over the goalie's blocker and scored for the win. Did the goalie have a chance? Final score: 3–2. Practice makes perfect.

References

Ahissar, E., Haidarliu, S., & Zacksenhouse, M. (1997). Decoding temporally encoded sensory input by cortical oscillations and thalamic phase comparators. *Proceedings of the National Academy of Sciences of the United States of America, 94,* 11633–11638.

Allen, G., Buxton, R. B., Wong, E. C., & Courchesne, E. (1997). Attentional activation of the cerebellum independent of motor involvement. *Science, 275,* 1940–1943.

Allen, G. I., & Tsukahara, N. (1974). Cerebrocerebellar communication systems. *Physiological Reviews, 54,* 957–1006.

Bares, M., Lungu, O. V., Liu, T., Waechter, T., Gomez, C. M., & Ashe, J. (2011). The neural substrate of predictive motor timing in spinocerebellar ataxia. *Cerebellum, 10,* 233–244.

Bastian, A. J. (2006). Learning to predict the future: the cerebellum adapts feedforward movement control. *Current Opinion in Neurobiology, 16,* 645–649.

Bell, C. C., Bodznick, D., Montgomery, J. C., & Bastian, J. (1997). The generation and subtraction of sensory expectations within cerebellum-like structures. *Brain, Behavior and Evolution, 50,* 17–31.

Bell, C. C., & Dow, R. S. (1967). Cerebellar circuitry. *Neurosciences Research Program Bulletin, 5,* 121–222.

Bell, C. C., & Grimm, R. J. (1969). Discharge properties of Purkinje cells recorded on single and double microelectrodes. *Journal of Neurophysiology, 32,* 1044–1055.

Bell, C. C., Han, V., & Sawtell, N. B. (2008). Cerebellum-like structures and their implications for cerebellar function. *Annual Review of Neuroscience, 31,* 1–24.

Bhanpuri, N. H., Okamura, A. M., & Bastian, A. J. (2013). Predictive modeling by the cerebellum improves proprioception. *Journal of Neuroscience, 33,* 14301–14306.

Bhanpuri, N. H., Okamura, A. M., & Bastian, A. J. (2014). Predicting and correcting ataxia using a model of cerebellar function. *Brain, 137,* 1931–1944.

Blenkinsop, T. A., & Lang, E. J. (2006). Block of inferior olive gap junctional coupling decreases Purkinje cell complex spike synchrony and rhythmicity. *Journal of Neuroscience, 26,* 1739–1748.

Bower, J. M., Beerman, D. H., Gibson, J. M., Shambes, G. M., & Welker, W. (1981). Principles of organization of a cerebro-cerebellar circuit: mapping the projections from cerebral (SI) to cerebellar (granule cell layer) tactile areas of rats. *Brain, Behavior and Evolution, 18,* 1–18.

Bower, J. M., & Schmahmann, J. D. (1997). Control of sensory data acquisition. In *The cerebellum and cognition–international review of neurobiology* (Vol. 41) (pp. 489–513). San Diego: Academic Press.

Bower, J. M., de Zeeuw, C. I., Strata, P., & Voogd, J. (1997). Is the cerebellum sensory for motor's sake, or motor for sensory's sake: the view from the whiskers of a rat? In *Progress in brain research the cerebellum: From structure to function* (pp. 463–496). Amsterdam: Elsevier Science B.V.

Brand, S., Dahl, A. L., & Mugnaini, E. (1976). The length of parallel fibers in the cat cerebellar cortex. An experimental light and electron microscopic study. *Experimental Brain Research, 26,* 39–58.

Bullock, T. H. (1997). Signals and signs in the nervous system: the dynamic anatomy of electrical activity is probably information-rich. *Proceedings of the National Academy of Sciences of the United States of America, 94*, 1–6.

Buzsaki, G. (2004). Large-scale recording of neuronal ensembles. *Nature Neuroscience, 7*, 446–451.

Buzsaki, G. (2006). *Rhythms of the brain*. New York: Oxford University Press.

Buzsaki, G., Logothetis, N., & Singer, W. (2013). Scaling brain size, keeping timing: evolutionary preservation of brain rhythms. *Neuron, 80*, 751–764.

Buzsaki, G., & Moser, E. I. (2013). Memory, navigation and theta rhythm in the hippocampal-entorhinal system. *Nature Neuroscience, 16*, 130–138.

Cardin, J. A., Carlen, M., Meletis, K., Knoblich, U., Zhang, F., Deisseroth, K., et al. (2009). Driving fast-spiking cells induces gamma rhythm and controls sensory responses. *Nature, 459*, 663–667.

Chen, G., Popa, L. S., Wang, X., Gao, W., Barnes, J., Hendrix, C. M., et al. (2009). Low-frequency oscillations in the cerebellar cortex of the tottering mouse. *Journal of Neurophysiology, 101*, 234–245.

Cheron, G., Servais, L., & Dan, B. (2008). Cerebellar network plasticity: from genes to fast oscillation. *Neuroscience, 153*, 1–19.

Chorev, E., Yarom, Y., & Lampl, I. (2007). Rhythmic episodes of subthreshold membrane potential oscillations in the rat inferior olive nuclei in vivo. *Journal of Neuroscience, 27*, 5043–5052.

Courchesne, E., & Allen, G. (1997). Prediction and preparation, fundamental functions of the cerebellum. *Learning & Memory, 4*, 1–35.

Courtemanche, R., Chabaud, P., & Lamarre, Y. (2009). Synchronization in primate cerebellar granule cell layer local field potentials: basic anisotropy and dynamic changes during active expectancy. *Frontiers in Cellular Neuroscience, 3*.

Courtemanche, R., & Lamarre, Y. (2005). Local field potential oscillations in primate cerebellar cortex: synchronization with cerebral cortex during active and passive expectancy. *Journal of Neurophysiology, 93*, 2039–2052.

Courtemanche, R., Pellerin, J. P., & Lamarre, Y. (2002). Local field potential oscillations in primate cerebellar cortex: modulation during active and passive expectancy. *Journal of Neurophysiology, 88*, 771–782.

Courtemanche, R., Robinson, J. C., & Aponte, D. I. (2013). Linking oscillations in cerebellar circuits. *Frontiers in Neural Circuits, 7*, 125.

Crapse, T. B., & Sommer, M. A. (2008). Corollary discharge across the animal kingdom. *Nature Reviews: Neuroscience, 9*, 587–600.

Cullen, K. E., & Brooks, J. X. (2015). Neural correlates of sensory prediction errors in monkeys: evidence for internal models of voluntary self-motion in the cerebellum. *Cerebellum, 14*, 31–34.

D'Angelo, E. (2008). The critical role of Golgi cells in regulating spatio-temporal integration and plasticity at the cerebellum input stage. *Frontiers in Neuroscience, 2*, 35–46.

D'Angelo, E., Koekkoek, S. K., Lombardo, P., Solinas, S., Ros, E., Garrido, J., et al. (2009). Timing in the cerebellum: oscillations and resonance in the granular layer. *Neuroscience, 162*, 805–815.

D'Angelo, E., Mazzarello, P., Prestori, F., Mapelli, J., Solinas, S., Lombardo, P., et al. (2011). The cerebellar network: from structure to function and dynamics. *Brain Research Reviews, 66*, 5–15.

D'Angelo, E., Nieus, T., Maffei, A., Armano, S., Rossi, P., Taglietti, V., et al. (2001). Theta-frequency bursting and resonance in cerebellar granule cells: experimental evidence and modeling of a slow k+-dependent mechanism. *Journal of Neuroscience, 21*, 759–770.

D'Angelo, E., Solinas, S., Mapelli, J., Gandolfi, D., Mapelli, L., & Prestori, F. (2013). The cerebellar Golgi cell and spatiotemporal organization of granular layer activity. *Frontiers in Neural Circuits, 7*, 93.

D'Angelo, E., & de Zeeuw, C. I. (2009). Timing and plasticity in the cerebellum: focus on the granular layer. *Trends in Neurosciences, 32*, 30–40.

Dalal, S. S., Osipova, D., Bertrand, O., & Jerbi, K. (2013). Oscillatory activity of the human cerebellum: the intracranial electrocerebellogram revisited. *Neuroscience and Biobehavioral Reviews, 37*, 585–593.

De Gruijl, J. R., Hoogland, T. M., & De Zeeuw, C. I. (2014). Behavioral correlates of complex spike synchrony in cerebellar microzones. *Journal of Neuroscience, 34*, 8937–8947.

De Montigny, C., & Lamarre, Y. (1973). Rhythmic activity induced by harmaline in the olivo-cerebello-bulbar system of the cat. *Brain Research, 53*, 81–95.

De Zeeuw, C. I., Hoebeek, F. E., Bosman, L. W., Schonewille, M., Witter, L., & Koekkoek, S. K. (2011). Spatiotemporal firing patterns in the cerebellum. *Nature Reviews: Neuroscience, 12*, 327–344.

Devor, A., & Yarom, Y. (2002). Generation and propagation of subthreshold waves in a network of inferior olivary neurons. *Journal of Neurophysiology, 87*, 3059–3069.

Dieudonné, S., & Dumoulin, A. (2000). Serotonin-driven long-range inhibitory connections in the cerebellar cortex. *Journal of Neuroscience, 20*, 1837–1848.

Dugué, G. P., Brunel, N., Hakim, V., Schwartz, E. J., Chat, M., Lévesque, M., et al. (2009). Electrical coupling mediates tunable low-frequency oscillations and resonance in the cerebellar Golgi cell network. *Neuron, 61*, 126–139.

Duhamel, J. R., Colby, C. L., & Goldberg, M. E. (1992). The updating of the representation of visual space in parietal cortex by intended eye movements. *Science, 255*, 90–92.

Ebner, T. J., Wang, X., Gao, W., Cramer, S. W., & Chen, G. (2012). Parasagittal zones in the cerebellar cortex differ in excitability, information processing, and synaptic plasticity. *Cerebellum, 11*, 418–419.

Eccles, J. C., Ito, M., & Szentágothai, J. (1967). *The cerebellum as a neuronal machine*. New York: Spinger-Verlag.

Engel, A. K., Friston, K., Kelso, J. A. S., König, P., Kovàcs, I., MacDonald, A., III, et al. (2010). Coordination in behavior and cognition. In C. von der Marlsburg, et al. (Ed.), *Dynamic coordination in the brain: From neurons to mind* (pp. 267–299). Cambridge, MA: MIT Press.

Forti, L., Cesana, E., Mapelli, J., & D'Angelo, E. (2006). Ionic mechanisms of autorhythmic firing in rat cerebellar Golgi cells. *The Journal of Physiology (London), 574*, 711–729.

Frederick, A., Bourget-Murray, J., & Courtemanche, R. (2013). Local field potential, synchrony of. In D. Jaeger, & R. Jung (Eds.), *Encyclopedia of computational neuroscience*. Berlin Heidelberg: SpringerReference. Springer-Verlag www.springerreference.com.

Fries, P. (2009). Neuronal gamma-band synchronization as a fundamental process in cortical computation. *Annual Review of Neuroscience, 32*, 209–224.

Galliano, E., Mazzarello, P., & D'Angelo, E. (2010). Discovery and rediscoveries of Golgi cells. *Journal of Physiology, 588*, 3639–3655.

Gao, J. H., Parsons, L. M., Bower, J. M., Xiong, J., & Fox, P. T. (1996). Cerebellum implicated in sensory acquisition and discrimination rather than motor control. *Science, 272*, 545–547.

Gao, Z., van Beugen, B. J., & De Zeeuw, C. I. (2012). Distributed synergistic plasticity and cerebellar learning. *Nature Review: Neuroscience, 13*, 619–635.

Geurts, F. J., De Schutter, E., & Dieudonne, S. (2003). Unraveling the cerebellar cortex: cytology and cellular physiology of large-sized interneurons in the granular layer. *Cerebellum, 2*, 290–299.

Gross, J., Timmermann, L., Kujala, J., Dirks, M., Schmitz, F., Salmelin, R., et al. (2002). The neural basis of intermittent motor control in humans. *Proceedings of the National Academy of Sciences of the United States of America, 99*, 2299–2302.

Hartmann, M. J., & Bower, J. M. (1998). Oscillatory activity in the cerebellar hemispheres of unrestrained rats. *Journal of Neurophysiology, 80*, 1598–1604.

Hartmann, M. J., & Bower, J. M. (2001). Tactile responses in the granule cell layer of cerebellar folium crus IIa of freely behaving rats. *Journal of Neuroscience, 21*, 3549–3563.

Hawkes, R., de Zeeuw, C. I., Strata, P., & Voogd, J. (1997). An anatomical model of cerebellar modules. In C. I. de Zeeuw, et al. (Ed.), *Progress in brain research the cerebellum: From structure to function* (pp. 39–52). Amsterdam: Elsevier Science B.V.

Heckroth, J. A., & Eisenman, L. M. (1988). Parasagittal organization of mossy fiber collaterals in the cerebellum of the mouse. *The Journal of Comparative Neurology, 270*, 385–394.

Heck, D. H., Thach, W. T., & Keating, J. G. (2007). On-beam synchrony in the cerebellum as the mechanism for the timing and coordination of movement. *Proceedings of the National Academy of Sciences of the United States of America, 104*, 7658–7663.

Herrup, K., & Kuemerle, B. (1997). The compartmentalization of the cerebellum. *Annual Reviews of Neuroscience, 20*, 61–90.

Huang, C. C., Sugino, K., Shima, Y., Guo, C., Bai, S., Mensh, B. D., et al. (2013). Convergence of pontine and proprioceptive streams onto multimodal cerebellar granule cells. *eLife, 2*, e00400.

Imamizu, H., Kuroda, T., Miyauchi, S., Yoshioka, T., & Kawato, M. (2003). Modular organization of internal models of tools in the human cerebellum. *Proceedings of the National Academy of Sciences of the United States of America, 100*, 5461–5466.

Ito, M. (2006). Cerebellar circuitry as a neuronal machine. *Progress in Neurobiology, 78*, 272–303.

Ito, M. (2010). Cerebellar cortex. In G. M. Shepherd, & S. Grillner (Eds.), *Handbook of brain microcircuits* (pp. 293–300). New York, NY: Oxford University Press.

Jacobson, G. A., Lev, I., Yarom, Y., & Cohen, D. (2009). Invariant phase structure of olivo-cerebellar oscillations and its putative role in temporal pattern generation. *Proceedings of the National Academy of Sciences of the United States of America, 106*, 3579–3584.

Jacobson, G. A., Rokni, D., & Yarom, Y. (2008). A model of the olivo-cerebellar system as a temporal pattern generator. *Trends in Neuroscience, 31*, 617–625.

Keating, J. G., & Thach, W. T. (1995). Nonclock behavior of inferior olive neurons: interspike interval of Purkinje cell complex spike discharge in the awake behaving monkey is random. *Journal of Neurophysiology, 73*, 1329–1340.

Keating, J. G., & Thach, W. T. (1997). No clock signal in the discharge of neurons in the deep cerebellar nuclei. *Journal of Neurophysiology, 77*, 2232–2234.

King, V. M., Armstrong, D. M., Apps, R., & Trott, J. R. (1998). Numerical aspects of pontine, lateral reticular, and inferior olivary projections to two paravermal cortical zones of the cat cerebellum. *Journal of Comparative Neurology, 390*, 537–551.

Lainé, J., & Axelrad, H. (1996). Morphology of the Golgi-impregnated Lugaro cell in the rat cerebellar cortex: a reappraisal with a description of its axon. *Journal of Comparative Neurology, 375*, 618–640.

Lakatos, P., Chen, C. M., O'Connell, M. N., Mills, A., & Schroeder, C. E. (2007). Neuronal oscillations and multisensory interaction in primary auditory cortex. *Neuron, 53*, 279–292.

Lamarre, Y., De Montigny, C., Dumont, M., & Weiss, M. (1971). Harmaline-induced rhythmic activity of cerebellar and lower brain stem neurons. *Brain Research, 32*, 246–250.

Lang, E. J. (2002). GABAergic and glutamatergic modulation of spontaneous and motor-cortex-evoked complex spike activity. *Journal of Neurophysiology, 87*, 1993–2008.

Lang, E. J., Sugihara, I., & Llinás, R. (1996). GABAergic modulation of complex spike activity by the cerebellar nucleoolivary pathway in rat. *Journal of Neurophysiology, 76*, 255–275.

Lang, E. J., Sugihara, I., Welsh, J. P., & Llinás, R. (1999). Patterns of spontaneous Purkinje cell complex spike activity in the awake rat. *Journal of Neuroscience, 19*, 2728–2739.

Laurent, G. (1996). Dynamical representation of odors by oscillating and evolving neural assemblies. *Trends in Neuroscience, 19*, 489–496.

Lisberger, S. G., & Thach, W. T. (2013). The cerebellum. In E. R. Kandel, et al. (Ed.), *Principles of neural science* (pp. 960–981). New York, NY: McGraw-Hill.

Llinás, R. R. (2009). Inferior olive oscillation as the temporal basis for motricity and oscillatory reset as the basis for motor error correction. *Neuroscience, 162*, 797–804.

Llinás, R. R., Brookhart, J. M., & Mountcastle, V. B. (1981). Electrophysiology of the cerebellar networks. In *Handbook of physiology–The nervous system II* (pp. 831–876). Bethesda, Maryland: American Physiological Society.

Llinás, R. R., Humphrey, D. R., & Freund, H. J. (1991). The noncontinuous nature of movement execution. In *Motor control: Concepts and issues* (pp. 223–242). Chichester, England: John Wiley and Sons.

Llinás, R. R., & Sugimori, M. (1992). The electrophysiology of the cerebellar Purkinje cell revisited. In R. R. Llinás, & C. Sotelo (Eds.), *The cerebellum revisited* (pp. 167–181). New York: Springer-Verlag.

Llinás, R., & Volkind, R. A. (1973). The olivo-cerebellar system: functional properties as revealed by harmaline-induced tremor. *Experimental Brain Research, 18*, 69–87.

McCloskey, D. I., & Brooks, V. B. (1981). Corollary discharges: motor commands and perception. In *Handbook of physiology section I: The nervous system vol. II: Motor control part 2* (pp. 1415–1447). Baltimore: Waverly Press Inc.

Middleton, S. J., Racca, C., Cunningham, M. O., Traub, R. D., Monyer, H., Knopfel, T., et al. (2008). High-frequency network oscillations in cerebellar cortex. *Neuron, 58*, 763–774.

Morissette, J., & Bower, J. M. (1996). Contribution of somatosensory cortex to responses in the rat cerebellar granule cell layer following peripheral tactile stimulation. *Experimental Brain Research, 109*, 240–250.

Moser, E., Corbetta, M., Desimone, R., Frégnac, Y., Fries, P., Graybiel, A. M., et al. (2010). Coordination in brain systems. In C. von der Marlsburg, et al. (Ed.), *Dynamic coordination in the brain: From neurons to mind* (pp. 193–214). Cambridge, MA: MIT Press.

Nikonov, A. A., Parker, J. M., & Caprio, J. (2002). Odorant-induced olfactory receptor neural oscillations and their modulation of olfactory bulbar responses in the channel catfish. *Journal of Neuroscience, 22*, 2352–2362.

O'Connor, S., Berg, R. W., & Kleinfeld, D. (2002). Coherent electrical activity between vibrissa sensory areas of cerebellum and neocortex is enhanced during free whisking. *Journal of Neurophysiology, 87*, 2137–2148.

Paulin, M. G. (1993). The role of the cerebellum in motor control and perception. *Brain, Behavior and Evolution, 41*, 39–50.

Pellerin, J. P., & Lamarre, Y. (1997). Local field potential oscillations in primate cerebellar cortex during voluntary movement. *Journal of Neurophysiology, 78*, 3502–3507.

Person, A. L., & Raman, I. M. (2012). Synchrony and neural coding in cerebellar circuits. *Frontiers in Neural Circuits, 6*, 97.

Peterburs, J., Thurling, M., Rustemeier, M., Goricke, S., Suchan, B., Timmann, D., et al. (2015). A cerebellar role in performance monitoring–evidence from EEG and voxel-based morphometry in patients with cerebellar degenerative disease. *Neuropsychologia, 68*, 139–147.

Popa, L. S., Hewitt, A. L., & Ebner, T. J. (2014). The cerebellum for jocks and nerds alike. *Frontiers in System Neuroscience, 8*, 113.

Proville, R. D., Spolidoro, M., Guyon, N., Dugue, G. P., Selimi, F., Isope, P., et al. (2014). Cerebellum involvement in cortical sensorimotor circuits for the control of voluntary movements. *Nature Neuroscience, 17*, 1233–1239.

Requarth, T., Kaifosh, P., & Sawtell, N. B. (2014). A role for mixed corollary discharge and proprioceptive signals in predicting the sensory consequences of movements. *Journal of Neuroscience, 34*, 16103–16116.

Ros, H., Sachdev, R. N., Yu, Y., Sestan, N., & McCormick, D. A. (2009). Neocortical networks entrain neuronal circuits in cerebellar cortex. *Journal of Neuroscience, 29*, 10309–10320.

Rossiter, H. E., Worthen, S. F., Witton, C., Hall, S. D., & Furlong, P. L. (2013). Gamma oscillatory amplitude encodes stimulus intensity in primary somatosensory cortex. *Frontiers in Human Neuroscience, 7*, 362.

Ruigrok, T. J. (2011). Ins and outs of cerebellar modules. *Cerebellum, 10*, 464–474.

Sasaki, K., Bower, J. M., & Llinás, R. (1989). Multiple Purkinje cell recording in rodent cerebellar cortex. *The European Journal of Neuroscience, 1*, 572–586.

Sasaki, K., & Massion, J. (1979). Cerebro-cerebellar interconnections in cats and monkeys. In *Cerebro-cerebellar interactions* (pp. 105–124). Amsterdam: Elsevier/North-Holland Biomedical Press.

Sasaki, K., Oka, H., Matsuda, Y., Shimono, T., & Mizuno, N. (1975). Electrophysiological studies of the projections from the parietal association area to the cerebellar cortex. *Experimental Brain Research, 23*, 91–102.

Scheffer, M., Carpenter, S. R., Lenton, T. M., Bascompte, J., Brock, W., Dakos, V., et al. (2012). Anticipating critical transitions. *Science, 338*, 344–348.

Scheibel, A. (1977). Sagittal organization of mossy fiber terminal system in the cerebellum of the rat: a Golgi study. *Experimental Neurology, 57*, 1067–1070.

Schweighofer, N., Arbib, M. A., & Kawato, M. (1998). Role of the cerebellum in reaching movements in humans. I. Distributed inverse dynamics control. *The European Journal of Neuroscience, 10*, 86–94.

Schweighofer, N., Lang, E. J., & Kawato, M. (2013). Role of the olivo-cerebellar complex in motor learning and control. *Frontiers in Neural Circuits, 7*, 94.

Sillitoe, R. V., Chung, S. H., Fritschy, J. M., Hoy, M., & Hawkes, R. (2008). Golgi cell dendrites are restricted by Purkinje cell stripe boundaries in the adult mouse cerebellar cortex. *Journal of Neuroscience, 28*, 2820–2826.

de Solages, C., Szapiro, G., Brunel, N., Hakim, V., Isope, P., Buisseret, P., et al. (2008). High-frequency organization and synchrony of activity in the Purkinje cell layer of the cerebellum. *Neuron, 58*, 775–788.

Sperry, R. W. (1950). Neural basis of the spontaneous optokinetic response produced by visual inversion. *Journal of Comparative and Physiological Psychology, 43*, 482–489.

Traub, R. D., & Whittington, M. A. (2010). *Cortical oscillations in health and disease.* New York, NY: Oxford University Press.

Voogd, J., & Glickstein, M. (1998). The anatomy of the cerebellum. *Trends in Neuroscience, 21*, 370–375.

Voogd, J., Ruigrok, T. J. H., de Zeeuw, C. I., & Strata, P. (1997). Transverse and longitudinal patterns in the mammalian cerebellum. In *Progress in brain research the Cerebellum: From structure to function* (pp. 22–37). Amsterdam: Elsevier Science B.V.

Vranesic, I., Iijima, T., Ichikawa, M., Matsumoto, G., & Knopfel, T. (1994). Signal transmission in the parallel fiber-Purkinje cell system visualized by high-resolution imaging. *Proceedings of the National Academy of Sciences of the United States of America, 91*, 13014–13017.

Welsh, J. P., Ahn, E. S., & Placantonakis, D. G. (2005). Is autism due to brain desynchronization? *International Journal of Developmental Neuroscience, 23*, 253–263.

Welsh, J. P., Lang, E. J., Sugihara, I., & Llinás, R. (1995). Dynamic organization of motor control within the olivocerebellar system. *Nature, 374*, 453–457.

Welsh, J. P., & Llinas, R. (1997). Some organizing principles for the control of movement based on olivocerebellar physiology. *Progress in Brain Research, 114*, 449–461.

Wolpert, D. M., Miall, R. C., & Kawato, M. (1998). Internal models in the cerebellum. *Trends in Cognitive Sciences, 2*, 338–347.

Yarrow, K., Brown, P., & Krakauer, J. W. (2009). Inside the brain of an elite athlete: the neural processes that support high achievement in sports. *Nature Reviews: Neuroscience, 10*, 585–596.

de Zeeuw, C. I., Hoebeek, F. E., & Schonewille, M. (2008). Causes and consequences of oscillations in the cerebellar cortex. *Neuron, 58*, 655–658.

Single-Neuron and Network Computation in Realistic Models of the Cerebellar Cortex

Egidio D'Angelo[1,2], Stefano Masoli[1],
Martina Rizza[1], Stefano Casali[1]

[1]Department of Brain and Behavioral Sciences, University of Pavia, Pavia, Italy; [2]Brain Connectivity Center, C. Mondino National Neurological Institute, Pavia, Italy

INTRODUCTION

Largely inspired by the regular internal connectivity and the limited number of neuronal types (Fig. 1), cerebellar investigation has been constellated by several theories and models. Another issue fueling the effort was the attempt to explain the cerebellar function as that of a forward controller embedded into the sensorimotor control system and capable of correcting errors on the basis of internal memory. The theories that are worth being mentioned, since they have driven experimental and modeling investigations in the past few decades, have seen the cerebellum as a learning machine (motor learning theory: Albus, 1971; Marr, 1969) or as a timing machine (Eccles, 1973; Eccles, Ito, & Szentagothai, 1967, Eccles, Sabah, Schmidt, & Táboríková, 1972). Whereas in the Marr–Albus theory the core intuition was based on connection statistics, in the Eccles theory the geometry of connectivity played a major role in determining the spatiotemporal reorganization of signals in the circuit. The concept of time was further developed by considering the parallel fibers (pf's) as delay lines (delay-line theory: Braitenberg, 1967; Braitenberg, Heck, & Sultan, 1997). Finally, abstract models have been developed and used to show how forward controllers inspired by the cerebellum could intervene in sensorimotor control and mental activity (Ito, 1972, 1984, 2006, 2008),

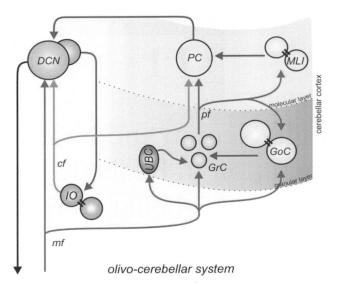

FIGURE 1   The olivocerebellar circuit. This schematic view shows the main architecture of the olivocerebellar circuits. Inputs from mossy fibers (mf), parallel fibers (pf), and inferior olive (IO) projections (climbing fibers, cf) provide the excitatory drive, while the inhibitory connections are shown in blue. In particular, the granular layer and the molecular layer include an inhibitory loop mediated by local interneurons (Golgi cell, GoC, and molecular layer interneuron, MLI, respectively), while the whole cerebellar cortex acts as the inhibitory loop to the deep cerebellar nuclei (DCN) neurons, through the Purkinje cell (PC) connection. DCN neurons project to the IO through inhibitory connections. The mfs and cfs project both to the cerebellar cortex and to the DCN neurons. The mf's contact granule cells (GrC's) and send collaterals to GoC's. The pfs originating from GrCs make synaptic contact with PCs, MLIs, and GoC's (defining a granular layer feedback loop). IO neurons, GoCs, and MLIs are connected through gap junctions (shown in black). UBC, unipolar brush cell.

leading to robotic implementations (Imamizu & Kawato, 2009; Kawato & Gomi, 1992; Kawato et al., 2003; Kawato, Kuroda, & Schweighofer, 2011; Schweighofer, Arbib, & Kawato, 1998, Schweighofer, Spoelstra, Arbib, & Kawato, 1998; Wolpert, Miall, & Kawato, 1998). However, the effective implementation of circuit models of the cerebellar circuit based on neuronal biophysical properties had to wait until recently, when developments in informatics and computational sciences allowed intensive simulations to be performed.

Modern models can be broadly divided between those designed to solve specific computational questions and those based on neuronal biophysics and aiming at a realistic reconstruction of the electrophysiological and biochemical properties of the neurons. Clearly, tailoring the model around the problem to be solved by using a minimal parameter set has the advantage of elegance and simplicity but faces the risk of missing the complex interactions and the flexibility of biological systems. Conversely, the detailed reproduction of membrane biophysics and electrotonic neuronal structure requires extensive knowledge and setting of many parameters, a procedure that may appear troublesome but that can be made much simpler and handy by following a set of fundamental rules of neuronal reconstruction (Koch, 1999; Koch & Segev, 1998). The implementation of these rules is now facilitated by using specific modeling platforms such as NEURON (Hines & Carnevale, 1997, 2001, 2008; Hines, Davison, & Muller, 2009; Hines, Morse, & Carnevale, 2007; Migliore, Cannia, Lytton, Markram, & Hines, 2006) and GENESIS (Bower & Beeman, 1998). The philosophy of realistic neuronal and network reconstruction has been embraced by worldwide modeling initiatives such as the Human Brain Project (https://www.humanbrainproject.eu/) and Open Source Brain (opensourcebrain.org/). Automatic parameter-setting routines have been developed to allow parameter optimization based on genetic algorithms (Druckmann, Banittet, 2007; Druckmann, Berger, Hill, 2008; Druckmann, Berger, Schürmann, 2011).

At present, the cerebellum is second only to the cerebral cortex in terms of realistic model development. Here, the most relevant realistic models of neurons and microcircuits of the cerebellum will be considered in view of the predictions they have provided about cerebellar functioning. These models are helping us understand the structure–function relationship in neurons, the impact of membrane properties on spike timing, the role of synaptic dynamics in the expression of short- and long-term plasticity, and eventually the impacts of various input parameter sets on neuronal computation, signal coding, and information transfer.

The other main question that realistic models can help to answer is how neurons and neuronal mechanisms take part in computation in a system dynamically controlled by the behavioral consequences of its activity. In this case the question is not just how the neurons work but rather how their mechanisms are engaged in a biologically relevant, dynamically evolving context. Clearly, investigating neuronal biophysics in vivo during behavior is out of reach in most cases and the modeling approach provides an alternative way to face the issue. Simplified versions of cerebellar models have been designed to run in real time and have been embedded into closed-loop robotic systems. In this way, the feedback and feed-forward controller operations of the cerebellum can be tested and the impact of elementary mechanisms on the whole system can be investigated. Although this operation is still under development, the first results have shown that cerebellar spiking networks can actually be embedded into robotic controllers and that appropriate learning rules can generate the timing and learning properties that the cerebellum is expected to perform.

BIOPHYSICALLY DETAILED MODELS OF THE CEREBELLAR NEURONS AND MICROCIRCUITS

A remarkable series of biophysically detailed models of neurons and synapses of the cerebellum was originally motivated by the need to understand the complex dynamics of these neurons in terms of ionic channel and distributed membrane properties. However, these models soon became the basis for the construction of realistic networks of the cerebellum and to explore synaptic and microcircuit dynamics in an unprecedented way. Through these models, all ionic channel and synaptic receptor parameters are available and can be analyzed during simulated network responses to specific input stimuli. Moreover, the immense parameter space of the network can be carefully explored and unique predictions on how molecular and cellular mechanisms influence cerebellar network functions and computation can be made.

Modeling One of the Simplest Neurons: The Granule Cell

The granular layer has surely been the most deeply investigated area of the cerebellum in terms of detailed modeling. The models have been used to face a series of critical physiological issues and have exploited some special properties of the neurons and synapses to raise cases of general interest.

The granule cell (GrC) merits a special place. This small neuron is unique not just for its impressive number of elements (on the order of 10^{11} in humans) but also for its architectural simplicity, which has allowed a very precise physiological and computational analysis, making it a prototype for the understanding of brain neuronal properties. Following the first attempt using a composite selection of ionic channels (Gabbiani, Midtgaard, & Knopfel, 1994), the GrC was the first neuron to be fully modeled based on a direct determination of most of its own ionic conductances (D'Angelo et al., 2001). In that work, a monocompartmental GrC model predicted the existence of an M-type current, which was subsequently demonstrated experimentally. Moreover the model incorporated a complex Na current composed of transient, persistent, and resurgent components, which all proved necessary to explain near-threshold oscillations and other electroresponsive aspects of the neuron. The 2001 model was followed by a series of extensions. The Na currents were subsequently investigated in specific electrophysiological works and a 13-state model has been adopted. Moreover, to account for certain properties of synaptic transmission and spike generation, the model was made multicompartmental to include the dendrites and axon (Diwakar et al., 2009). The main outcome was to demonstrate that the dendrites have a very short electrotonic length and conduct synaptic current with minimal decrement to the soma, that action potentials are generated in the axon initial segment (AIS) and then back-propagate to the soma and dendrites, and that therefore the

GrC behaves as a perfect time integrator retransmitting signal to Purkinje cells (PCs) with minimal delay (0.3 ms). Improvements in the modeling of ionic channel properties, ionic channel balancing, axon properties, and intracellular biochemical mechanisms are still ongoing.

A major step forward was to incorporate dynamic models of synaptic transmission. This was done by implementing a three-state vesicular cycle in the presynaptic terminal (Tsodyks & Markram, 1997), equations for neurotransmitter diffusion in the glomerulus, and kinetic schemes for α-amino-3-hydroxy-5-methyl-4-isoxazolepropionic acid (AMPA), N-methyl-D-aspartate (NMDA), and gamma-aminobutyric acid (GABA) postsynaptic receptors (Nieus, Sola, 2006, Nieus, Mapelli, & D'Angelo, 2014). The models faithfully reproduced postsynaptic excitatory postsynaptic currents and inhibitory postsynaptic currents and their dynamic changes in response to mossy fiber (mf) stimulus trains. The neurotransmission models have also been transformed into stochastic versions to simulate quantal release and synaptic noise in order to estimate information transfer through the GrC relay (Arleo et al., 2010).

These models have allowed some major predictions about the functions of the cerebellar granular layer. The introduction of excitatory synaptic mechanisms has allowed us to predict how the NMDA and AMPA currents regulate spike firing in GrCs: the AMPA current controls the precise time of occurrence of the first spike, while the NMDA current controls the subsequent burst discharge. In particular, during long-term potentiation (LTP) the increase in glutamate release causes a specific effect on spike discharge: while changing release probability controls the time-to-first spike by modifying short-term vesicle release dynamics, changing postsynaptic receptor density simply scales the average frequency of GrC responses. Therefore, the model predicts that two different regimens of potentiation coexist and are separately regulated by presynaptic and postsynaptic mechanisms (Nieus et al., 2006).

A stochastic version of the model was used for extensive calculations of mutual information (MI) transfer through the mf–GrC relay (Arleo et al., 2010). This calculation exploited the unique property of GrCs to have a small number of synaptic inputs and allowed therefore the only case of full computation of MI in a central neuron. This work demonstrated that half of the MI during an mf burst is transferred by the time delay of the first spike, the rest by the following tail discharge. This is again a remarkable indication that the GrC operates as a precise time integrator. The stochastic GrC model has been used to evaluate the impact of anesthetics, revealing reduced MI transfer under desflurane (Mapelli et al., 2015).

The multicompartmental version of the model was used to reconstruct the local field potentials in the cerebellar granular layer. This was used in turn to predict, through a reconvolution process, the composition of discharging GrC clusters in vivo. This allowed the determination that granular layer activation in response to punctuate facial stimulation occurs in dense clusters with a proportion of about 10% discharging GrCs and that this proportion modifies consistently during long-term synaptic plasticity (Diwakar, Lombardo, Solinas, Naldi, & D'Angelo, 2011).

The investigation of the interplay of both excitatory and inhibitory synapses has allowed an extensive analysis of the input–output space of the GrCs and of their excitatory/inhibitory balance (Nieus et al., 2014). This analysis has demonstrated a critical role for phasic inhibition in regulating the timing and composition of output spike patterns from the GrCs and has at the same time demonstrated a minor contribution of tonic inhibition to dynamic spike processing.

Modeling Special Properties in Granular Layer Interneurons: The Golgi Cell and Unipolar Brush Cell

Two other neurons that required accurate modeling to understand their intrinsic electroresponsiveness are the Golgi cell (GoC) and unipolar brush cell (UBC).

The GoC is a complex neuron, which is thought to play a critical role in regulating signal transfer in the granular layer. GoCs have been modeled on the basis of detailed information on intrinsic electroresponsiveness and pharmacology, thereby selecting and tuning a corresponding set of ionic conductances (Solinas et al., 2007a,b). The model reproduced all the complex series of nonlinear behaviors revealed experimentally, including pacemaking, resonance, and phase reset. This GoC model is an integral part of the cerebellar microcircuit model (see below) and has been connected into a GoC network through gap junctions (Vervaeke et al., 2010). The impact of channel distribution across soma, axon, and dendrites remains to be modeled, as well as the complex arrangement of its synaptic inputs (D'Angelo et al., 2013).

The UBC is a recently discovered neuron, which is thought to play a critical role in regulating signal amplification and delay in the granular layer, especially in the vestibulocerebellum. UBCs have been modeled on the basis of detailed information on intrinsic electroresponsiveness and pharmacology, thereby selecting and tuning a corresponding set of ionic conductances (Subramaniyam et al., 2014). The model reproduced all the complex series of nonlinear behaviors of the neuron, including bursts and rebounds, and in particular the late-onset burst response, which is thought to make an important contribution to generating delay lines in the circuit. Interestingly, this model coupled synaptic receptor activation with an intracellular signaling cascade modulating gating of H-channels and TRP-channels in a way that accurately predicted the mechanisms of generation of the late-onset response. A spiking model implementing synaptic transmission mechanisms has also been used to explain transmission delays in the network, suggesting that multiple mechanisms (synaptic and nonsynaptic) contribute to regulating delay lines in the vestibulocerebellum (van Dorp & De Zeeuw, 2014). The UBC model still remains to be integrated into the spiking cerebellar circuit model. Nonetheless, UBCs have been considered to lie at the core of relevant computational processes by using simplified large-scale cerebellar network models (Kennedy et al., 2014).

The First Detailed Network Model of Cerebellar Microcircuits: The Granular Layer

The granular cell and GoC models with all the synapses in between have been assembled into the first biophysically detailed large-scale granular layer model (Solinas, Nieus, & D'Angelo, 2010). This model provided a demonstration of the impact of circuit wiring in response to specific stimulus patterns, that is, background noisy mf activity and bursts in defined mf bundles.

Background mf activity caused the model to oscillate at frequencies lower than (but increasing with) the average frequency of the input. Importantly, this granular layer circuit oscillation was due to GrC–GoC feedback inhibition, as predicted previously (Maex & De Schutter, 1998, 2005), but disappeared when mf–GoC feed-forward inhibition was turned on. In turn, the granular layer demonstrated marked resonant properties in the theta band and therefore is prone to oscillating when this frequency pattern is conveyed through the mfs (Gandolfi, Lombardo, Mapelli, Solinas, & D'Angelo, 2013). It seems therefore improbable that the granular layer generates autonomous oscillations under the pressure of random mf activity, while it is more plausible that it is entrained into specific input rhythms through a resonance mechanism (see also Kistler & De Zeeuw, 2003).

In response to mf bursts, the granular layer model showed a characteristic spatiotemporal structure of activity. The response was organized into center-surround patterns exploiting the lateral inhibition of GoCs, consistent with experimental observations (Gandolfi et al., 2013). This structure implements a differential frequency-dependent gain controller, which can channel input signals with higher gain and broader bandwidth in the center compared to the surround (Mapelli, Gandolfi, & D'Angelo, 2010a,b). Moreover, the response showed a time-windowing effect, in which the feedback and feed-forward inhibitory GoC circuits blocked the tail of GrC spike discharge, making the bursts well timed and short. The model therefore demonstrates that the combination of center-surround and time-windowing generates a spatiotemporal filter sharpening the incoming response in space and time, generating effective transmission channels. In addition, long-term synaptic plasticity was shown to tune these spatiotemporal filtering properties, effectively regulating signal transmission through the granular layer.

Other granular layer models have been constructed using simplified neuron models and used to explore the impact of neuronal synchronization through gap junctions (Billings, Piasini, Lorincz, Nusser, & Silver, 2014; Dugue et al., 2009; Vervaeke et al., 2010).

Modeling One of the Most Complex Neurons: The Purkinje Cell

The PC is one of the most complex neurons in the brain and has provided a workbench for the development of single-neuron models (Bower, 2013). The PC was first observed in 1837 by Jan Evangelista Purkyně who, using the microscopes available at that time and without tissue staining, described the pear-shaped soma and just a limited number of dendrites. The impressive extension of the dendritic tree was seen by Camillo Golgi using his Golgi staining method and then by Ramon Y Cajal using a revised Golgi method (DeFelipe, 2015). The presence of highly bifurcated dendrites with a total area of more than $10,000\,\mu m^2$ was the first obstacle for modelers, since it required a huge computational power to solve the cable equations. The idea that PC dendrites could have active conductances was promoted at the end of the 1960s (Llinas, Nicholson, Freeman, Hillman, & 1968), opposing the initial hypothesis of a passive structure (Calvin & Hellerstein, 1969) purely based on the Rall cable theory (see Koch & Segev, 1998). This debate led to critical tests comparing active with passive computational models (Zucker, 1969) until the demonstration that ionic channels were indeed located in PC dendrites (Llinas & Sugimori, 1980).

The first active PC model (Pellionisz & Szentàgothai, 1974) had four dendrites able to respond independently to simple synaptic stimuli. The only active properties were the synaptic inputs, since there were no other channels along the dendrites and soma. A step forward was reported 2 years later (Llinas & Nicholson, 1976), showing the responses to climbing fiber (cf) activation. Even in that case the dendrites had no active conductances except for synaptic inputs but, for the first time, the soma contained channels based on the Hodgkin-Huxley(HH) equations. The first modern model (Pellionisz, Llinás, & Perkel, 1977) was composed of 62 compartments divided into a branched dendritic tree, a soma, the AIS, and a part of the axon. All the sections, except the dendrites, were endowed with active conductances based on the HH equations. This model was able to demonstrate the absence of spike back-propagation from the soma to apical dendrites, the near-perfect forward propagation of synaptic inputs from distal dendrites to the soma, and the complex response of the neuron to cf activity. Until that time, the structure of the neuronal compartments was based on equivalent morphologies.

The first model of a dendritic tree based on the morphology of a real rat PC (though still passive) appeared in 1985 (Shelton, 1985). That was the first case of a model specifically designed to be reused by other modelers as a base for further expansion. The basis for the best known PC models of all times was set in 1992 (Rapp, Segev, & Yarom, 1994; Rapp, Yarom, & Idan, 1992) when three different morphologies were reconstructed from the guinea pig cerebellum with the purpose of investigating the specific passive properties of this morphology in conjunction with experimental recordings. Then, a major step forward was the reconstruction of 10 specific ionic channels, based on the HH equations, and their distribution in the soma and in the entire dendritic tree (De Schutter & Bower, 1994b,c). This model was able to cover a wider range of parameters with respect to previous models, including a broader range of stimuli generated by current injections and synaptic activity, confirming the reliability of this approach and the need for an explicit representation of multiple ionic channel conductances distributed over multiple compartments to reproduce the functional properties of a complex neuron. This model has been adapted and used to explain experimental results both in vivo and in vitro (for a list of the papers published using modification of the original model, see Bower, 2013) and was fundamental to promoting further PC modeling. Soon thereafter, based on the morphology of Shelton and a series of improvements to ionic channel properties obtained from new experiments done with ion channel blockers, a new PC model was built to test intracellular calcium dynamics (Miyasho et al., 2001). The only drawback was the absence of the AIS and the axon.

In a historical perspective, as much as the 1960s and 1970s were dominated by morphological passive models and the 1980 and 1990s saw the introduction of active membrane properties and realistic morphologies, in the new-century ionic channels have established their importance in the modeling process. The most complete reproduction of the typical PC sodium channel based on careful experimental determinations (Nav1.6) was introduced and tested in a monocompartmental model (Khaliq, Gouwens, & Raman, 2003). This Nav1.6 was composed of 13 different states, including closed, inactivated, opened, and blocked states, and was able to reproduce the persistent, transient, and resurgent sodium current, explaining specific electro-responsive properties of the PC. Another PC monocompartmental model was generated to improve the effectiveness of Na channels at physiological temperature (Akemann & Knopfel, 2006) and investigate their interaction with a subfamily of Kv3 channels in generating the action potentials. In yet another model, a Markovian calcium buffer (CDP5) was used in association with two new reconstructions of the main PC high-voltage activated (HVA) calcium channel (Cav2.1—P/Q type) and low-voltage activated (LVA) calcium channel (Cav3.1—T type) (Anwar, Sungho, & De Schutter, 2012).

In 2014 and 2015, three new models of PCs were published to address specific properties of the neuron. The first one (Couto, Linaro, De Schutter, & Giugliano, 2015) was based on previous models (De Schutter & Bower, 1994b,c; Khaliq et al., 2003) and was used to investigate the phase-response curves of firing rate dependency of rat PCs in vitro. The second one (Forrest, 2014) was also based on previous models for morphology (Shelton, 1985), for ionic channels (Khaliq et al., 2003), and for intracellular calcium dynamics (Miyasho et al., 2001) and was used to study the impact of the sodium pumps on PC information-encoding ability. The last model was intended to integrate available experimental knowledge, which in the meanwhile had revealed several properties not yet accounted for and for which the impact had to be tested (Masoli, Solinas, & D'Angelo, 2015). The morphology was taken from the 1993 model (De Schutter & Bower, 1994b,c) and extended to include the AIS, a 400-μm-long axon, and an axonal collateral. Most of the effort has been devoted to active properties. All the channels originally used in previous models have been substituted with 15 channels that were chosen based on recent immunohistochemical and biomolecular papers and located accordingly in seven different active regions. The resulting model was able to extend even more the biological realism, reproducing multiple properties of PCs including pacemaking, burst–pause behaviors, and complex firing at high input intensities. This new model predicted generation of spikes in the AIS with amplified back-propagation in the soma and decremental diffusion in the dendrites. Forward propagation in the axon occurred through the nodes of Ranvier causing low-pass filtering and limiting the maximum transmitted frequencies. One of the still unresolved issues for PC models is the absence of spines on the dendrites, which have been considered in specific modeling efforts (Antunes & De Schutter, 2012) but have not been incorporated into the entire neuron model for the investigation of synaptic inputs.

Modeling the impact of PCs in the whole cerebellar cortex or even only in the molecular layer depends not just on these neurons but also on precise modeling of molecular layer interneurons (MLIs), the stellate and basket cells. No detailed biophysical models of these neurons are available yet and simplified versions of the MLI–PC interaction have been proposed in large-scale models of the cerebellum (Lennon, Hecht-Nielsen, & Yamazaki, 2014; Santamaria, Tripp, & Bower, 2007; see below).

Models of the Deep Cerebellar Nuclei and Inferior Olivary Cells

While the largest effort has been devoted to model neurons and microcircuits of the cerebellar cortex, interest is now rising in models of the two other main structures of the olivocerebellar system, the deep cerebellar nuclei (DCN), and the inferior olive (IO).

The DCN are placed at the exit points of the cerebellar cortex and sample, retransmit, and store information conveyed through the cerebellar circuit. There are six different types of DCN neurons subdivided into three main categories: the big glutamatergic neurons, which transmit to the red nucleus and thalamus; the medium/small GABAergic interneurons;

and the small GABAergic neurons which project to the IO (Uusisaari & De Schutter, 2011). A model of the glutamatergic neurons was created to investigate the interaction between PCs and DCN cells. The model was based on a realistic morphological reconstruction with active channels in the dendrites, soma, AIS, and axon (Steuber, Schultheiss, Silver, De Schutter, & Jaeger, 2011) and was used to analyze synaptic integration and DCN rebound firing after inhibition. In an advanced version, the model was used to study the dependence of neuronal encoding on short-term synaptic plasticity in the afferent synapses (Luthman et al., 2011). A further version was specifically adapted to study the impact of Kv1 channels on the spontaneous generation of spikes and in their ability to regulate the output (Ovsepian et al., 2013). The electrophysiological properties of GABAergic neurons have not been fully characterized (Najac & Raman, 2015) and no models are available yet.

The IO has been intensely investigated, since, by integrating information coming from higher centers and the sensory system and then projecting cfs to the PCs, it is considered a key element for the functioning of the whole olivocerebellar system. The cf's in turn generate a powerful excitatory input for the PCs, the complex spike followed by a pause in spontaneous firing, and also project to the DCN. A monocompartmental model of IO neurons was built to investigate the interaction of ionic currents characterized through direct recordings in these same neurons (Manor, Rinzel, Segev, & Yarom, 1997). This model was able to show modification to subthreshold oscillations (STOs) when two neurons were connected through gap junctions and was subsequently expanded in a second, more advanced version (Torben-Nielsen, Segev, & Yarom, 2012). The first bicompartment model (Schweighofer, Doya, & Kawato, 1999) was able to reproduce the typical STOs and the particular spikes generated by the interaction of sodium and calcium currents in the soma/dendritic compartments. A three-compartment model was then built to account for the interactions between the dendrites, soma, and AIS in generating the STOs and spike output of the IO neurons (De Gruijl, Bazzigaluppi, de Jeu, & De Zeeuw, 2012). The AIS improved the mechanism of spike generation.

Therefore, as of this writing, neuronal interactions within the DCN and their connections with other structures of the olivocerebellar system are only incompletely resolved at the modeling as well as the experimental level.

LARGE-SCALE SPIKING MODELS OF THE OLIVOCEREBELLAR NETWORK

The reconstruction of a single-cell model normally proceeds in four steps: construction (use of fundamental data on membrane channels and neuronal passive structure), validation (against data not used for reconstruction), testing (under different functional conditions), and propagation (into the local network). The effort is remarkable and is amplified when trying to simulate an entire network of neurons with the correct proportion of cells and connections. To mitigate this requirement, many network reconstructions have been built with simplified monocompartmental or even integrate-and-fire (I&F) neurons, allowing one to explore high-level questions in a way that may not be achieved in a reasonable time with more complex (yet more realistic) neuronal models. Large-scale spiking networks of the cerebellum have been built until now using I&F neuron models and simplified synapses.

One of the first examples of a detailed cerebellar spiking network using biophysically inspired monocompartmental neurons was built to investigate GrC activity driven by mfs and the associated inhibitory GoC control (Maex & De Schutter, 1998). This model revealed oscillatory granular layer activity when mfs were stimulated randomly. An evolution of this first network was obtained by connecting a multicompartmental model of the PC (De Schutter & Bower, 1994a,b) to a new multicompartmental model of the GrC built with ascending axons and pfs (Santamaria et al., 2007). The GoCs were not present and the MLIs were not explicitly modeled but their activity was integrated in the synaptic responses on PCs. This model provided insight into the interaction between the pf's and PCs under control of MLIs, predicting that PC beams could be switched off by the concomitant pf activation of feed-forward molecular layer inhibition.

A model including both the cerebellar cortex and the DCN neurons was developed to explain eyeblink conditioning experiments (Medina, Garcia, Nores, Taylor, & Mauk, 2000; Medina & Mauk, 1999, 2000). This model was based on simplified conductance-based spiking neurons and included plasticity at the mf–DCN synapse. By using the model, three forms of plasticity at mf synapses in the cerebellar nucleus were tested to determine the prerequisites of persistent memory storage. Results suggested that only a plasticity rule controlled by the activity of the PC allowed formation of a stable memory trace.

A different model incorporating simplified spiking neurons with specific excitable properties, notably postinhibitory rebound in DCN cells, was developed to investigate the dynamics developing in a circuit including the cerebellar cortex, the IO, the DCN, and a precerebellar nucleus (the reticular formation) (Kistler & De Zeeuw, 2003). In this model, activity generated by the mf's and IO reverberated through the loop, generating a theta-band network oscillation that spread over the granular and molecular layer and DCN. More specifically, GoCs controlled the ring time of GrCs rather than their ring rate, and PCs triggered precisely timed rebound spikes in neurons of the DCN. These oscillatory dynamics may have implications for synaptic plasticity and timing.

REAL-TIME MODELS FOR CLOSED-LOOP ROBOTIC SIMULATIONS OF CEREBELLAR LEARNING AND CONTROL

A critical application of modeling is that of providing information about the dynamic behavior of a complex system operating in a natural context while keeping all the relevant parameters measured and controllable, that is, doing an operation that is impossible to perform in biological experiments. There have been several attempts at modeling in an efficient way the olivocerebellar system to investigate its circuit timing and plasticity. This approach proved especially useful for the investigation of the impact of the multiple synaptic plasticities reported in the cerebellar network (D'Angelo, 2014; Gao, van Beugen, & De Zeeuw, 2012; Hansel, Linden, & D'Angelo, 2001) and their relationship with the spike timing (D'Angelo & De Zeeuw, 2009; D'Angelo et al., 2009), though at the expense of some simplification required to reduce network complexity and computational load. The full integration of biophysically realistic neurons into a real-time robotic spiking network is still impractical as of this writing, but it is envisaged that the development of field programmable gate array (FPGA) and graphic processing unit (GPU) technologies will provide new efficient solutions.

Traditional Robotic Models

In a first model based on a classical implementation of the motor control system (Schweighofer et al., 1998a,b), an expanded representation of the granular layer was used to determine how plasticity impinging on GrCs could contribute to sensorimotor control. Indeed, mf–GrC and GoC–GrC plasticity played a critical role in regulating the number of active GrCs maintaining sparseness (Schweighofer, Doya, & Lay, 2001). This, in turn, by optimizing granular layer expansion recoding, improved cerebellar performance in complex tasks involving corrections of apparent forces and accelerations of robotic arms moving along the complex trajectories.

Liquid-State Machine Models

In a series of experiments, the cerebellum was modeled using a simplified version of spiking neurons and was subsequently implemented in FPGA and GPU modules (Honda, Yamazaki, Tanaka, Nagao, & Nishino, 2011; Lennon et al., 2014; Luo et al., 2014; Yamazaki & Igarashi, 2013; Yamazaki & Nagao, 2012; Yamazaki, Nagao, Lennon, & Tanaka, 2015; Yamazaki & Tanaka, 2007, 2009).

In the model, the granular layer generated a finite nonrecurrent sequence of active neurons representing the passage of time. This activity was evoked by mossy fiber patterns and generated various sequences of active neurons. The PCs in turn learned to stop firing at the timing instructed by the arrival of signals from the IO. In this scheme, the functional roles of the granular layer and PCs corresponded to a liquid-state generator coupled to readout neurons, suggesting that the cerebellum had to be considered as a liquid-state machine with powerful information processing capability going beyond that of a perceptron, as it was previously assumed.

The entire network with as many as 105,000 neurons has been optimized to run on a commercial graphics card GPU, which is up to 100 times faster than a multicore CPU. This extensive network is able to reproduce in real time the delayed eyeblink conditioning and has been used in a robotic arm with the ability to hit a ball after many sessions of learning (Yamazaki & Igarashi, 2013).

Closed-Loop Real-Time Robotic Simulations Using Spiking Cerebellar Networks

In a series of works, the impact of distributed cerebellar plasticity was investigated using a reverse engineering approach, that is, making a biologically plausible reconstruction of the olivocerebellar system and embedding it into a robotic controller connected to a simulated or to a real robot. This allowed for the first time the investigation of the internal mechanisms of function of the whole cerebellar network under dynamic behaviors in a closed loop, although some simplifications and assumptions had to be accepted and the models had to be developed and cross-checked along a complex series of tests.

In a first series of tests, analog models were designed to run in robotic simulators and real robots. In these models, firing frequency was the control variable but neurons were not spiking, emphasizing the introduction of multiple synaptic plasticity rules rather than the realism of neuronal firing mechanisms. Multiple plasticity rules were implemented in the molecular layer and DCN. The cfs provided a teaching signal driving long-term synaptic plasticity at the pf–PC synapses and both PC–DCN and mf–DCN synapses were made plastic. Finally, plasticity at the IO–DCN connection was predicted to have a critical role for cerebellar functioning too (Garrido, Luque, D'Angelo, & Ros, 2013; Luque, Garrido, Carrillo, D'Angelo, & Ros, 2014).

In a second series of tests, the cerebellar network models were constructed using spiking neurons and accelerated up to real time using a look-up table approach (Casellato, Antonietti, Garrido, Carrillo, 2014; Casellato, Antonietti, Garrido, Ferrigno, 2015; Garrido, Ros, & D'Angelo, 2013). These robotic simulations were still based on a spike-rate coding scheme since commands generated by the motor cortex of the robot were analog and translated into spikes by radial-basis functions. Correspondingly, neurons were of the I&F type and were appropriate to process the rate codes. These models were therefore inappropriate for resolving the nonlinear time-dependent dynamics imposed by neurons and synapses, but could be used to investigate the evolution of plasticity at multiple sites. The simulations indeed revealed the following:

- Multiple plasticities allow *scalable gain control* and prevent synapse saturation and loss of efficiency in the learning capabilities of the system.
- Multiple plasticities allow the implementation of multiple tunable forward and feedback loops inside the cerebellum and the whole sensorimotor system, improving the efficiency of learning, which accelerates and stabilizes rapidly.
- Pf–PC plasticity was fundamental to relate cerebellar plasticity to motor errors, but it proved insufficient per se to make the cerebellum an effective forward controller. At the pf–PC synapse, long-term adaptation (LTD) and LTP had to coevolve dynamically to control pf–PC transmission, making it reversible for resetting and reuse.
- The memory stored in the pf–PC synapse was rapidly transferred into DCN synapses allowing consolidation. This memory transfer was controlled by feedback signals arriving through extracerebellar loops and proved critical to allow self-rescaling and automatic gain adjustment, preventing pf–PC saturation. This operation required double adjustment of mf–DCN and PC–DCN synapses to balance memory deposition in DCN neurons.
- The memory deposition in DCN neurons was greatly accelerated and stabilized by IO–DCN plasticity. This action is remarkable at the beginning of the learning process but then becomes negligible.

These robotic simulations were successfully applied to various behaviors involving cerebellar learning, including VOR, EBCC, force-field correction, and arm trajectory control (Casellato et al., 2014, 2015; Garrido et al., 2013; Luque et al., 2014), suggesting that the implicit algorithm of the cerebellar network was of general applicability.

These models can now be implemented in several ways. First of all, they could include plasticity in the granular layer, which is expected to store the large variety of spatiotemporal patterns required for expansion recoding of mf signals. This aspect could become critical when multiple input signals from extended sensorimotor structures are considered. Second, neurons with realistic nonlinear firing patterns could be used to reveal the impact of their membrane properties on neuronal computations. However, this would require a radically new design, in which the whole system should embed nonlinear spiking neurons and temporal dynamics, a condition that is not yet at hand.

There are nonetheless some predictions that can be derived from these simulations and require now experimental verification. First, all plasticities should be reversible, so they should express both LTP and LTD. Second, since the memory transferred into downstream structures (e.g., from pf–PC into DCN) is controlled by feedback signals arriving through extracerebellar loops, understanding distributed plasticity requires the whole system to be working in a closed loop. Third, there are forms of plasticity that may not last for long during free behavior (e.g., pf–PC LTD itself) and this should be taken into account when searching for such plasticities experimentally. Fourth, there could be forms of plasticity that have not yet been identified experimentally but could have remarkable impact on cerebellar learning (e.g., the IO–DCN plasticity). Finally, DCN neurons could process not just two but even three forms of plasticity coming from mf–DCN, PC–DCN, and potentially also IO–DCN synapses. Therefore, further experimental investigation on the plasticity of synapses impinging on DCN neurons is needed.

CONCLUSIONS

Realistic models are contributing to our understanding of the biophysical properties of cerebellar neurons and synapses, unveiling the intimate relationships between multiple membrane and synaptic mechanisms. Moreover, once embedded into networks and connected synaptically, they are providing insights into microcircuit functions. It is envisaged that incorporation of sophisticated neuron models into spiking networks embedded into robotic controllers will allow us in the future to investigate the closed-loop behavior of brain circuits with potential applications not just in robotics but also in neurophysiology and neurorehabilitation.

LIST OF ABBREVIATIONS

cf Climbing fiber
DCN Deep cerebellar nuclei
EBCC Eyeblink classical conditioning
FPGA Field programmable gate array
GoC Golgi cell
GPU Graphic processing unit
GrC Granule cell
IO Inferior olive
mf Mossy fiber
MLI Molecular layer interneuron
PC Purkinje cell
pf Parallel fiber
UBC Unipolar brush cell
VOR Vestibulo-ocular reflex

References

Akemann, W., & Knopfel, T. (2006). Interaction of Kv3 potassium channels and resurgent sodium current influences the rate of spontaneous firing of Purkinje neurons. *Channels*, *26*, 4602–4612.

Albus, J. S. (1971). A theory of cerebellar function. *Mathematical Biosciences*, *10*, 25–61.

Antunes, G., & De Schutter, E. (2012). A stochastic signaling network mediates the probabilistic induction of cerebellar long-term depression. *Journal of Neuroscience*, *32*, 9288–9300.

Anwar, H., Sungho, H., & De Schutter, E. (2012). Controlling Ca^{2+}-activated K^+ channels with models of Ca^{2+} buffering in purkinje cells. *Cerebellum*, *11*, 681–693.

Arleo, A., Nieus, T., Bezzi, M., D'Errico, A., D'Angelo, E., & Coenen, O. J. (2010). How synaptic release probability shapes neuronal transmission: information-theoretic analysis in a cerebellar granule. *Neural Computation*, *22*, 2031–2058.

Billings, G., Piasini, E., Lorincz, A., Nusser, Z., & Silver, R. A. (2014). Network structure within the cerebellar input layer enables lossless sparse encoding. *Neuron*, *83*, 960–974.

Bower, J. M. (2013). The emergence of community models in computational neuroscience: the 40-year history of the cerebellar purkinje cell. In S. Science (Ed.), *20 years of computational neuroscience*. New York: Springer Science.

Bower, J., & Beeman, D. (1998). *The book of GENESIS: Exploring realistic neural models with the GEneral NEural SImulation System* (2nd ed.). New York: Springer-Verlag.

Braitenberg, V. (1967). Is the cerebellar cortex a biological clock in the millisecond range? *Progress in Brain Research*, *25*, 334–346.

Braitenberg, V., Heck, D., & Sultan, F. (1997). The detection and generation of sequences as a key to cerebellar function: experiments and theory. *Behavioral and Brain Sciences*, *20*, 229–245; discussion 245–277.

Calvin, W. H., & Hellerstein, D. (1969). Dendritic spikes versus cable properties. *Science*, *163*, 96–97.

Casellato, C., Antonietti, A., Garrido, J. A., Carrillo, R. R., Luque, N. R., Ros, E., et al. (2014). Adaptive robotic control driven by a versatile spiking cerebellar network. *PLoS One*, *9*, e112265.

Casellato, C., Antonietti, A., Garrido, J. A., Ferrigno, G., D'Angelo, E., & Pedrocchi, A. (2015). Distributed cerebellar plasticity implements generalized multiple-scale memory components in real-robot sensorimotor tasks. *Frontiers in Computational Neuroscience*, *9*, 24.

Couto, J., Linaro, D., De Schutter, E., & Giugliano, M. (2015). On the firing rate dependency of the phase response curve of rat Purkinje neurons in vitro. *PLoS Computational Biology*, *11*, e1004112.

D'Angelo, E. (2014). The organization of plasticity in the cerebellar cortex: from synapses to control. *Progress in Brain Research*, *210*, 31–58.

D'Angelo, E., & De Zeeuw, C. I. (2009). Timing and plasticity in the cerebellum: focus on the granular layer. *Trends in Neuroscience*, *32*, 30–40.

D'Angelo, E., Koekkoek, S. K. E., Lombardo, P., Solinas, S., Ros, E., Garrido, J., et al. (2009). Timing in the cerebellum: oscillations and resonance in the granular layer. *Neuroscience*, *162*, 805–815.

D'Angelo, E., Nieus, T., Maffei, A., Armano, S., Rossi, P., Taglietti, V., et al. (2001). Theta-frequency bursting and resonance in cerebellar granules: experimental evidence and modeling of a slow K+-dependent mechanism. *The Journal of Neuroscience*, *21*, 759–770.

D'Angelo, E., Solinas, S., Mapelli, J., Gandolfi, D., Mapelli, L., & Prestori, F. (2013). The cerebellar golgi cell and spatiotemporal organization of granular layer activity. *Frontiers in Neural Circuits*, *7*, 93.

De Gruijl, J. R., Bazzigaluppi, P., de Jeu, M. T., & De Zeeuw, C. I. (2012). Climbing fiber burst size and olivary sub-threshold oscillations in a network setting. *PLoS Computational Biology*, e1002814. USA.

De Schutter, E., & Bower, J. M. (1994a). An active membrane model of the cerebellar Purkinje cell II. Simulation of synaptic responses. *Journal of Neurophysiology, 71*, 401–419.

De Schutter, E., & Bower, J. M. (1994b). An active membrane model of the cerebellar Purkinje cell. I. Simulation of current clamps in slice. *Journal of Neurophysiology, 71*, 375–400.

De Schutter, E., & Bower, J. M. (1994c). Simulated responses of cerebellar Purkinje cells are independent of the dendritic location of granule synaptic inputs. *Proceedings of the National Academy of Sciences of the United States of America, 91*, 4736–4740.

DeFelipe, J. (2015). The dendritic spine story: an intriguing process of discovery. *Frontiers in Neuroanatomy, 9*, 14.

Diwakar, S., Lombardo, P., Solinas, S., Naldi, G., & D'Angelo, E. (2011). Local field potential modeling predicts dense activation in cerebellar granules clusters under LTP and LTD control. *PLoS ONE, 6*, e21928.

Diwakar, S., Magistretti, J., Goldfarb, M., Naldi, G., & D'Angelo, E. (2009). Axonal Na+ channels ensure fast spike activation and back-propagation in cerebellar granules. *Journal of Neurophysiology, 101*, 519–532.

van Dorp, S., & De Zeeuw, C. I. (2014). Variable timing of synaptic transmission in cerebellar unipolar brush cells. *Proceedings of the National Academy of Sciences of the United States of America*, 5403–5408. USA.

Druckmann, S., Banitt, Y., Gidon, A., Schürmann, F., Markram, H., & Segev, I. (2007). A novel multiple objective optimization framework for constraining conductance-based neuron models by experimental data. *Frontiers in Neuroscience, 1*, 7–18.

Druckmann, S., Berger, T. K., Hill, S., Schürmann, F., Markram, H., & Segev, I. (2008). Evaluating automated parameter constraining procedures of neuron models by experimental and surrogate data. *Biological Cybernetics, 99*, 371–379.

Druckmann, S., Berger, T. K., Schürmann, F., Hill, S., Markram, H., & Segev, I. (2011). Effective stimuli for constructing reliable neuron models. *PLoS Computational Biology, 7*, e1002133 e1002133.

Dugue, G. P., Brunel, N., Hakim, V., Schwartz, E., Chat, M., Levesque, M., et al. (2009). Electrical coupling mediates tunable low-frequency oscillations and resonance in the cerebellar golgi cell network. *Neuron, 61*, 126–139.

Eccles, J. C. (1973). The cerebellum as a computer: patterns in space and time. *The Journal of Physiology, 229*, 1–32.

Eccles, J. C., Ito, M., & Szentagothai, J. (1967). *The cerebellum as a neural machine*. Berlin, Heidelberg, New York: Springer-Verlag.

Eccles, J. C., Sabah, N. H., Schmidt, R. F., & Táboríková, H. (1972). Mode of operation of the cerebellum in the dynamic loop control of movement. *Brain Research, 40*, 73–80.

Forrest, M. D. (2014). The sodium-potassium pump is an information processing element in brain computation. *Frontiers in Physiology, 5*, 472.

Gabbiani, F., Midtgaard, J., & Knopfel, T. (1994). Synaptic integration in a model of cerebellar granules. *Journal of Neurophysiology, 72*, 999–1009.

Gandolfi, D., Lombardo, P., Mapelli, J., Solinas, S., & D'Angelo, E. (2013). Theta-frequency resonance at the cerebellum input stage improves spike timing on the millisecond timescale. *Frontiers in Neural Circuits, 7*, 64.

Gao, Z., van Beugen, B. J., & De Zeeuw, C. I. (2012). Distributed synergistic plasticity and cerebellar learning. *National Reviews Neuroscience, 13*, 619–635.

Garrido, J. A., Luque, N. R., D'Angelo, E., & Ros, E. (2013). Distributed cerebellar plasticity implements adaptable gain control in a manipulation task: a closed-loop robotic simulation. *Frontiers in Neural Circuits, 7*, 159.

Garrido, J. A., Ros, E., & D'Angelo, E. (2013). Spike timing regulation on the millisecond scale by distributed synaptic plasticity at the cerebellum input stage: a simulation study. *Frontiers in Computational Neuroscience, 7*, 64.

Hansel, C., Linden, D. J., & D'Angelo, E. (2001). Beyond parallel fiber LTD: the diversity of synaptic and non-synaptic plasticity in the cerebellum. *Nature Neuroscience, 4*, 467–475.

Hines, M. L., & Carnevale, N. T. (1997). The NEURON simulation environment. *Neural Computation, 9,* 1179–1209.

Hines, M. L., & Carnevale, N. T. (2001). NEURON: a tool for neuroscientists. *Neuroscientist, 7,* 123–135.

Hines, M. L., & Carnevale, N. T. (2008). Translating network models to parallel hardware in NEURON. *Journal of Neuroscience Methods, 169,* 425–455.

Hines, M. L., Davison, A. P., & Muller, E. (2009). NEURON and python. *Frontiers in Neuroinformatics, 3,* 1.

Hines, M. L., Morse, T. M., & Carnevale, N. T. (2007). Model structure analysis in neuron. *Methods in Molecular Biology, 401,* 91–102.

Honda, T., Yamazaki, T., Tanaka, S., Nagao, S., & Nishino, T. (2011). Stimulus-dependent state transition between synchronized oscillation and randomly repetitive burst in a model cerebellar granular layer. *PLoS Computational Biology,* e1002087. United States.

Imamizu, H., & Kawato, M. (2009). Brain mechanisms for predictive control by switching internal models: implications for higher-order cognitive functions. *Psychological Research, 73,* 527–544.

Ito, M. (1972). Neural design of the cerebellar motor control system. *Brain Research, 40,* 81–84.

Ito, M. (1984). *The cerebellum and neural control.* New York: Raven Press.

Ito, M. (2006). Cerebellar circuitry as a neuronal machine. *Progress in Neurobiology, 78,* 272–303.

Ito, M. (2008). Control of mental activities by internal models in the cerebellum. *Nature Reviews Neuroscience, 9,* 304–313.

Kawato, M., & Gomi, H. (1992). A computational model of four regions of the cerebellum based on feedback-error learning. *Biological Cybernetics, 68,* 95–103.

Kawato, M., Kuroda, T., Imamizu, H., Nakano, E., Miyauchi, S., & Yoshioka, T. (2003). Internal forward models in the cerebellum: fMRI study on grip force and load force coupling. *Progress in Brain Research, 142,* 171–188.

Kawato, M., Kuroda, S., & Schweighofer, N. (2011). Cerebellar supervised learning revisited: biophysical modeling and degrees-of-freedom control. *Current Opinion in Neurobiology.*

Kennedy, A., Wayne, G., Kaifosh, P., Alvina, K., Abbott, L. F., & Sawtell, N. B. (2014). A temporal basis for predicting the sensory consequences of motor commands in an electric fish. *Nature Neuroscience,* 416–422. United States.

Khaliq, Z. M., Gouwens, N. W., & Raman, I. M. (2003). The contribution of resurgent sodium current to high-frequency firing in Purkinje neurons: an experimental and modeling study. *The Journal of Neuroscience, 23,* 4899–4912.

Kistler, W. M., & De Zeeuw, C. I. (2003). Time windows and reverberating loops: a reverse-engineering approach to cerebellar function. *Cerebellum, 2,* 44–54.

Koch, C. (1999). *Biophysics of computation: Information processing in single neurons.* New York: Oxford University Press.

Koch, C., & Segev, I. (1998). *Methods in neural modeling: From ions to networks* (2nd ed.). Cambridge, MA: The MIT Press.

Lennon, W., Hecht-Nielsen, R., & Yamazaki, T. (2014). A spiking network model of cerebellar Purkinje cells and molecular layer interneurons exhibiting irregular firing. *Frontiers in Computational Neuroscience, 8,* 157.

Llinas, R., Nicholson, C., Freeman, J. A., & Hillman, D. E. (1968). Dendritic spikes and their inhibition in alligator purkinje cells. *Science, 160,* 1132–1135.

Llinas, R., & Nicholson, C. (1976). Reversal properties of climbing fiber potential in cat Purkinje cells: an example of a distributed synapse. *Journal of Neurophysiology, 39,* 311–323.

Llinas, R., & Sugimori, M. (1980). Electrophysiological properties of in vitro Purkinje cell dendrites in mammalian cerebellar slices. *The Journal of Physiology, 305,* 197–213.

Luo, J., Coapes, G., Mak, T., Yamazaki, T., Tin, C., & Degenaar, P. (2014). A scalable FPGA-based cerebellum for passage-of-time representation. *Conference Proceedings: Annual International Conference of the IEEE Engineering in Medicine and Biology Society, 2014,* 3102–3105.

Luque, N. R., Garrido, J. A., Carrillo, R. R., D'Angelo, E., & Ros, E. (2014). Fast convergence of learning requires plasticity between inferior olive and deep cerebellar nuclei in a manipulation task: a closed-loop robotic simulation. *Frontiers in Computational Neuroscience*, *8*, 97.

Luthman, J., Hoebeek, F. E., Maex, R., Davey, N., Adams, R., De Zeeuw, C. I., et al. (2011). STD-dependent and independent encoding of input irregularity as spike rate in a computational model of a cerebellar nucleus neuron. *Cerebellum*, *10*, 667–682.

Maex, R., & De Schutter, E. (1998). Synchronization of golgi and granule firing in a detailed network model of the cerebellar granule layer. *Journal of Neurophysiology*, *80*, 2521–2537.

Maex, R., & De Schutter, E. (2005). Oscillations in the cerebellar cortex: a prediction of their frequency bands. *Progress in Brain Research*, *148*, 181–188.

Manor, Y., Rinzel, J., Segev, I., & Yarom, Y. (1997). Low-amplitude oscillations in the inferior olive: a model based on electrical coupling of neurons with heterogeneous channel densities. *Journal of Neurophysiology*, *77*, 2736–2752.

Mapelli, J., Gandolfi, D., & D'Angelo, E. (2010a). High-pass filtering and dynamic gain regulation enhance vertical bursts transmission along the MfPathway of cerebellum. *Frontiers in Cellular Neuroscience*, *4*, 14.

Mapelli, J., Gandolfi, D., & D'Angelo, E. (2010b). Combinatorial responses controlled by synaptic inhibition in the cerebellum granular layer. *Journal of Neurophysiology*, *103*, 250–261.

Mapelli, J., Gandolfi, D., Giuliani, E., Prencipe, F. P., Pellati, F., Barbieri, A., et al. (2015). The effect of desflurane on neuronal communication at a central synapse. *PLoS One*, e0123534. United States.

Marr, D. (1969). A theory of cerebellar cortex. *The Journal of Physiology*, *202*, 437–470.

Masoli, S., Solinas, S., & D'Angelo, E. (2015). Action potential processing in a detailed Purkinje cell model reveals a critical role for axonal compartmentalization. *Frontiers in Cellular Neuroscience*, *9*, 47.

Medina, J. F., Garcia, K. S., Nores, W. L., Taylor, N. M., & Mauk, M. D. (2000). Timing mechanisms in the cerebellum: testing predictions of a large-scale computer simulation. *The Journal of Neuroscience*, *20*, 5516–5525.

Medina, J. F., & Mauk, M. D. (1999). Simulations of cerebellar motor learning: computational analysis of plasticity at the mfto deep nucleus synapse. *The Journal of Neuroscience*, *19*, 7140–7151.

Medina, J. F., & Mauk, M. D. (2000). Computer simulation of cerebellar information processing. *Nature Neuroscience*, *3*(Suppl.), 1205–1211.

Migliore, M., Cannia, C., Lytton, W. W., Markram, H., & Hines, M. L. (2006). Parallel network simulations with NEURON. *Journal of Computational Neuroscience*, *21*, 119–129.

Miyasho, T., Takagi, H., Suzuki, H., Watanabe, S., Inoue, M., Kudo, Y., et al. (2001). Low-threshold potassium channels and a low-threshold calcium channel regulate Ca2+ spike firing in the dendrites of cerebellar Purkinje neurons: a modeling study. *Brain Research*, *891*, 106–115.

Najac, M., & Raman, I. M. (2015). Integration of Purkinje cell inhibition by cerebellar nucleo-olivary neurons. *The Journal of Neuroscience*, *544*–549. United States: 2015 the authors 0270-6474/15/350544-06$15.00/0.

Nieus, T. R., Mapelli, L., & D'Angelo, E. (2014). Regulation of output spike patterns by phasic inhibition in cerebellar granules. *Frontiers in Cellular Neuroscience*, *8*, 246.

Nieus, T., Sola, E., Mapelli, J., Saftenku, E., Rossi, P., & D'Angelo, E. (2006). LTP regulates burst initiation and frequency at mossy fiber-granule synapses of rat cerebellum: experimental observations and theoretical predictions. *Journal of Neurophysiology*, *95*, 686–699.

Ovsepian, S. V., Steuber, V., Le Berre, M., O'Hara, L., O'Leary, V. B., & Dolly, J. O. (2013). A defined heteromeric KV1 channel stabilizes the intrinsic pacemaking and regulates the output of deep cerebellar nuclear neurons to thalamic targets. *The Journal of Physiology*, 1771–1791. England.

Pellionisz, A., & Szentàgothai, J. (1974). Dynamic single unit simulation of a realistic cerebellar network model. II. Purkinje cell activity within the basic circuit and modified by inhibitory systems. *Brain Research, 68,* 19–40.

Pellionisz, A., Llinás, R., & Perkel, D. H. (1977). A computer model of the cerebellar cortex of the frog. *Neuroscience, 2,* 19–35.

Rapp, M., Segev, I., & Yarom, Y. (1994). Physiology, morphology and detailed passive models of guinea-pig cerebellar Purkinje cells. *The Journal of Physiology, 474,* 101–118.

Rapp, M., Yarom, Y., & Idan, S. (1992). The impact of parallel fiber background activity on the cable properties of cerebellar Purkinje cells. *Neural Computation, 4,* 518–533.

Santamaria, F., Tripp, P. G., & Bower, J. M. (2007). Feedforward inhibition controls the spread of granule-induced Purkinje cell activity in the cerebellar cortex. *Journal of Neurophysiology, 97,* 248–263.

Schweighofer, N., Arbib, M. A., & Kawato, M. (1998). Role of the cerebellum in reaching movements in humans. I. Distributed inverse dynamics control. *European Journal of Neuroscience, 10,* 86–94.

Schweighofer, N., Doya, K., & Kawato, M. (1999). Electrophysiological properties of inferior olive neurons: a compartmental model. *Journal of Neurophysiology, 82,* 804–817.

Schweighofer, N., Doya, K., & Lay, F. (2001). Unsupervised learning of granule sparse codes enhances cerebellar adaptive control. *Neuroscience, 103,* 35–50.

Schweighofer, N., Spoelstra, J., Arbib, M. A., & Kawato, M. (1998). Role of the cerebellum in reaching movements in humans. II. A neural model of the intermediate cerebellum. *European Journal of Neuroscience, 10,* 95–105.

Shelton, D. P. (1985). Membrane resistivity estimated for the Purkinje neuron by means of a passive computer model. *Neuroscience, 14,* 111–131.

Solinas, S., Forti, L., Cesana, E., Mapelli, J., Schutter, E. D., & D'Angelo, E. (2007a). Computational reconstruction of pacemaking and intrinsic electroresponsiveness in cerebellar golgi cells. *Frontiers in Cellular Neuroscience, 1,* 2.

Solinas, S., Forti, L., Cesana, E., Mapelli, J., Schutter, E. D., & D'Angelo, E. (2007b). Fast-reset of pacemaking and theta-frequency resonance patterns in cerebellar golgi cells: Simulations of their impact in vivo. *Frontiers in Cellular Neuroscience, 1,* 1–9.

Solinas, S., Nieus, T., & D'Angelo, E. (2010). A realistic large-scale model of the cerebellum granular layer predicts circuit spatio-temporal filtering properties. *Frontiers in Cellular Neuroscience, 4,* 12.

Steuber, V., Schultheiss, N. W., Silver, R. A., De Schutter, E., & Jaeger, D. (2011). Determinants of synaptic integration and heterogeneity in rebound firing explored with data-driven models of deep cerebellar nucleus cells. *Journal of Computational Neuroscience, 30,* 633–658.

Subramaniyam, S., Solinas, S., Perin, P., Locatelli, F., Masetto, S., & D'Angelo, E. (2014). Computational modeling predicts the ionic mechanism of late-onset responses in unipolar brush cells. *Frontiers in Computational Neuroscience, 8,* 237.

Torben-Nielsen, B., Segev, I., & Yarom, Y. (2012). The generation of phase differences and frequency changes in a network model of inferior olive subthreshold oscillations. *PLoS Computational Biology,* e1002580. USA.

Tsodyks, M. V., & Markram, H. (1997). The neural code between neocortical pyramidal neurons depends on neurotransmitter release probability. *Proceedings of the National Academy of Sciences of the United States of America, 94,* 719–723.

Uusisaari, M., & De Schutter, E. (2011). The mysterious microcircuitry of the cerebellar nuclei. *The Journal of Physiology.*

Vervaeke, K., Lorincz, A., Gleeson, P., Farinella, M., Nusser, Z., & Silver, R. A. (2010). Rapid desynchronization of an electrically coupled interneuron network with sparse excitatory synaptic input. *Neuron, 67,* 435–451.

Wolpert, D. M., Miall, R. C., & Kawato, M. (1998). Internal models in the cerebellum. *Trends in Cognitive Sciences, 2,* 338–347.

Yamazaki, T., & Igarashi, J. (2013). Realtime cerebellum: a large-scale spiking network model of the cerebellum that runs in realtime using a graphics processing unit. *Neural Networks, 47*, 103–111.

Yamazaki, T., & Nagao, S. (2012). A computational mechanism for unified gain and timing control in the cerebellum. *PLoS One*, e33319. USA.

Yamazaki, T., Nagao, S., Lennon, W., & Tanaka, S. (2015). Modeling memory consolidation during posttraining periods in cerebellovestibular learning. *Proceedings of the National Academy of Sciences of the United States of America*, 3541–3546. USA.

Yamazaki, T., & Tanaka, S. (2007). The cerebellum as a liquid state machine. *Neural Networks*, 290–297. United States.

Yamazaki, T., & Tanaka, S. (2009). Computational models of timing mechanisms in the cerebellar granular layer. *Cerebellum, 8*, 423–432.

Zucker, R. S. (1969). Field potentials generated by dendritic spikes and synaptic potentials. *Science, 165*, 409–413.

Index

Printed in the United States
By Bookmasters